Doctors and Medicine in Early Renaissance Florence

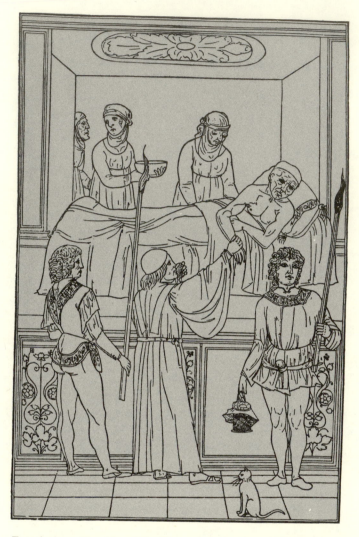

Frontispiece: Physician taking the pulse of a plague victim. From
Fasciculo di medicina vulgare, tr. Ioannis de Ketham, Venice, 1493.

Doctors and Medicine in Early Renaissance Florence

KATHARINE PARK

PRINCETON UNIVERSITY PRESS
PRINCETON, NEW JERSEY

Copyright © 1985 by Princeton University Press
Published by Princeton University Press,
41 William Street, Princeton, New Jersey 08540
In the United Kingdom:
Princeton University Press, Guildford, Surrey

All Rights Reserved
Library of Congress Cataloging in Publication Data will be
found on the last printed page of this book

ISBN 0-691-08373-8

Publication of this book has been aided by a grant from
The Andrew W. Mellon Foundation

This book has been composed in Linotron Galliard

Clothbound editions of Princeton University Press books
are printed on acid-free paper, and binding materials are
chosen for strength and durability

Printed in the United States of America by
Princeton University Press
Princeton, New Jersey

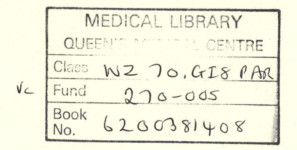

To my teachers

Contents

Tables

Tables

Acknowledgments

I AM GRATEFUL to all those who have helped me transform this study from a graduate research project into the present book. Among many others, Melissa Chase, Gino Corti, Riccardo Fubini, Philip Gavitt, David Hubel, Bill Kent, Elaine Rosenthal, Paul Starr, and Ronald Weissman took time from their own work in Florence and at Harvard to supply me with references, information, ideas, and moral support. Anthony Molho and Charles Schmitt provided valuable advice during the formative stages of my research, while John Murdoch and Barbara Rosenkrantz directed the dissertation on which this book is based. I owe a special debt, finally, to the various friends and scholars who read and criticized part or all of the intermediate manuscript: Nancy Siraisi, Jonathan Knudsen, David Park, John Henderson, Jill Kraye, Anthony Grafton, Davis Dyer, and John Najemy. *Sine quibus non.*

On the material plane, I have received generous financial support from the Danforth Foundation, the American Council of Learned Societies, the Renaissance Society of America, Wellesley College, and above all the Society of Fellows of Harvard University. I owe much to the staffs of the various archives and libraries which I used in the course of my research: the state archives of Florence, Prato, Pistoia, and Lucca; the Biblioteca Nazionale, Biblioteca Laurenziana, and Biblioteca Riccardiana in Florence; the Biblioteca Apostolica Vaticana; the Wellcome Institute for the History of Medicine, the Warburg Institute, and the British Library in London; and Countway, Widener, and Houghton libraries at Harvard.

Abbreviations and Note
Concerning Transcriptions

AIMSSF   *Annali dell'Istituto e museo di storia della scienza di Firenze.*

Annales   *Annales: Economies, sociétés, civilisations.*

ASI   *Archivio storico italiano.*

Atti XXI *Atti del XXI Congresso internazionale di storia della medicina.* 2 vols. Siena, 1968.

BDSPU   *Bollettino della Deputazione di storia patria per l'Umbria.*

BHM   *Bulletin of the History of Medicine.*

Delizie   *Delizie degli eruditi toscani.* Ed. Ildefonso di San Luigi. 24 vols. Florence, 1770-89.

JHM   *Journal of the History of Medicine and Allied Sciences.*

RIS   *Rerum italicarum scriptores.* Ed. Lodovico Antonio Muratori. 34 vols. Bologna, 1900-17.

RSSMN *Rivista di storia delle scienze mediche e naturali.*

For additional abbreviations referring to archival and manuscript material, see the first section of the Bibliography.

I have included in the notes to each chapter transcriptions of unpublished sources and early printed sources cited in translation or referred to prominently in the text. In both cases I have modernized punctuation but not spelling. Where I have had to change the text to produce a comprehensible reading (for example, where a manuscript has holes or lacunae), I have so indicated by the use of square brackets.

Doctors and Medicine in Early
Renaissance Florence

Introduction

IN 1346, wrote the Florentine chronicler Matteo Villani, Mars, Jupiter, and Saturn conjoined in Aquarius. In the same year a wave of pestilence appeared in the East, "toward Cathay and northern India," and began to spread westward.

It was a plague which touched people of every condition, age, and sex. They began to spit blood and then they died—some immediately, some in two or three days, and some in a longer time. And it happened that whoever cared for the sick caught the disease from them or, infected by the same corrupt air, became rapidly ill and died in the same way. Most had swellings in the groin, and many had them in the left and right armpits and other places; one could almost always find an unusual swelling somewhere on the victim's body.[1]

This disease—bubonic or pneumonic plague—had been unknown in Europe since the early Middle Ages.[2] By 1347, carried on Italian galleys fleeing the eastern Mediterranean, it reached the ports of Messina, Genoa, and Pisa. In the spring of the following year it spread throughout Italy, sparing only Milan.

When the plague arrived in Florence in late March of 1348, its inhabitants were already weakened by two years of famine and disease.[3] Nonetheless, the city reacted quickly to the challenge of this new

[1] Matteo Villani, *Cronica*, I, 2; 1:9-10. On the chronology and geography of the epidemic of 1348 see Dols, *Black Death*, 35-56, and Biraben, *Les hommes et la peste*, 1:71-105. Other contemporary descriptions of the Black Death in Florence appear in Boccaccio, *Decameron*, proemium; Stefani, *Cronaca fiorentina*, 230-33; and Morelli, *Ricordi*, 287-301.

[2] For a modern medical analysis of the disease in its various forms see Dols, *Black Death*, 68-74; Gottfried, *Epidemic Diseases*, 58-62; and Biraben, *Les hommes et la peste*, vol. 1, chap. 1. Bibliography on the early medieval epidemics in Dols, *Black Death*, 14n.

[3] Pinto, "Firenze e la carestia"; Corradi, *Annali delle epidemie*, 1:477-78; Carabellese, *La peste del 1348*, 2-3, 10-11; Carpentier, *Une ville*, 79-83. On the link between famines and epidemics in this period see Carpentier, "Autour de la peste noire," 1074-81.

epidemic. On April 3 a series of regulations was promulgated to stem its spread: no infected traveler from Pisa, Genoa, or elsewhere was to be given hospitality, and no cloth or bedclothes belonging to the infected were to be kept or sold; prostitution and the emptying of privies were restricted to certain times and places.[4] A week later, on April 11, the legislative councils of the Florentine republic appointed a commission of eight citizens to regulate matters of public health. In June the city treasurers paid for medical autopsies of the bodies of several plague victims "in order to know their illness more clearly." These administrative and hygienic measures were supplemented by acts of communal charity and piety. The priors took part in several religious processions, and on the feast of Saint Anne a number of prisoners were released from the city jail "on account of the infection of the air," as the provision read, "which is worse there than elsewhere."[5] A number of measures were voted in favor of Florence's most important pious associations—including the companies of Or. San Michele and the Misericordia as well as the hospitals of Santa Maria Nuova and San Gallo—to aid them in feeding and treating the sick and the poor.[6]

Despite the best efforts of public and private medicine and hygiene, however, the plague could not be broken. "All over the world," according to Villani,

> doctors found no remedy or true cure for this pestilential disease, whether in philosophy, medical theory, or astrology. Some, driven by greed, went about seeing patients and prescribing treatment, but the failure of such measures showed their art to be feigned and not true. Many, stricken by conscience, left their unjustly earned profits to be restored after their deaths.

In Florence alone, between April and September, when cooler autumn weather began to slow the spread of the disease, "at least three-fifths of the population died, of all ages and both sexes. The lower and middle orders suffered more than the upper classes, because they were weaker to begin with, because they were hit first and hardest, and because they had less aid and lived in poorer conditions. . . ."[7]

Recent research has borne out much of Villani's account, and in

---

[4] Carabellese, *La peste del 1348*, 44. The sources for this and other measures described by Carabellese were damaged in the flood of 1966 and are presently inaccessible.

[5] PR-36, fol. 133v (public health commission); del Badia, *Miscellanea fiorentina*, 1:158 (autopsies); LF-28, fol. 138r (prisoners). For a list of abbreviations used in references to sources in the Archivio di stato di Firenze see the first section of the Bibliography.

[6] Carabellese, *La peste del 1348*, 64-66.

[7] Matteo Villani, *Cronica*, I, 2; 1:11-12.

particular his estimates of the total mortality and the greater suffering of the poor. The death rate may have been somewhat lower in the countryside, but in the close quarters of the city the population seems to have dropped from well over a hundred thousand to less than half that number in the early 1350s. Furthermore, the plague did not disappear after its initial outbreak but returned in waves of varying severity over a period of three hundred years. In the fourteenth and fifteenth centuries alone, Florence witnessed epidemics in 1363 (Villani already referred to it as the "accustomed" disease), 1374, 1383, 1390, 1399-1400 (a devastating plague, which killed a quarter of the remaining inhabitants), 1411, 1417, 1430, 1448, 1456, 1478, and throughout the later 1490s. Florence's population continued to decline through the first quarter of the fifteenth century, and it took another fifty years to show any net gain.[8]

If the effects of plague on the Florentine population are clear, those on the city's economy and on its politics and society are harder to discern. In the later fourteenth and early fifteenth centuries, as a hundred years before, Florence's considerable economic prosperity continued to be based both on the agricultural and fiscal exploitation of its subject territories and on international trade, banking, and the textile industry, although there are signs of a reduction in the scale and security of such enterprises.[9] The government of the city—the Florentine commune—continued to function as a republic, dominated for the most part by the social and economic elites of the greater, or commercial and professional, guilds. The high mortality in 1348 and the epidemics immediately following may have encouraged a limited form of social mobility by bringing new individuals and new families to the fore and by fostering a wave of immigration into the depopulated city from the surrounding countryside, but these effects seem to have been relatively short-lived, and they did not radically alter either the structure of the Florentine social hierarchy or the composition of its ruling groups.[10]

---

[8] Ibid., X, 103; 2:299. For a synthesis of research on Florentine demography in this period see Herlihy and Klapisch-Zuber, *Les toscans*, 165-83. Note that the population of Florence and the surrounding district had already begun to decline several decades before 1348; for the significance of this fact see Herlihy, "Population, Plague and Social Change." See also Carmichael, "Epidemic Diseases," esp. chap. 2.

[9] For an introduction to Florentine history in this period see Brucker, *Renaissance Florence*. See Becker, *Florence in Transition*, 2:25-26, for a summary discussion and bibliography concerning the economic effects of the plague in Florence.

[10] The lack of precise recent studies of the nondemographic effects of plague in Florence is itself testimony to the difficulty of the problem. The recent work on Florentine politics and social life in the late fourteenth century by Gene Brucker, John Najemy, and others makes little or no reference to the subject: Brucker, *Florentine Politics and*

Even in the area of mentality and religious sentiment, it is difficult to find clear evidence of signally changed attitudes or expectations.[11]

There was, however, one area which saw immediate and important changes attributable directly to the plague: as Villani's account implies and as common sense argues, the epidemics placed new emphasis and new demands on public and private medical care; in the process they affected both the nature and the scale of medical organization in the city. Over the century before 1348 Florence, like other north Italian city-states, had evolved a large and complex set of institutions which cooperated in looking after the health of its inhabitants. The commune itself, the hospitals, the Guild of Doctors, Apothecaries, and Grocers, and many of the city's religious companies and orders concerned themselves with various aspects of the problem. These groups were among the first to respond to the medical crisis of 1348 and the succeeding waves of plague. Even as the population of Florence dropped, its hospitals increased in size and number, its medical profession expanded, and the state budget for poor-doctors, army doctors, and prison doctors grew.

One of my principal concerns in this book will be to analyze the effect of plague on Florence's medical organization and medical profession after the Black Death. In the process, however, I will be exploring the entire world of medical practitioners and medical practice in Florence in the century after 1348. In the course of this exploration I will return frequently to three main themes. In the first place, I will emphasize the variety of medical care available to the city population and its relative accessibility; I will show in particular that many attitudes, practices, and institutions often assumed to be the product of a more recent period—neighborhood clinics, for example, early forms of health insurance, publicly subsidized medicine, hospitals with a sophisticated medical organization—were already discernible in early Renaissance Italy. In the second place, I will argue that these attitudes, practices,

---

Society and *Civic World*; Najemy, *Corporatism and Consensus*; Becker, *Florence in Transition*, vol. 2, chap. 3; Molho, "Politics and the Ruling Class." But cf., for Siena, Bowsky, "Impact of the Black Death." Much remains to be done on this topic.

[11] Several historians have argued for a transformation in this area; see, for example, Meiss, *Painting in Florence and Siena*. Recently, however, the tendency has been to emphasize the existence of such tendencies even before 1348, although it is plausible that the advent of plague confirmed the preoccupation with collective sin and salvation as well as an inclination toward coercive patterns of thought; see Van Os, "Black Death and Sienese Painting," and Becker, *Florence in Transition*, 1:60-61. Most recent works on Florentine religious life in this period either ignore the effects of the plague or treat them as diffuse and indirect: see, for example, Becker, "Aspects of Lay Piety," 177-81, and Weissman, *Ritual Brotherhood*.

and institutions formed part of the corporate culture of the north Italian city-states and are best studied in that context. If we wish to understand developments rooted in the corporate and commercial culture of the high Middle Ages, we must look to the societies which created them and examine the cultural needs and assumptions which they reflected. The city-states of northern Italy were certainly not the only areas experimenting with such forms of medical organization, but they were arguably the most advanced, and Italian models were often adopted by more backward countries such as England.[12] In the third place, I will show that the plague represented a crisis in the history of the Italian medical profession, challenging the competence of doctors and undermining their social and political authority by disrupting the established patterns of recruitment to the profession. Thus the decades after 1348 saw the virtual collapse of the native Florentine medical profession as members of established families chose other careers. Their places were filled by immigrant doctors from the countryside and other, smaller towns, who lacked the social connections and political power of their predecessors. More than two centuries passed before these effects of plague began to reverse themselves and doctors emerged once again as an important force in the life of the city and their guild.

I have chosen to write on Florence both because it typifies in many ways the state of affairs in other Italian cities[13] and because the extraordinary range of documentation in the Tuscan archives has yielded a large body of good secondary literature on various aspects of Florentine history—literature upon which I have drawn heavily for background in my own account. My plan of research was twofold. On the one hand, I combed the archives of Florence and its subject towns for information about the various institutions that structured the medical profession and defined its functions and limits; these included the Guild of Doctors, Apothecaries, and Grocers, the communal government, and many of the city's hospitals, monasteries, and confraternities. On the other hand, I used guild matriculation lists, electoral records, tax rolls, and university documents to compile a roughly complete list of doctors practicing in Florence between the mid-fourteenth and the

---

[12] See Pelling and Webster, "Medical Practitioners," 165. For English reliance on the Italian model of the College of Physicians: Webster, "Thomas Linacre." For English interest in Florentine hospital organization: Passerini, *Storia degli stabilimenti*, 304, and (for revised dating) Somerville, *The Savoy*, 9-10.

[13] In Bologna, on the other hand, the university faculty of medicine dominated the city's procedures for medical licensing and medical regulation in a way that was uncharacteristic of most other areas; see Kibre, *Scholarly Privileges*, 50. The Florentine *studio* was neither large nor important enough to exert this kind of influence.

mid-fifteenth centuries. I then used what manuscript and archival sources were available to study the lives and careers of these men and women. On the basis of this research I have tried to sketch a balanced and comprehensive picture of the medical profession and medical practice in early Renaissance Florence, and to show their relationship to the nonmedical culture of the period.

A note concerning terminology: I have included in my list of doctors those who, when asked their occupation, identified themselves as doctors—*medici* or *medicae*—or who were so identified by others. According to contemporary definitions, this group embraced three main types of practitioner. Physicians (*fisici*) possessed a doctorate in medicine from a recognized university and usually practiced what we would call internal medicine. Surgeons (*chirurghi*) could learn their trade either at a university or by apprenticeship to a recognized surgeon; they treated external conditions such as rashes, fractures, and wounds. In Italy, as opposed to England or France, surgery was an academic discipline. Like physicians, surgeons were doctors; they were not associated with barbers, who performed certain medical operations, such as cupping and bleeding, but were considered a distinct occupational group. Finally, empirics (*empirici*) were less formally trained or self-taught and tended to specialize in particular (usually surgical) diseases, including cataracts, fractures, and hernias. In general, I have excluded from my study barbers, midwives, and others whose functions overlapped those of the medical profession without being equivalent. My definition of "doctor" thus corresponds to that given by the Guild of Doctors, Apothecaries, and Grocers in its statute of 1349 (see Chapter One). I use the term "medical profession" to refer to this group of practitioners; it corresponds effectively to the members of the "branch of doctors" in the guild.

My book falls into six chapters. The first three deal primarily with the institutional context of medical practice. Chapter One sets out the formal and informal organization of the medical profession within the Guild of Doctors, Apothecaries, and Grocers. Chapter Two provides a census of the doctors active in Florence and describes the various levels of practitioner represented within the legally constituted profession. Chapter Three takes up the complexities of medical practice and discusses the attitudes toward medical treatment and the relationships between client and practitioner that shaped the marketplace within which the Florentine doctor sold his services. The remaining chapters deal more directly with the doctors themselves. The fourth outlines the types of careers open to a Florentine doctor, the decisions he and his family would have had to make at various points in his career, and the considerations which motivated such decisions. The fifth treats the social and economic rewards and liabilities of practice and details the place of doctors in contemporary Florentine society. Chapter Six, finally, examines their intellectual and cultural interests and places these within the broader framework of the early Florentine Renaissance.

In this way my study cuts across several historical fields and intersects several historiographical traditions. I have, as I have already mentioned, drawn heavily on the work of other scholars of Florentine social and cultural history. As a study of a particular occupation my work is tied most closely to that of Lauro Martines on lawyers and, most recently, Richard A. Goldthwaite on masons and builders as well as to Raffaele Ciasca's important older book on the Guild of Doctors, Apothecaries, and Grocers.[14] Like Martines and Goldthwaite, I have been concerned to place my findings in the context of Florentine society as a whole and to describe the ways in which the experience of doctors confirms or contradicts recent findings concerning family structure, social identity, and access to political power. In choosing to write about doctors I have produced an account of a social group which is in some ways typical and in some ways highly unusual. Economically comfortable but for the most part socially obscure and politically insignificant, doctors had much in common with the broad middle orders of the Florentine population—a group which, unlike the patriciate or the working classes, has yet to find its historian.[15] At the same time, however, doctors stood apart from many of their contemporaries because so many of them were recent immigrants to the city. As the work of Charles de la Roncière, Johan Plesner, and others has shown, immigration was crucial to the growth of Florence, like other cities of the later Middle Ages and Renaissance, but I know of no detailed studies of the human motivations, costs, and benefits which lay behind such immigration.[16] The experiences of Florence's doctors

[14] Martines, *Lawyers*; Goldthwaite, *Building of Renaissance Florence*, esp. chaps. 5-7; Ciasca, *L'arte*.

[15] Most recent work in Florentine social history has focused on the patriciate. See, for example, F. W. Kent, *Household and Lineage*; Goldthwaite, *Private Wealth*; and Martines, *Social World*. The principal recent studies of the *popolo minuto* are Cohn, *Laboring Classes*, and de la Roncière, "Pauvres et pauvreté," which supplement and transform the older work of Rodolico, *Il popolo minuto*. The work of Anthony Molho and Julius Kirshner on the *Monte delle doti* promises to shed light on the social history of the middle orders of Florentine society; see their "Dowry and Marriage." The most important book in general Florentine social and demographic history to come out in recent years is Herlihy and Klapisch-Zuber, *Les toscans*, which I have used throughout as a source of comparative statistics.

[16] De la Roncière, *Florence*, 2:679-96; Plesner, *L'émigration*; Luzzato, "L'inurba-

illuminate the related processes of geographical and social mobility in vivid detail.

In the field of Florentine intellectual history also, doctors occupy a telling position. Scholars such as Eugenio Garin and Cesare Vasoli have begun to emphasize the links between the vigorous tradition of scholastic learning located in the Florentine *studio* and the early circles of Florentine humanists.[17] Trained in the scholastic tradition but allied by background and intellectual interests to the early humanists, Florentine physicians could act as mediators between university and non-university culture. Their activities as readers, writers, teachers, patrons of the arts, and practicing scientists can help us to appreciate the variety and richness of contemporary Florentine culture—too often reduced to the literary culture of humanism—and to examine its social and ideological functions.

My work also falls within the tradition of recent writing on the history of the plague. The last decades have seen a number of important new studies on the demographic, social, and economic effects of plague in late medieval and Renaissance Europe.[18] Yet very few of these have investigated the role of contemporary medicine in the epidemics and the peculiar effects of the Black Death on doctors and medical organization. Historians have tended to focus either on governmental regulations concerning public health[19] or on the contemporary medical analysis (and its defects) as contained in a handful of theoretical treatises.[20] Neither approach sheds much light on the upheaval the plague caused in the medical profession or on the reaction

---

mento"; Fiumi, "Fioritura e decadenza," 116:497-504; Herlihy and Klapisch-Zuber, *Les toscans*, 301-25. These studies have tended to emphasize the statistical phenomenon and its economic implications rather than the experience of individual immigrants.

[17] For instance, Garin, "Cultura fiorentina," and Vasoli, "Polemiche occamiste." This interpretation replaces that proposed by historians like Hans Baron, who see a radical break between scholastic and humanist scholars and tradition; cf. his *Humanistic and Political Literature*, 27-34.

[18] There are too many to list in detail. Among the most comprehensive are Biraben, *Les hommes et la peste*, esp. vol. 1, chap. 4, and Ziegler, *Black Death*. Gottfried, *The Black Death*, appeared too recently to be of use to me. Recent local studies for northern Italy in the fourteenth and early fifteenth centuries include Carpentier, *Une ville*; Herlihy, "Population, Plague and Social Change" and *Medieval and Renaissance Pistoia*, 104-20; and Bowsky, "Impact of the Black Death."

[19] The literature for Renaissance Italy alone is impressive in quantity and quality. Most relevant for this study are Carabellese, *La peste del 1348*; Chiappelli, "Ordinamenti sanitari"; Coturri, "Più antichi provvedimenti"; and Cipolla, *Public Health*. See Cipolla's bibliography for further references.

[20] For instance, Gottfried, *Epidemic Diseases*, chap. 3.

of the medical community in the area of practice.[21] My study of doctors and medicine in the century after 1348 addresses these issues and attempts to deal with these questions.

In the field of the history of medicine proper, my work has strong affinities with that of Danielle Jacquart, C. H. Talbot, E. A. Hammond, and Edward J. Kealey, who have studied the history of medieval medicine in France and England through the collective biographies of its practitioners—although the richness of the Italian archives has let me present more detailed results.[22] Like those writers, I have found that the picture of the medical profession and medical practice yielded by archival sources is often very different from that suggested by theoretical treatises; I have nonetheless benefited greatly from the recent studies of late thirteenth- and fourteenth-century medical doctrine and academic life by Nancy G. Siraisi and others, which my work complements rather than contradicts.[23] Like most recent historians of medicine, I have also had to reject the mythical history of the early medical profession constructed for the most part by the doctors who were its first students and whose unconscious impulses seem to have been, on the one hand, to celebrate their own achievements by exaggerating the obscurantism of medieval doctors and the superstitions of their patients and, on the other, to safeguard their own status and prestige by denying the artisanal component in their own history.[24] As I will argue in the case of Italy—and as has been recently shown

---

[21] Dols, *Black Death*, 268-69, and Thrupp, "Plague Effects," 480-81, indicate the interest of these questions but offer no information concerning them. Carpentier notes briefly the problems of medical recruitment during and after the plague of 1348; see *Une ville*, 146-47, 191; see also the older study of Campbell, *Black Death*, 119-20. The only treatment I know which touches on one aspect of the subject in more detail is Amundsen, "Medical Deontology."

[22] Jacquart, *Le milieu médical*, based on the earlier work of Wickersheimer, *Dictionnaire biographique*, and Jacquart, *Supplément*; Talbot and Hammond, *Medical Practitioners*; Kealey, *Medieval Medicus*. See also Lehoux, *Le cadre de vie*; Pelling and Webster, "Medical Practitioners"; and Roberts, "Personnel and Practice," I and II. Richard Palmer is taking a similar approach for Renaissance Venice; see his "Physicians and Surgeons." For Italy the other recent discussions of the medical profession are Ruggiero, "Status of Physicians and Surgeons," on Venice, and Cipolla, *Public Health*, which deals primarily with later sixteenth- and seventeenth-century Florence. There are also a number of more dated and antiquarian but still useful studies of doctors in various Italian towns: on Pistoia, Chiappelli, *Medici e chirurghi pistoiesi* and "Antichi medici"; on Pisa, Brugaro, "Contributo"; on Lucca, Ceccarelli, *La tradizione*; on Volterra, Battistini, *Medici in Volterra*; on Venice, Cecchetti, *Medicina in Venezia.*

[23] Siraisi, *Taddeo Alderotti* and *Arts and Sciences at Padua*, chap. 5. See also references to Michael McVaugh and Luke Demaitre in the Bibliography.

[24] This interpretation marks even the more recent and much more valuable study of Bullough, *Development of Medicine.*

for England[25]—university-trained physicians represented only a minority of established medical practitioners in the late Middle Ages and Renaissance, and private practice only one (and not necessarily the most important) sector of medical care.

The mythical version of medical history finds echoes, however, in the writings of sociologists on the early history of the professions, the last and least satisfactory of the historiographical traditions to which this book speaks. There is a tendency among Anglo-American students of the professions—the field is dominated by English and American scholars—to concentrate largely or entirely on English models for the premodern period.[26] This has led them to focus on university education as the principal source of those attributes usually taken to distinguish the professions from other kinds of occupations: controlled access, stringent licensing procedures, effective monopoly of the services rendered, and technical autonomy, as well as the derived features of social status and prestige.[27] Another misconception, which touches medicine in particular, is the common conviction that the theory and practice of the medical profession before the end of the nineteenth century was wholly inadequate and could not have inspired widespread public confidence. Thus the legally constituted body of premodern practitioners could not have enjoyed a monopoly rigorous enough to qualify them as a profession in the strictest sense.[28] This misconception then fits with the common assumption that the most

[25] See Pelling and Webster, "Medical Practitioners," esp. 165-66, 232-35.

[26] This is not in itself surprising; the concept of profession, in the strict sense of the "liberal" professions (medicine, law, and divinity in the early modern period), is to a large degree an invention and reflection of English society and culture; see Carr-Saunders and Wilson, *The Professions*; Geoffrey Holmes, *Augustan England*; and Reader, *Professional Men*. Europeans and students of Continental history have tended to use the term to encompass much broader social realities; see, for example, Rosenberg, *Bureaucracy, Aristocracy and Autocracy*, chap. 1. The best general introduction to the early history of the professions is Cipolla, "The Professions."

[27] See Geoffrey Millerson's analytical table of the traits proposed by various sociologists as basic to the idea of profession, in *Qualifying Associations*, 4-5. The two most compelling sociological discussions of these issues are Johnson, *Professions and Power*, 45-46, and Freidson, *Profession of Medicine*, 23, 82. For the most cogent historical statement of the university thesis as applied to medicine see Bullough, *Development of Medicine*, esp. chap. 5.

[28] For instance Freidson, *Profession of Medicine*, 12-15; cf. the more shaded argument of William J. Goode in his "Encroachment, Charlatanism and the Emerging Profession," 904, where he argues that the social and political institutionalization of a profession depends not on any empirical test of effectiveness but on public perception of that effectiveness. For recent literature relating to the problem of medical effectiveness and the placebo effect see Freidson, *Profession of Medicine*, 265-67.

important precondition for the rise of the professions was industrialization.[29]

My study of medical practice and medical practitioners in early Renaissance Florence challenges these ideas. It is important to remember that England in this period was socially and economically isolated and backward and that, at least as far as medicine was concerned, it relied in important areas on continental and Italian models of organization. It seems reasonable, therefore, to look to those models as they originally evolved rather than to the imported English forms. What can the Florentine example tell us about the emergent medical profession in Italy? In the first place, we find that except in atypical towns such as Bologna it was not the university which licensed doctors and established standards for their practice; as Chapter One will show, this function was reserved for the guild, an institution shared by many commercial and artisanal occupations. Thus any analysis of the origins of the profession of medicine must focus on the guild as the primary form of organization or at the very least must take as its subject the complex interaction of university and guild. In the second place, as we will see in the second and third chapters, doctors in the Florentine medical guild enjoyed a monopoly of medical practice justified by generally accepted claims of technical competence. In fact, by the middle of the fourteenth century the Florentine doctors, as organized in their guild, seem to have possessed all the formal hallmarks, enumerated above, of a fully constituted profession.

Thus I would argue that the modern professions are the outcome of a continuous historical development which had its roots in the European "commercial revolution" of the twelfth and thirteenth centuries and which flowered in the social and secular context of the growth of cities associated with the rise of that economy.[30] The surplus labor and capital generated in the great towns of the later Middle Ages allowed the formation of large numbers of specialized and highly organized occupations, including several we now identify as professions. Furthermore, their particular forms of occupational control and autonomy—and to a remarkable extent even the arguments for that autonomy and that control—were a product of the late medieval urban environment.

I do not mean by this that the medical profession in early Renaissance Florence was a mirror image of the modern medical profession,

[29] For example Larson, *Rise of Professionalism*, xvi-xx, and Haskell, *Emergence of Social Science*, 26-44. Reader makes a similar point in his otherwise well considered *Professional Men*, e.g., 2.

[30] See Lopez, *Commercial Revolution*.

nor do I mean that medical organization remained static in Europe between the fourteenth and the late nineteenth centuries. Such a claim flies in the face of what we would expect and what we know. To accept the continuities between late medieval institutions and their modern counterparts, however, deepens our understanding of both. On the one hand, it encourages us to see the modern medical order as the product of a long historical evolution which has left its marks on both practice and the profession. On the other, it encourages us to interest ourselves in the early institutions and the ways in which they were shaped to fit the peculiar contours of the societies which produced them. A case in point is the Florentine Guild of Doctors, Apothecaries, and Grocers.

· I ·

The Guild

THE SOCIETY of early Renaissance Florence, like that of the other
north Italian city-states, functioned less as a collection of individuals than as a network of overlapping collectivities.[1] Some of
these collectivities, like families, served a multitude of public and private purposes. Some, like guilds or partnerships, were primarily economic in character, while others met needs of political organization or
defense; among these were neighborhood militias, parties or factions,
and the communal government itself. Still others embodied religious
ties—parish churches, monasteries, hospitals, confraternities. Although
such groups differed in size, permanence, cohesiveness, and legal status, they all represented, formally or informally, an ideal of solidarity
and mutual aid or protection. Medicine, too, was ordered by its corporate structures and cannot be understood in isolation from them.

The community of medical practitioners and the practice of medicine, like most of the other nonmenial occupations in Renaissance
Florence, was defined and regulated by its guild, the Guild of Doctors,
Apothecaries, and Grocers; this body established licensing requirements and standards which the profession was expected to observe.
Thus the statutes and matriculation lists of the guild represent the
official framework within which the Florentine doctor exercised his
trade. But the guild was much more than a simple regulatory body:
embedded in Florence's corporate order, it reflected changing economic, social, and political conditions in the city. In this way it serves
as a microcosm of the forces which shaped the lives of doctors in the
fourteenth and fifteenth centuries.

The Guild of Doctors, Apothecaries, and Grocers was one of the
twenty-one corporations of masters established in 1293 by the Ordi-

[1] On corporatism in Renaissance Florence and the problem of individualism see Brucker,
Civic World, chap. 1; Weissman, *Ritual Brotherhood*, 2-35; and the references in F. W.
Kent, *Household and Lineage*, 289n. For a general discussion of corporations in medieval
language and law see Michaud-Quantin, *Universitas*.

nances of Justice. It belonged to the group of the seven "greater guilds," which also governed law, banking, the cloth industry, and international trade. There were in addition fourteen lesser guilds with jurisdiction over the more traditional crafts and the food trade, none of which, as a rule, offered the status and income of banking, commerce, and the professions.[2] Like other medieval craft and merchant corporations, the Florentine guilds had originated as protective associations of workers in allied trades, asserting a monopoly over those trades and aiming at the defense of common economic interests. At the same time they also had a social component; their members were bound by ties of acquaintance and kinship, and these ties were expressed in their statutory obligations to observe the funerals of colleagues, to provide for the needs of less fortunate brethren, and to support joint religious works.

The guilds also functioned as political bodies. Each had its own power structure and political constitution. Furthermore, by the late thirteenth century the twenty-one corporations defined by the Ordinances of Justice had been established as the foundation of the city's electoral system; guild membership was required for the most important communal offices. The political power of the guilds was progressively, if intermittently, eroded beginning in the late 1320s. Nonetheless, the guilds continued to perform a variety of functions: they supplied a proving ground for political hopefuls, provided fraternal support, and regulated the many occupations on which the commercial economy of Florence depended.[3]

These multiple functions are reflected in the statutes of the Guild of Doctors, Apothecaries, and Grocers, which in turn shaped (and were shaped by) the conditions of medical practice. The statutes illuminate not only the specific licensing requirements and regulations which governed the professional life of Florence's doctors but also the nature and limits of the more intangible sense of cohesion which bound them together and gave them a group identity. Furthermore, the various

[2] The best general introduction to the Florentine guilds is Doren, *Le arti fiorentine*; see also his *Entwicklung*. The fundamental study of the Guild of Doctors, Apothecaries, and Grocers is Ciasca, *L'arte*. Ciasca has also edited the statutes of this guild; see his *Statuti*. The number and constellation of guilds varied greatly among northern Italian towns; doctors did not always appear allied with apothecaries, but might form part of another merchant guild or have their own organization; see Ciasca, *L'arte*, 198-209, and La Sorsa, *L'arte dei medici*, esp. xv-xvii.

[3] On legal, economic, social, and religious aspects of guild organization in medieval Europe as a whole see Michaud-Quantin, *Universitas*, 167-74, and the survey and bibliography in Thrupp, "Gilds." For an account of the changing position of the guilds in Florentine politics see Najemy, "Guild Republicanism" and *Corporatism and Consensus*.

amendments to the statutes passed in the years after 1348 show in detail how the plague affected the Florentine medical profession. But statutes and amendments alone offer at best a rather abstract picture of the aspirations of the profession and the way it attempted to realize them through the guild; they must be supplemented by a variety of other archival material to yield a clear sense of how important the guild actually was in the life of the medical profession and how it made its influence felt. In this chapter we will be shifting back and forth from the ideal to the real, from statute to enforcement. The evidence is often frustratingly incomplete; nonetheless it allows us to assemble at least a fragmentary portrait of the formal and informal organization of the Florentine medical profession.

Doctors in the Constitution of the Guild

As the name of the Guild of Doctors, Apothecaries, and Grocers suggests, medical practitioners were only one of the occupational groups it governed. Most Florentine guilds shared this heterogeneous character to some degree,[4] but the Guild of Doctors, Apothecaries, and Grocers was perhaps the most extreme example. Originally an association of spice and drug merchants, it had come to encompass a number of related trades by the end of the thirteenth century, including not only the other two eponymous groups, doctors (who also handled drugs) and grocers (who sold various other sorts of dry goods), but also a miscellaneous lot of chandlers, painters, stationers, leatherworkers, and metalworkers. Over the course of the fourteenth century a number of new occupations, including barbers and gravediggers, also made their appearance in its rolls.[5]

The heterogeneity of its members determined to some extent the character of the guild. By the mid-fourteenth century it was probably the largest of the greater guilds, boasting a membership of roughly six hundred.[6] Furthermore, its internal history was particularly turbulent, as its various constituent occupations jockeyed for power. The product of these struggles was a federation of diverse occupational groups with

---

[4] Goldthwaite, *Building of Renaissance Florence*, 249-51.

[5] On its internal divisions and early history see Doren, *Entwicklung*, 51-59; Najemy, "*Audiant omnes artes*," 78-80; and esp. Ciasca, *L'arte*, 1-90 (list of constituent occupations on 60-61n). The three main branches are defined in the statute of 1349, II, 23 (Ciasca, *Statuti*, 132-35).

[6] Najemy, "*Audiant omnes artes*," 69. Goro Dati specifically mentions the great size of the guild at the beginning of the fifteenth century; see *L'istoria di Firenze*, 142.

varying degrees of authority and autonomy. By 1314, the year of the guild's first surviving statute, the three subcorporations or branches (*membri*) of doctors, apothecaries, and grocers had assumed autonomous and equal status in its constitution. They presided in turn over an elaborate hierarchy of subordinate occupations; among these the saddlers, incorporated as a subgroup of the grocers, and the painters, a subgroup of the apothecaries, had their own statutes, although none was represented in the central administration of the guild.[7] The federative structure of the Guild of Doctors, Apothecaries, and Grocers was confirmed in the revised statute of 1349, which, with subsequent amendments, was to govern its activities, and by extension those of the medical profession, during the entire Renaissance period.[8]

The statute of 1349 defined both the corporate nature of Florence's medical profession (the guild's branch of doctors) and its relationship to the broader guild community. In some respects, doctors shared the general privileges and obligations of all members of the Guild of Doctors, Apothecaries, and Grocers. They participated in its common ceremonial life, attending the religious observances and banquet associated with the feasts of Mary and St. Barnabas.[9] Like other members, they joined the guild by paying a matriculation fee and swearing an oath of obedience to the consuls, its chief officers. Like other members, they benefited from the guild's claim to monopolize the practice of their occupation in the Florentine territories.[10] They were required to observe the common regulations concerning treatment of apprentices, rental of shops, and general honesty which governed the guild membership as a whole; accused of infractions, they were tried by the guild's six consuls in its *palazzo* on the Via Sant'Andrea.[11] In case of

[7] Ciasca, *L'arte*, 31-64.

[8] Ciasca's edition of the statutes and amendments, which I will use for all references, is based on the contemporary Italian translations of the original Latin texts. For a description of the various codices extant in the Florentine archives see his *Statuti*, ix-xxv.

[9] Ciasca, *L'arte*, 253-55.

[10] Statute of 1349, I, 3; II, 23, 38, 90 (Ciasca, *Statuti*, 106-7, 131, 145-48, 199-200). See Doren, *Le arti fiorentine*, 1:120-62, and Ciasca, *L'arte*, 165-73. Guild organization was in conception monopolistic: Thrupp, "Gilds," 247-53. On the monopolistic claims of Florentine guilds in particular see Camagna, "L'organizzazione interna," 184-89, and Doren, *Le arti fiorentine*, 1:77-78, 97-108. For those masters who refused to join, the statute prescribed a number of fines and penalties, the most effective of which was probably the provision that the unmatriculated practitioner be shunned, both professionally and personally, by the matriculants of the guild; see statute of 1349, II, 38 (Ciasca, *Statuti*, 147).

[11] For example statute of 1349, II, 21, 24, 37, 60-62 (Ciasca, *Statuti*, 129-30, 136, 144, 181). On the judicial functions of the guild consuls see Camagna, "L'organizzazione interna," 194-99; Doren, *Le arti fiorentine*, vol. 2, chaps. 6-7; Ciasca, *L'arte*, 151-54.

need, doctors were eligible for the material aid which the guild offered, at least in theory, to members who had fallen on hard days, and their funerals were to be attended by a delegation of the consuls and representatives of the guild as a whole.[12] Like the members of the other principal branches, finally, doctors were eligible for the consulship and other guild offices—as councilors, syndics, arbiters, and special consular appointees (*arroti*)—although by 1349, because their numbers were so much smaller than those of the apothecaries and grocers, the proportion of offices assigned to them was the smallest of the three.[13]

In addition to these common rights and obligations, however, the statute of 1349 also contains provisions specific to particular subject trades. Chandlers had to use wax of a certain quality, for example; apothecaries could not sell or administer various dangerous drugs; stationers could not erase entries for clients seeking to falsify contracts and records.[14] Furthermore, a special kind of social solidarity existed— or was supposed to exist—among workers in the same occupation. Thus, for example, when a painter, pursemaker, or scabbardmaker died, each workshop of his colleagues was to send a mourner to his funeral.[15]

The rubrics of the statute of 1349 governing medical practitioners encouraged a similar but heightened sense of community among Florentine doctors. Alone of all the members of the Guild of Doctors, Apothecaries, and Grocers, for example, doctors were expected to attend the funerals not only of their colleagues but also of their colleagues' wives. Unlike other guild members, they were forbidden to speak ill of one another, either publicly or in private.[16] This solidarity extended also to their work. A doctor could be fined for treating another's patient before the first had been paid in full.[17] A surgeon attending a patient suffering from a cranial fracture or other life-threatening condition was required to consult a colleague. A physician called on by the communal authorities to make a forensic judgment concern-

---

[12] Statute of 1349, II, 35-36 (Ciasca, *Statuti*, 143-44).

[13] Ciasca, *L'arte*, 149-64; statute of 1349, I, 1-4, 6, 8, 10; II, 17 (Ciasca, *Statuti*, 97-116, 126-127). For the changes in the representation among the three principal branches see Ciasca, *L'arte*, 25-28, 91-94.

[14] Statute of 1349, II, 46-47, 59, 76, 91 (Ciasca, *Statuti*, 158-65, 180, 189, 200).

[15] Ibid., II, 35 (143-44).

[16] Ibid. and II, 71 (186-87): "Niuno medico ardisca o presumma dire d'alcun altro medico secretamente o palesemente rusticità o parole ingiuriose. E contra faccenti pe' consoli in soldi cento di f. p. sieno condempnati, e tante volte."

[17] Ibid., II, 71 (187n; MS B only): "Ordinamus quod nullus medicus, cuiuscumque condictionis fuerit, audeat vel presumat medicare aliquem infirmum quem alter medicus primo curasset, nisi tali medico qui primo curasset satisfiat de suo labore, . . . sub pena soldorum quadraginta f. p."

ing cause of death was to seek a second opinion from a surgeon, and vice versa.[18]

Such special protective regulations, different in degree though not in kind from the regulations governing other occupations within the guild, encouraged close collegial bonds. They also reflected the special licensing requirements placed on doctors by the guild. Doctors were alone among its members in having to prove their competence before being allowed to matriculate and enter practice. The statute of 1349 spelled out the requirements. "And so that no doubt can arise over who are doctors," it read,

> we declare that all persons in the city or countryside of Florence who practice physic or surgery, set bones, and treat mouths, whether they use writing or not, are understood to be doctors, and are to be held and considered doctors, and must swear obedience and submit to the guild and its consuls.[19]

Furthermore, the statute stipulated,

> no new doctor, whether physician or surgeon, who does not have a doctorate may practice the art of medicine or heal in physic or surgery in the city or district of Florence, unless he has been examined by those consuls who are doctors, along with four doctors selected for the purpose by the consuls who are doctors, and approved as competent by those consuls and the four other doctors in a secret vote conducted by the guild notary.[20]

[18] Ibid., II, 69 (184-85). The penalty was £50, waivable at the request of the judicial official.

[19] Ibid., II, 23 (132): "Et acciò che niuno dubbio possa nascere di quegli che sono medici, spetiali e merciai, dichiariamo che tucti e ciascuni medicanti in phisica o cerusica, e aconcianti ossa, e medicanti bocche nella città o contado di Firenze, quandunche aranno medicato con scriptura o senza, s'intendino medici e per medici sieno avuti e reputati, e giurare et essere sotto posti all'arte predetta e a' consoli della detta arte." After 1384 this rubric was amended to include the barbers, whose own short-lived guild had been a product of the Ciompi revolt in 1378 and a casualty of the subsequent political reaction; see Ciasca, L'arte, 125-28, and amendment of 1384 (Ciasca, Statuti, 320-21).

[20] Statute of 1349, II, 70 (Ciasca, Statuti, 185-86): "Niuno medico nuovo, o fisico o cerusico, possa, debba o presumma exercitare l'arte della medicina in fisica o in cirusica nella città o distrecto di Firenze, il quale non sarà conventato, se prima non sarà examinato pe' consoli medici con quattro medici, quali a queste cose essi consoli medici avere vorranno, e aprovati per essi consoli medici e quattro altri medici, quali a queste cose vorranno avere a secreto scruptineo, il quale si debba fare col notaio della detta arte, per sufficiente." The fine prescribed for the illegal practitioner was £25; that for guild members who trafficked with him, £10.

As in the case of the other principal occupations over which they had jurisdiction, the consuls were to discourage unregulated medical practice by fining illegal practitioners and any guild member who had dealings with them; the fine of twenty-five lire (£) prescribed for unmatriculated doctors was, however, considerably larger than the forty soldi with which the other groups were threatened. (For a sketch of the Florentine monetary system, see Appendix I.)

The requirement of either a doctorate or a practical examination set medicine apart from the other occupations governed by the Guild of Doctors, Apothecaries, and Grocers, and indeed from most of the occupations governed by the other Florentine guilds. A number of guilds imposed special conditions for admission, but these generally concerned only the moral charater of the candidate or, in the case of the Guild of Bankers and Moneylenders, his residence and solvency.[21] The only other greater guild to ask for a demonstration of technical competence from some or all of its prospective matriculants was the Guild of Lawyers and Notaries, which required from the former proof of a university degree and from the latter satisfactory performance on three examinations.[22] Furthermore, by 1349 approval of the prospective doctor, like that of the prospective lawyer or notary, was entirely in the hands of his own profession—of the medical professors who voted the degree, in the case of the university-trained physician or surgeon, and of the examining doctors chosen by the guild, in the case of practitioners without a degree. This was a relatively new development, since as recently as 1314 the examining board had included all six of the guild's consuls (only two of whom were doctors) in addition to "two Franciscan and two Dominican friars selected by the priors or guardians of their orders."[23]

Thus the only two guilded occupations in Florence to demand a demonstration of competence (besides the craft of armormaking) were law and medicine. In both cases the justification was couched in terms of the elevated nature of the calling and the need to protect the public

[21] On admission requirements in general see Doren, *Le arti fiorentine*, 1:130-36. The masterpiece, commonly required for matriculation in the craft guilds of northern Europe, seems to have been unknown in Florence, at least by this period.

[22] Guild of Lawyers and Notaries: statute of 1344, I, 7; IV, 4, in Calleri, *L'arte dei giudici e notai*, 29-34, and see 102-21 for documents relating to notarial examinations given in 1337. Also Martines, *Lawyers*, chap. 2. Alone of all the minor guilds, the Guild of Armorers also provided for its candidates to be examined for proof of competence; see Guild of Armorers: statute of 1321, in Marri, *Statuti*, 28-29. Various other guilds, like the Linen Merchants or the Butchers, required a certain number of years of apprenticeship but no demonstration of competence; see Doren, *Le arti fiorentine*, 1:134.

[23] Statute of 1314, III, 55 (Ciasca, *Statuti*, 49).

in such crucial and delicate domains; in both cases the existence of a university curriculum and a special title for its masters expressed the selective nature of the profession. Lawyers and doctors did not differ from the rest in enjoying a legal monopoly on the practice of their trades; that was the assumption which underlay the entire guild system. Their distinction was, rather, that by the middle of the fourteenth century they had gained both the right to require certain technical qualifications for guild membership and the exclusive responsibility for setting, verifying, and enforcing those qualifications. (The commune itself did not license medical practitioners, although by 1415 the Florentine statutes explicitly recognized the rights of the guild in this matter.) These privileges of monopoly and of autonomy in setting licensing requirements are usually identified by Anglo-American scholars as the hallmarks of a profession and associated with the attainment of a university degree.[24] The Florentine case suggests a more complicated dynamic: the development of a body of sophisticated theory embedded in a university curriculum may have allowed the branch of doctors to argue for special, more stringent licensing requirements; nonetheless, the institution which enforced these requirements was not the university but the guild, and the requirements did not exclude empirically trained doctors of proven competence.

Medical licensing in fourteenth-century Florence differed from later and northern European forms in setting a broad set of qualifications for legal admission to the profession.[25] Candidates could choose between two entirely different criteria: the university degree and the guild examination. Once deemed qualified, however, all were matriculated without distinction in the books of the guild and granted the honorific title of master (*maestro* or *magister*).[26] As a result, the guild's branch

[24] See, for example, the argument of Bullough in *Development of Medicine*, esp. 4, 108-11.

[25] Many other Italian cities also used a qualifying examination for doctors; see Ciasca, *L'arte*, 268n. The situation was very different in England and France, for example, where physicians and surgeons belonged to different organizations and where empirics, although legion, were not given legal recognition by being allowed to matriculate as doctors; see Pelling and Webster, "Medical Practitioners," esp. 165-88, and Kibre, "Faculty of Medicine."

[26] The title itself deserves clarification. In the earlier period (thirteenth and early fourteenth centuries) doctors were addressed either as maestro (abbreviated M°) or with the notarial title ser; by 1350 the latter was no longer used for doctors. Others called maestro included university students, university lecturers in arts or theology, private teachers in subjects like arithmetic or grammar, and occasional performers, like some fencing masters or musicians. On the whole, however, the overwhelming majority of men with the prefix maestro in this period can be assumed to be doctors. A very few empirical practitioners appear in the matriculation lists of the guild without the title;

of doctors included people of widely differing social classes and medical training, from the physician with a doctorate from Padua to the shoemaker who couched cataracts; all, however, were fully licensed practitioners.

Thus Florentine doctors, bolstered by the sensitivity and prestige of their art as well as by their relative overrepresentation in the power structure of the guild before 1349, managed to incorporate into the new statute of that year a number of special provisions designed to protect the profession's livelihood and reputation. These provisions aimed to reduce competition, establish licensing requirements and standards for practice, and multiply opportunities for consultation. In the process, they also aimed to promote a closer sense of community than obtained among the other occupations governed by the guild. In practical terms, however, the very breadth of the licensing requirements must have served to limit medical collegiality. We know, for example, that university-trained physicians sometimes objected to working with empirics; it is also hard to believe that Florentine physicians would have mustered much enthusiasm at the funeral of the wife of an illiterate tooth-doctor. Even in the ideal world of the statute of 1349, moreover, there was a rubric hinting at a special solidarity restricted to the higher ranks of medical practitioners: all physicians were required to attend disputations on medical topics at the University of Florence, if so notified by the guild.[27] Since the university was established only in 1348, this provision did not appear in the earlier statute of 1314; it represents the beginning of a process of differentiation which was to culminate in 1392 with the foundation of a separate corporation of university-educated doctors within the guild.

We will discuss this process in more detail in the third section of this chapter. Here, however, we need to look more closely at the actual

---

this would seem to indicate a very low level of practice, on a par with that of barbers. Usually, however, a doctor denied the title in guild records acquired it in other communal documents, like treasury accounts or tax rolls. Otherwise it is impossible to distinguish between different types of doctors on the basis of the forms of their names in contemporary documents. The only legal distinction between university- and empirically trained doctors in this period was in sumptuary regulation. Physicians and surgeons with university degrees were accorded a number of special privileges in dress and funeral pomp; see Corsini, *Il costume*, 3-7 (on dress); Statuti-11 (Statuto del Capitano, 1355), fols. 150r-53v; and *Statuta populi et communis Florentiae*, IV, 13-16; 2:374-77 (on funerals).

[27] Statute of 1349, II, 70 (Ciasca, *Statuti*, 186): "Ordinanti che ogni fisico sia tenuto ire in ogni disputatione, la quale si facesse d'alcuna questione medicinale nelle scuole de' medici per lo comune di Firenze a llui, se a llui sarà notificato o sarà richiesto o amonito, sotto la pena di soldi .xl. di f. p. . . . ."

nature and extent of the corporate ties which bound Florentine doctors to one another and to other members of their·guild. The statute of 1349 embodied an ideal of community sealed with a degree of exclusivity. How potent was this ideal in practice? How effectively did the guild enforce its monopoly of medical practice? What proportion of doctors actually matriculated in the guild? The statutory material cannot answer such questions, and the guild's books of deliberations and condemnations from the fourteenth and early fifteenth centuries have not survived. Thus we must look at other archival sources—tax lists, political records, legislation—to judge the degree to which the guild's statutes expressed the actual nature of the medical profession and of medical practice in Florence.

The Guild and Professional Life

One would expect a reasonably high rate of matriculation among doctors. The two main barriers to guild membership—the licensing examination, for candidates without a university degree, and the matriculation fee and other moneys exacted by the guild—do not seem to have been insurmountable for most members of the profession. The examination, as various amendments to the statute of 1349 complained, was required only sporadically, and even when administered seems to have been little more than a formality, as an amendment from 1422 indicates: "no one in the past has ever been refused," it reads, "but everyone has always been admitted and accepted."[28] (The matriculation list for that year bears this out, including as it does the name of one Paolo di Ricco di Paolo, "blacksmith and doctor.")[29] The matriculation fee itself was reasonable. The sum of 4 florins (fl.) for natives of the Florentine territories and fl. 8 for foreigners, raised in 1404 to fl. 6 and fl. 12 respectively, was low compared with that of the other greater guilds, even in theory.[30] (Most doctors enjoyed an an-

[28] Amendment of 1422, V (Ciasca, Statuti, 422). Note that this amendment did not refer specifically to the branch of doctors but to the guild membership in general.

[29] AMS-21, ad annum 1421.

[30] Amendment of 1404, I (Ciasca, Statuti, 378); on Florentine matriculation fees see Doren, Le arti fiorentine, 1:136-40. The fees for the Guild of Lawyers and Notaries were fl. 16 (lawyers) and fl. 8 (notaries), according to their statute of 1344: Calleri, L'arte dei giudici e notai, 31. By 1400 lawyers were paying fl. 25; Martines, Lawyers, 31. The Lana, Cambio, and Calimala guilds all set their fees in the fl. 20 range; see Doren, Le arti fiorentine, 1:137n. In comparison, fees for the lesser guilds were considerably lower: for example new matriculants in the Guild of Carpenters after 1346 paid £10, as did those in the Guild of Leatherworkers after 1338; Morandini, Statuti, 149, and Marri, Statuti, 33-35.

nual income of between fl. 100 and fl. 400, while a typical unskilled laborer made about fl. 40 a year; see Appendix I.) In practice, only a small minority of matriculants paid even those amounts. Children (male and female), grandchildren, and sons-in-law of guild members matriculated free, while brothers, nephews, and uncles paid half price.[31] More to the point, many of the nonprivileged matriculants defaulted after paying no more than a fraction of the two-installment entrance fee, as various amendments to tighten the matriculation procedure testify.[32]

The frequency of these reforms indicates that they were not very successful; this impression is confirmed in the day-by-day list of new matriculants between 1409 and 1444, which includes the fees due and the installments as they were paid.[33] In general the schedule of payments depended on the wealth of the doctor and on the length of his stay in Florence. A few rich immigrant doctors, including some readers in medicine at the university, managed to pay even their relatively high sum of fl. 12 in a short period, while some local doctors of more modest means paid in full by spreading out their payments in many installments over a number of years.[34] But most doctors registered in the book escaped full payment. Some enjoyed a total exemption be-

---

[31] Statute of 1349, II, 38 (Ciasca, Statuti, 147); amendment of 1404, I (378).

[32] An amendment from 1392 stipulated that no one was to matriculate without paying in full, while allowing the consuls to make exceptions for the poor (Ciasca, Statuti, 345-46). In 1404 an amendment raising fees removed this power from the consuls and required back dues to be paid within six months if the member was to be "really" (realmente e veramente) matriculated (ibid., 378-80). An amendment of 1468 specified that doctors and apothecaries, as the members of the guild most able to afford it, should pay their fees in full at the time of matriculation (ibid., 498-99).

[33] AMS-21. The matriculation lists which survive from this period in the archive of the Guild of Doctors, Apothecaries, and Grocers are of three kinds: day-by-day records of new matriculants (AMS-21 and parts of AMS-9); cumulative lists of current members (AMS-8 and parts of AMS-9); and an alphabetical and chronological compilation from earlier rolls covering the years between the end of the thirteenth century and 1444 (AMS-7). For a more detailed description of the various sections of these lists see Ciasca, L'arte, 173n. The basic list (AMS-7), while remarkably accurate, is not always complete, occasionally omitting names—particularly for the years around 1350—and toponymics. I have crosschecked it throughout with the original records in AMS-8 (for the period before 1353), AMS-9 (for 1353-86), and AMS-21 (1409-44). The only period for which an original is entirely missing is 1386-1408; the information on matriculations from those years is correspondingly less complete and less reliable.

[34] An example of the first is M° Ventura Venturelli da Pesaro, who taught at the studio from 1413 to 1415; he paid his fee of fl. 12 in eight installments between the end of January 1414/5, when he matriculated, and August 1415. For purposes of comparison the annual salary for his lectureship in medicine, which he doubtless supplemented with income from private practice, was fl. 100; see AMS-21, ad annum 1415, and Park, "Readers," 272-73. An example of the latter is M° Agnolo di Cristofano dal contado di Arezzo, who settled permanently in Florence, paying his fee of fl. 6 in six payments over seven years beginning in 1415 (AMS-21, ad annum 1415).

cause their fathers or grandfathers were members; others left the city before completing payment or (in the case even of permanent residents) simply gave up on their installments. Of the fourteen doctors recorded in the *catasto* (wealth tax) of 1427 whose matriculation records are contained in the day-by-day list, for example, seven were exempted as relatives and five paid a third or less of the amount due, while only two paid in full.[35]

We can only guess at the reasons for this laxity. The guild seems to have been caught in a dilemma between an exclusive and an inclusive model of operation. The arguments for the former, which would have been expressed in stiff entrance requirements and high matriculation fees, included the wish to restrict licensed competition as much as possible. The arguments for the latter, expressed in a tendency to apply matriculation requirements loosely, included the wish to swell the guild's authority, and its treasury, by bringing the maximum number of medical practitioners under guild control; this alternative must have appealed also because it would have been impossible to enforce the strict licensing procedures without investing inordinate amounts of the guild's time and money. Amendments adopted during the later fourteenth and the fifteenth centuries testify to a continuing tug of war between these alternatives: fees and examinations were waived and reinstated for various groups at irregular intervals.

On the whole, however, the inclusive model seems to have prevailed in Florence, as it did in many other Italian cities. This sets the Florentine profession apart from its English counterpart, which is too often taken as the norm by historians and sociologists of early medicine. Whereas in England most medical practitioners operated outside the very narrow institutional framework of the profession, in Florence the matriculation rate was extremely high.[36] Although the period after the plague saw periodic complaints about the incidence of unlicensed heal-

---

[35] The breakdown is as follows (dates in parentheses refer to the year in which the matriculation record appears in AMS-21): Mᵒ Angelo di Cristofano dal contado di Arezzo, fl. 6, in full (1415); Mᵒ Luca di mᵒ Antonio, exempt (1433); Mᵒ Bartolomeo di mᵒ Antonio, exempt (1433); Mᵒ Giovanni di mᵒ Antonio, exempt (1433); Mᵒ Bandino di mᵒ Giovanni Banducci, exempt (1418); Mᵒ Paolo di mᵒ Domenico, exempt (1425); Mᵒ Piero di mᵒ Domenico, exempt (1425); Mᵒ Giovanni di Bartolomeo da Montecatini, fl. 2 paid out of fl. 6 owed (1417); Mᵒ Guasparre di ser Matteo da Radda, £4 paid out of fl. 6 owed (1421); Mᵒ Iacopo di ser Antonio da Poppi, fl. 2 paid out of fl. 6 owed (1423); Mᵒ Iacopo di Martino da Spoleto, no record of any payment (1424); Mᵒ Ridolfo di Francesco da Cortona, fl. 6, in full (1423); Mᵒ Salvadore di mᵒ Niccolò da Catania, no record of any payment (1425); Mᵒ Taddeo di Cambino, exempt (1423).

[36] Cf. Pelling and Webster, "Medical Practitioners," 232-35.

ers, the overwhelming majority of medical practitioners were matriculated as doctors and therefore operated lawfully and within the officially constituted profession. The picture is clear if one compares the matriculation lists with the names of doctors appearing in sample tax rolls or granted explicit tax exemptions by the commune.[37]

As table 1-1 shows, the proportion of unmatriculated doctors who had settled in Florence long enough (often only a few months) to appear in the communal tax records was small in relation to the profession as a whole. Even at its largest, in the decades immediately after the plague of 1348, this group was relatively small, and by the end of the fourteenth century it had, in effect, disappeared. Unmatriculated doctors in the earlier tax lists represent almost exclusively empirics, who were to a certain extent marginal members of the profession even though many of their number belonged to the guild. Matriculation levels would certainly have been lower among (untaxed) transients and those not legally resident in the city; this group included some readers in arts and medicine at the university as well as traveling empirics, but even among these doctors the matriculation rate was extremely high.

TABLE 1-1
Unmatriculated Doctors and the Guild

Year	Doctors in Tax List (or exempt)	Number Matriculated	No Record of Matriculation	Identity Unclear
1359	27	23	4	—
1369	40	35	1	4
1379	49	44	3	2
1390	38	38	—	—
1399	45	44	1	—
1406	37	37	—	—
1427	36	36	—	—

SOURCES: Prestanze-5, 143, 144, 146, 156, 367, 368, 369, 1262, 1263, 1264, 1265, 1787, 1788, 1789, 1790, 2386, 2387, 2388, 2389; Catasto-65 to 83 and Catasto-Campioni del Monte-San Giovanni-1427. For details see note 37.

[37] Figures from the records of selected *prestanze* and the *catasto* of 1427, as follows: Prestanze-5 (1359); Prestanze-143, 144, 146, 156 (1369, quarter of Santa Maria Novella from same distribution in January 1369/70); Prestanze-367, 368, 369 (1379, not including quarter of Santo Spirito); Prestanze-1262, 1263, 1264, 1265 (1390, quarter of Santo Spirito from same distribution in 1392); Prestanze-1787, 1788, 1789, 1790 (1399); Prestanze-2386, 2387, 2388, 2389 (1406); Catasto-65 to 83 and Catasto-Campioni del Monte-San Giovanni-1427. For more information on the various kinds of taxes levied in Florence see Appendix I. Note that the figures from the *prestanze* can be taken only as minimum numbers for practicing doctors, since they did not include transients or dependents.

Thus by the end of the fourteenth century the guild's monopoly on medical practice in Florence, even if only a de facto monopoly, was more or less complete. This impression is borne out by the single book of guild deliberations surviving from this period; compiled in the mid-1470s, it includes no complaints about unlicensed practice or encroachment by apothecaries or others.[38]

In order to understand what guild membership meant to a Florentine doctor, however, we must look beyond the rates of matriculation for medical practitioners. Matriculation corresponded chronologically to the young doctor's entry into independent practice. In this connection, probably the most important legal benefit it conferred was the right to bring suit before the guild court to recover money owed by patients or guild members. For those who met the citizenship and residency requirements, it also granted general political eligibility for the whole gamut of communal offices and particular access to the various guild positions which formed the first step in the *cursus honorum* of Florentine public life.[39] At least as important as these formal benefits of guild membership, however, were the informal ones. The more one studies the records of doctors' personal and professional lives, the more one realizes that the Guild of Doctors, Apothecaries, and Grocers was not just a corporation regulating the economic and political life of a number of related occupational groups; it corresponded, rather, to an intricate social world whose members, both as families and as individuals, were knit together by a dense network of varied ties: indebtedness, partnership, contract, kinship, marriage, and friendship.

These ties were particularly close among doctors and between doctors and apothecaries. To begin with purely financial dealings, even a quick glance at the lists of debtors and creditors in doctors' declarations for the *catasto* of 1427 reveals a high proportion of apothecaries and fellow doctors.[40] The money owed or lent doctors and relatives of doctors probably reflected the normal relations of acquaintance or kinship found within any occupational group. These tended to be strongest among practitioners of the same geographical origin. The declaration of Maestro Iacopo di maestro Antonio da Montecatini, for

[38] AMS-49, unpag. What complaints there are concern not breaches of doctors' monopoly by apothecaries and empirics but the facts that apothecaries were careless in filling doctors' prescriptions and that empirics were wearing the special insignia (long gown, gold buckle) reserved by sumptuary legislation to holders of the doctorate. The volume also contains a proposal to forbid nonuniversity-trained doctors from practicing medicine, but it was never passed.

[39] See Becker, *Florence in Transition*, 2:31n, 98.

[40] For the doctors in the *catasto* of 1427 see Appendix III.

example, indicates that he owned one-third of a house in Montecatini, the rest of which belonged to the two minor heirs of Maestro Ugolino di maestro Giovanni da Montecatini, an illustrious physician who had died in Florence shortly before. Maestro Iacopo further noted that he owed the heirs of Maestro Ugolino fl. 60—interest-free, by the terms of Maestro Ugolino's will—for a period of ten years. Finally, the tax official added, "the said Maestro Iacopo has no books, unless he buys some, and he has borrowed several of those which belonged to Maestro Ugolino, while or if it pleases his sons to let him have them."[41]

Debts between doctors and apothecaries usually represented more commercial arrangements, and such arrangements were common, given the mutual dependence of the two occupations. Doctors, according to their tax declarations and their diaries, invested in the drug and spice trade more frequently than in any other kind of business. Sometimes, like Maestro Paolo and Maestro Piero di maestro Domenico Toscanelli, they owned a company outright. Sometimes, like Maestro Iacopo di Coluccino da Lucca, they acted as freelance commercial middlemen, importing substances like pepper or saffron and wholesaling them to local shops. Sometimes they invested in an established concern; in 1451, for example, Maestro Ugolino di Piero recorded among the sums owed to him fl. 200 "on deposit in an apothecary's shop in the Mercato Vecchio."[42] Often doctors and apothecaries formed companies together as partners in the spice trade.[43]

An even more common arrangement was the contract by which a doctor (usually a physician), in return for a regular salary, agreed to see patients in a particular apothecary's shop for a certain number of hours a week, during which he wrote prescriptions to be filled on the premises. (Sometimes the doctor even slept above the shop.)[44] As a

[41] Catasto-83, fols. 123v-24r (declaration), and Catasto-296, fols. 79v-80r (*campione*, or official summary): "Libri nonn à il decto M° Iacopo se non ne compra, e à in presto parte di quegli furono del M° Ugolino mentre o se piacerà a' figliuoli lasciarlili tenere." There are many other examples of networks of debts between doctors; see, for example, the declaration of M° Ridolfo di Francesco da Cortona in Catasto-74, fol. 201r-v. On the form of Florentine names in this period see Appendix I.

[42] Uzielli, *Toscanelli*, 504-11; *ricordanza* of M° Iacopo di Coluccino Bonavia da Lucca (ASL: Ospedale di S. Luca, fols. 7r, 13r, 19v); declaration of M° Ugolino di Piero (Catasto-709, fol. 391r).

[43] This arrangement was legal in Florence, although prohibited in some other Italian cities, presumably as a form of conflict of interest; for an example see the *ricordanza* of M° Iacopo di Coluccino Bonavia da Lucca, fol. 27v. The Guild of Doctors, Apothecaries, and Grocers did forbid doctors to accept kickbacks from apothecaries on the price of medicines prescribed; statute of 1349, II, 72 (Ciasca, *Statuti*, 187).

[44] This arrangement was apparently common all over Tuscany and almost certainly elsewhere in Italy. It is frequently referred to in doctors' diaries and account books, as

result of such agreements, certain apothecaries came to be identified with certain doctors; a typical entry in the accounts of the hospital of Santa Maria Nuova reads, "To the apothecary of Maestro Fruosino for the electuary he made up for Ghita, s. 11, d. 8."[45] In the course of things this kind of contract tended to generate debts between doctors and apothecaries, since, as *catasto* declarations show, doctors commonly answered to apothecaries for money owed by patients who had had prescriptions made up on credit. Maestro Giorgio di Niccolò, for example, recorded a debt of fl. 24 (a considerable amount in comparison to his net worth of fl. 73) "for medicines, and as security for medicines ordered for others."[46] As one of the offshoots of this kind of arrangement, doctors often appointed apothecaries—presumably apothecaries with whom they had invested or to whom they were under contract—as their procurators, or legal and financial agents.[47]

These formal and contractual ties among members of occupational groups associated within the guild were supplemented by a number of miscellaneous financial dealings, often involving the rent or sale of houses, shops, and land.[48] As was common in Florence, such transactions often reflected social ties of kinship, marriage, or friendship. Again, these ties were particularly dense within the medical profession and between physicians and apothecaries. Sylvia Thrupp points out in her general discussion of European guilds that guilds governing highly monopolistic groups—like doctors, given their special licensing requirements, or apothecaries, given the relatively few sources of supply—tend to show strong social solidarity, most notably in the form

---

noted below in Chapter Three. The parties involved were often related by blood or marriage.

[45] SMN-4408, fol. 46r: "A lo speziale del Maestro Fruosino per latovare ch'egli fecie per la Ghita."

[46] Catasto-49, fol. 1552r: "per medicine e per sechurtà di medicine fatte dare ad altrui." See also the entry in the declaration of M° Francesco di ser Conte Mini, in Catasto-53, fol. 925r: "Ugho di Niccholò Vecchietti de' dare [fl. 10], i quali promissi per lui alla bottegha d'Agnolo Grifi spetiale, per medicine e zuchero e confetti quando medichai Monna Marta sua donna del ghavociolo a Sa' Moro nel '23."

[47] See, for example, the records of salary payments for readers in medicine at the University of Florence, including M° Andrea dalla Pergola, M° Antonio Roselli da Arezzo, and M° Giovanni di m° Piero da Sermoneta, all of whom were listed as having apothecaries as procurators: Monte-1604, fol. 129v; 1605, fol. 131r; 1595, fol. 95r.

[48] In 1369, for example, M° Tommaso Del Garbo sold a house for fl. 420. Among the witnesses to the agreement were M° Falcone di Donato da Radda and M° Banco di m° Latino, both Florentine doctors, and the latter—according to the seventieth novella of Tommaso Sacchetti—a special friend of M° Tommaso; see Corsini, "Nuovo contributo," 275.

of occupational inheritance and intermarriage.[49] This pattern certainly holds for the guilds of Florence, which encouraged the growth of strong family traditions by eliminating or reducing matriculation fees for relatives and in-laws of past and present members. Within the guild of Doctors, Apothecaries, and Grocers in particular there was a high degree of occupational inheritance. Of the thirty-seven doctors appearing in the *catasto* as either dependents or heads of household, for example, fifteen had doctors for fathers, and at least four were sons of apothecaries.

This is not to say that the medical profession was a closed caste in Florence, as it tended to be in some other Italian cities,[50] or that the same was true of the guild. Doctors' families were also frequently linked to the notariate and to law (the two other proto-professions of the Renaissance) as well as to the textile business, Florence's largest industry. Five of the doctors in the 1427 *catasto* were sons of notaries. Furthermore, in most families there seems to have been a conscious attempt to diversify employment, within and even between generations, to assure the family's financial security while keeping strong links to its principal occupation.[51] Of the four sons of Maestro Lodovico di Bartolo da Gubbio, for example, Maestro Bartolomeo became a physician, Batista an apothecary, Messer Guasparre a lawyer, and Piero a cloth retailer after he abandoned a brief university career.[52]

But even though the tendency of doctors' families to choose occupations governed by their guild remained strong, the pattern varied over time. Through the mid-fourteenth century, sons of doctors often followed in their fathers' footsteps. For example, both the father and the grandfather of Maestro Iacopo di maestro Bartolo Novellucci da Prato, who immigrated to Florence in the 1340s, were doctors. His two sons, Maestro Giovanni and Maestro Agnolo, became physicians, and Maestro Agnolo's sons Maestro Lorenzo and Maestro Niccolò

---

[49] Thrupp, "Gilds," 247-49. On family traditions within the Florentine guilds see Doren, *Le arti fiorentine*, 1:141-49. Such traditions account to a large extent for the fact that doctors from better families matriculated in more than one guild. M° Cristofano di Giorgio, M° Galileo di Giovanni Galilei, and M° Piero de' Pulci, for example, all joined the Silk Guild—to which their fathers' belonged—as well as the Guild of Doctors, Apothecaries, and Grocers: Seta-7, fols. 40v, 79r, 157v.

[50] Compare, for example, Parma and Padua; see Ciasca, *L'arte*, 309.

[51] This was in accordance with the advice of contemporary writers and moralists, such as Paolo da Certaldo, *Libro di buoni costumi*, 193. For a more detailed discussion of these kinds of career choices see Chapter Four.

[52] The sources of this and similar statements are to be found in the various matriculation lists of the Guild of Doctors, Apothecaries, and Notaries, supplemented by the lists of other greater guilds, and the *fondi* of Prestanze and Tratte.

also went into medicine and matriculated in the guild. This pattern became increasingly rare during the century after the coming of the plague, for reasons which will be discussed in Chapter Five, but there was a compensatory rise in the number of sons of doctors becoming apothecaries and the number of apothecaries' sons becoming doctors. Thus Tommaso, Luigi, and Bartolo, the three sons of Maestro Niccolò di Bonaventura da Mantova, a reader in medicine at the *studio* and a naturalized Florentine citizen, all matriculated in the guild as apothecaries in the second half of the fourteenth century.

Families of doctors and apothecaries could also be joined by marriage. Doctors' daughters often married doctors or apothecaries.[53] Sometimes the bonds were even more complex, as is evident in the (partial) genealogies of two Florentine families prominent in the fifteenth-century Guild of Doctors, Apothecaries, and Grocers: the Cini and the Toscanelli (see table 1-2). Such family associations were often cemented by business arrangements. Doctors and apothecaries related by blood or marriage entered into the contractual clinical arrangements described above or formed companies with each other. Bartolomea, daughter of the Florentine doctor Maestro Niccolò di Francesco Falcucci, for instance, married the apothecary Giovanni di Ristoro; their son Ristoro also became an apothecary and entered into a partnership with his grandfather Maestro Niccolò.[54]

Finally, guild members often shared bonds of acquaintance and friendship, as many documents show. For example, immigrants ac-

TABLE 1-2

The Cini and Toscanelli Families

M° Domenico di Piero Toscanelli (doctor)			
M° Paolo (doctor)	M° Piero (doctor)	Cinozzo di Giovanni Cini (apothecary)	
M° Lodovico (doctor)	Antonio (apoth.)	Ginevra = Ser Agnolo (notary)	M° Simone (doctor)
M° Oliviero = Dianora da Siena (doctor)	M° Domenico (doctor)	M° Girolamo (doctor)	

SOURCE: Uzielli, *Toscanelli*, 492-506 passim (based mainly on *catasto* records).

[53] Thus Lucrezia, daughter of M° Agnolo di Cristofano, married M° Teodorigo di Piero da Spilimbergo del Friuli, and the daughter of M° Niccolò Falcucci married Giovanni di Ristoro, apothecary; see Alessandro Gherardi, *Statuti*, 463-64, and Ristori, "Niccolò Falcucci," 262-63.

[54] Ristori, "Niccolò Falcucci," 280.

cepting Florentine citizenship were required to have a guarantor when they swore their oath to the city, and records of doctors' oaths show a high proportion of guarantors who were also doctors. Thus Maestro Francesco di ser Niccolò acted as guarantor to both Maestro Niccolò da Mantova and Maestro Filippo di maestro Giovanni da Milano when they were granted citizenship in 1368.[55] Furthermore, many doctors referred in their private correspondence to close friendships with others in their occupation—friendships often formed during the years at university. This was the case, for example, with Maestro Lorenzo Sassoli and Maestro Dino di Dino Del Garbo, a Pratese and a Florentine who had studied together at Bologna; in one letter Maestro Lorenzo recommended himself to his friend, adding, "Maestro Dino has always been a brother to me, and I am bound to him now more than ever."[56]

Perhaps the best records of all these relationships—personal, financial, and professional—are doctors' wills. Sometimes bequests went to other doctors, while apothecaries often figured as witnesses, executors, or legatees.[57] In 1478, for example, Maestro Iacopo da Bisticci (brother of the stationer Vespasiano, whose occupation also fell under the jurisdiction of the guild) made special mention in his will of his apothecary, Bartolomeo d'Antonio: "For eighteen years or thereabouts he has served Maestro Iacopo, especially in his illnesses, accepting both work and sleepless nights. He has looked after not only Maestro Iacopo but also his house and family with great diligence; he has governed and administered many of his affairs, has always rendered good account and service, and has been faithful."[58] For his pains, Maestro Iacopo left Bartolomeo several houses and stipulated that he was to live with the doctor's own family until he felt ready to set up his own household.

It is worth noting that the bonds we have been discussing were particularly dense among university-educated physicians and between physicians and the guild's dominant merchant group, apothecaries. This is not to say that surgeons and empirics did not form the same kinds

[55] LF-39, fol. 90r. See also LF-40, entry of 13.ii.1377/8, where M° Piero di Giovanni Benini stood as guarantor to M° Filippo di Stefano da Montesecco.

[56] ASP: Archivio Datini, Carteggio privato-1102 (Busta), letter of 15.xii.1403: "M° Dino senpre m'è stato fratello, e ora più che mai il tengo." (M° Dino, scion of Florence's most illustrious family of physicians in the fourteenth century, eventually went into his father's cloth business.)

[57] See, for example, the will of M° Antonio di m° Guccio da Scarperia, in Baccini, "Maestro Antonio di Guccio da Scarperia," 411-16, or the tangled financial obligations imposed on M° Lionardo di m° Agnolo as a condition of his inheritance from M° Nuto di Bandino da Bibbiena, in Catasto-25, fol. 96v.

[58] Notarile-D.89, fol. 286v; quoted in Cagni, *Vespasiano da Bisticci*, 28.

of attachments; although in this as in every other respect the documentation concerning surgeons and empirics is scarcer, what we can find out regarding the prevalence of intermarriage and occupational inheritance implies a similar pattern. Rather, it is to suggest that this corporate life had its roots less in the guild as a formal organization than in the social and economic activities which the guild governed and expressed, and that various groups within the guild, and even within a single occupational group, tended to form associations on the basis of shared background, expectations, and interests.

Despite this diversity, however, it is easy to see why doctors practicing in Florence, even for a relatively short time, almost invariably joined the Guild of Doctors, Apothecaries, and Grocers. A member of a guild family would have matriculated without charge as a matter of course. An immigrant doctor or a local doctor from a family not traditionally associated with the guild would have joined as a matter of choice; membership gave to the newcomer not only legal protection but also a sense of belonging, since it was within the guild network that the doctor's professional life, in the form of contracts, partnerships, and referrals, took its course.

DOCTORS AND PLAGUE

On one level, the Guild of Doctors, Apothecaries, and Grocers corresponded to a stable community, or group of communities, grounded in the rock of Florence's urban society and commercial economy; as that society and economy retained its shape throughout the early Renaissance, so did the network of relations which bound doctors to other guild members. But on another level, the period was one of disruption and substantial change for the city. The hundred years between the mid-fourteenth and mid-fifteenth centuries saw tumultuous political crises—the most dramatic being the despotic rule of the duke of Athens in the early 1340s and the revolt of the Ciompi in 1378—which pitted oligarchical against more democratic visions of republicanism. During the same period the city suffered at least five devastating epidemics; these reduced its population by more than 50 percent and began a time of demographic instability and renewed immigration.

These changes found their echoes within the community of the guild. Both the advent of plague in 1348 and the consolidation of a narrowly oligarchical form of government in the last decades of the fourteenth century had particular consequences for Florence's doctors—consequences which are clearly documented not only in amendments to the guild statute in the decades after 1349 but also in its lists of officers. These sources reflect a crisis in the life of the Florentine medical profession, affecting its organization, its composition, and its standing in the power structure of the guild.

In the first place, the plague challenged and weakened the profession by raising serious doubts about its competence and its superior ethic of charity and service. With each new epidemic doctors showed themselves inadequate to manage the disease, which quickly established itself as the leading cause of death.[59] This fact did not go unnoticed. Matteo Villani's criticisms of medical impotence, quoted in the Introduction, were echoed in many contemporary sources in the decades after 1348. Marchionne di Coppo Stefani made much the same complaint in his own chronicle:

> neither doctor nor medicine was of any use, either because the diseases were not yet known or because doctors had never studied them, and there did not appear to be any remedy. . . . There were no doctors to be had, because they died like everyone else. Those available wanted an exorbitant sum in hand before entering the patient's house, and once inside they felt his pulse with their faces turned away and inspected his urine from afar, holding strong-smelling substances to their noses.[60]

By the end of the fourteenth century these themes had become a literary commonplace. Writer after writer lamented the avarice and cowardice of doctors in times of plague and their inability to treat or prevent the disease. These criticisms were leveled particularly against physicians, that is, the upper level of the profession, both because they had resources to flee the city with the rest of the wealthier citizens and because their claims to special knowledge and special status, expressed in their occupational costume and their university degrees, made them more vulnerable to accusations of hypocrisy and deception. Many Florentines turned in reaction to popular remedies, as is evident in a

---

[59] On causes of death in Florence see Herlihy and Klapisch-Zuber, *Les toscans*, 463-67; in this period many more men, women, and children died of plague than of any other illness.

[60] Stefani, *Cronaca fiorentina*, 230. Note that in other respects general confidence in the competence of doctors was quite high and that, even with respect to plague, not all writers were as critical as Matteo Villani or Stefani. For example Morelli, in his *Ricordi*, 292-93, says that while no medical remedies or rules are fail-safe against plague, it is certainly best to do as the doctors say. He is, however, the only chronicler I have found to speak sympathetically about the medical profession in connection with plague.

letter of Ser Lapo Mazzei, a Florentine notary, written during the great epidemic of 1400:

> I'll tell you what our bishop said to me the other day. Finding no relief from all the doctors, he says a poor person gave him a remedy which cured him immediately; namely, take a well-cooked onion, crush it with butter, and apply it to the [bubo]. Don't fool around with pills, because Maestro Bernardino [di Ser Pistoia, a prominent Florentine physician] ate a bushel of them and died anyway. And Ser Vanni Stefani's brother, who took lots and lots, died the other day, because too many are bad for you.[61]

To the external threat was added a related internal one, as the Florentine profession found itself flooded by a wave of newcomers. Many were empirics, miscellaneously trained practitioners attracted by the growing market for medical services in an era of endemic plague; others were immigrant doctors from the countryside and elsewhere, who took part in the general demographic movement into cities depopulated by the disease. Even laymen like Boccaccio noticed the change, while amendments to the guild statute of 1349 complained repeatedly about the presence of "incompetent foreign doctors" and the large number of empirical practitioners who had slipped by the guild's lax licensing procedures.[62] "Through the neglect of the rectors of the guild," said one, "the form and order of the said statute has not been observed, especially since the time of the great plague and pestilence. As a result, many laymen and people completely ignorant of the art and science of healing, who previously worked as smiths or in other mechanical trades, have begun to practice medicine."[63]

The reaction to these challenges was quick and determined. Between 1351 and 1392 doctors with influence in the guild pushed through a

---

[61] Mazzei, *Lettere*, 1:259. See also 1:260 (letter of 24.viii.1400): "E rimanemmo che medico da Firenze non chiedesse, però che a questi mali non faceano nulla; e che se pur lo volesse, nol potrebbe avere."

[62] Boccaccio, proemium to *Decameron*; amendment of 1351, IX (Ciasca, *Statuti*, 231): "e con ciò sia cosa che, dal tempo della mortalità in qua, nella detta città di Firenze sia stato e ancora oggi sia gran difecto e piccola quantità di sofficienti medici, maximamente cirusichi, e spesse volte e medici forestieri insufficienti instantemente co' detti rectori e ufficiali procurano a lloro fare tale commissione di tali iudicii, e per la loro imperitia ne' detti loro iudicii evidentissimi e enormi errori e difecti spesse volte si commetta. . . ."

[63] Amendment of 1353, I (242-43): "per difecto de' rectori della dett'arte la forma e l'ordine del dicto statuto, maximamente dal tempo della gran mortalità e pestilenza in qua, non è stato osservato, per la qual cagione molti idioti e al tucto ignoranti l'arte e scientia del medicare cominc[i]orono a medicare e l'arte della medicina exercitare, che prima solevano l'arte de' fabri e l'altre arti mecchaniche operare. . . ."

variety of amendments to the statute in the area of medical practice; these culminated in the formation of the College of Doctors in 1392 and, in 1415, in the state's recognition of the medical monopoly and licensing requirements of the guild. Many of these reforms were of dubious effectiveness. Their intention, however, shines clear: by tightening discipline and standards for admission, guild doctors hoped to reduce competition from new practitioners outside the established profession; at the same time they aimed to restore their authority and reputation, along with the sense of cohesion and identity they had enjoyed before the disruptive advent of the Black Death.

Two such amendments, passed in 1353 and 1391, concerned medical licensing. The framers of the first began by complaining of the guild's laxity in admitting new doctors; they lamented the influx of "idiots and mechanicals" into the profession after the plague—a situation they described as dangerous to public health and safety, since "it frequently happens that patients treated by such pretenders are harmed and injured rather than helped or cured." On these grounds, the amendment reaffirmed the principle that no doctor was to practice unless matriculated, or to matriculate unless certified by a university or examined by a board of four doctors, including at least one surgeon, to be appointed by the consuls of the guild. To enforce this provision, it called for the appointment of one or more officials to search out unqualified practitioners who might have slipped into the guild's membership and report them to the consuls.[64] Apparently these measures were not fully effective, for they were confirmed forty years later in a new amendment, which noted that "some doctors have been examined and approved and others not, although they have nonetheless been matriculated and received and written down in the matriculation list."[65]

The second thrust of the guild's protective reaction was a series of reforms intended to restore public confidence in the medical profession by enforcing standards of conduct among doctors. The first of these amendments, passed in 1352, merely forbade doctors "of any condition whatsoever" to frequent brothels and taverns or to engage in "improper" (dishonesta) behavior.[66] The second, in 1372, was one of a group designed to "restore Florentine doctors subject to the guild to good habits, so that their knowledge may increase." But whereas the reform of 1352 was concerned with moral behavior and governed

---

[64] Ibid. (243-44).

[65] Amendment of 1391, IV (338). This amendment differed from that of 1353 in not requiring that unqualified practitioners be removed from the rolls.

[66] Amendment of 1352, XII (239).

all members of the medical profession, the amendments of 1372 focused specifically on the intellectual standards of those with university degrees. They created a new office, that of the provost of doctors, with responsibility for enforcing these standards. He was to ensure that the disputations on medical questions sponsored by the guild in accordance with the statute of 1349 were not neglected but took place twice a month, without "brawls or scandals," in the presence of all the guild's physicians, and he was to initiate and oversee a new guild activity: regular human anatomical dissections.[67]

Both disputations and dissections were activities traditionally associated with the medical faculties of Italian universities. In the past, guild physicians had been able to participate in those sponsored by the University of Florence. But the *studio* had effectively shut its doors in 1370, unable to compete with the fiscal demands of the revolt of San Miniato and the war with Milan.[68] Thus the professed intention of the reforms of 1372 was to raise the level of medical knowledge among the city's physicians by establishing the guild as an alternative center of medical education and research, and doubtless also to restore the physicians' somewhat tarnished claim to technical competence.

In response to repeated complaints that the relevant statutes were not being observed, to the detriment of the "honor of the doctors,"[69] subsequent amendments, in 1376 and 1388, saw a continuous enlargement of the provost's power. Finally, in 1392, he was made head of the College of Doctors, a new corporation within the Guild of Doctors, Apothecaries, and Grocers with its own matriculation list and matriculation fees (fl. 2 for natives of the city and countryside and fl. 4 for foreigners, in addition to the regular guild fees). At its foundation it was to include all doctors with a university doctorate (*conventus*); other members could be added later by a vote of two-thirds of the current membership.[70]

The College of Doctors in this period is a puzzling and underdocumented group; its matriculation list does not survive, and except

---

[67] Amendment of 1372, I (278); also III and IV (279-80). The medical guilds of other Italian towns also sponsored disputations and anatomical dissections in this period; see Ciasca, *L'arte*, 277-81.

[68] See Park, "Readers," 250-51, 264-67. It is possible that the dissections were supervised by M° Lodovico di Bartolo da Gubbio, who continued to lecture on surgery through 1380.

[69] Amendment of 1376, I (Ciasca, *Statuti*, 290), which allowed him to fine disobedient doctors, and amendment of 1388, I (328-329), which gave him authority to have them imprisoned and their goods confiscated.

[70] Amendment of 1392, VIII (347). The *Collegio de' medici* was actually mentioned for the first time in 1389 (334), although at that date it had no formal constitution.

for the amendment establishing it there are no documents before the later fifteenth century which give any sense of its activities or its importance in the lives of its members.[71] Unlike the Company of San Luca, the painters' confraternity founded within the guild at roughly the same time, the College of Doctors seems to have sponsored activities that were more intellectual and professional than social and religious.[72] The disputations and dissections overseen by the provost were carried out under its auspices, but the only provision detailing its operations concerns the examination of candidates for the doctorate in medicine at the University of Florence; here the amendment of 1392 specified that only inhabitants of the city might participate and that they should receive an emolument of up to one florin for their services, whether or not the degree was awarded. Another amendment from the same year stipulated that the provost of the College of Doctors could not be a reader at the university itself.[73]

It seems clear from these amendments that the college was not merely a fraternal organization but was intended to protect the interests of two groups within the Florentine medical profession: the university-trained physicians, who felt threatened by the increasing number of practitioners without degrees, and the native Florentine doctors, who feared a growing influx of immigrant competition. In this respect, the foundation of the college was merely the final step in a series of reforms aimed at buttressing the position of the established local profession in the wake of the plague. The response of the Florentine physicians was to establish an exclusive subgroup of the university-educated within the inclusive branch of doctors, probably in hopes of salvaging the reputation of at least their wing of the profession and distancing themselves from what they saw as a proliferation of charlatans taking

[71] The literature on the college perpetuates a number of completely erroneous ideas concerning its early history. Most of these were first advanced in Gatti, "Il Collegio medico fiorentino," and repeated by Panebianco in his "Contributo" and by Mannelli in "Il Collegio medico fiorentino." In general, these errors result from projecting the activities of the *collegio* after the reform of 1560 back on the fourteenth-century foundation. It is wrong, for example, to identify the earlier *collegio* with the group of doctors chosen by the guild to examine and license prospective matriculants in accordance with the statute of 1349 and the amendment of 1353, or with the completely independent *Collegio medico* of university readers in medicine at the *Studio fiorentino*, as described in the university statute of 1388, II, 73-74, in Alessandro Gherardi, *Statuti*, 81-82. For a general discussion of Italian medical colleges see Palmer, "Physicians and the State," 49-53, and Webster, "Thomas Linacre," 213-18.

[72] On the activities of the Company of San Luca see amendment of 1406, I-III (Ciasca, *Statuti*, 392-94).

[73] Amendment of 1392, IX and X (348).

advantage of the medical crisis of the Black Death to insinuate themselves into the guild. It was above all in the higher-paid levels of medical practice that the competition for patients was acute, and the doctors of the college hoped to stake out that market for themselves.

Similar motives inform the provisions governing the apparently strained relations between the College of Doctors and the medical faculty at the University of Florence, which represented the other main source of competition for the physicians of the guild. The university, or *Studio fiorentino*, had been founded immediately after the plague in 1349 as part of a communal effort to repopulate the city. Publicly funded, its size and vitality waxed and waned with the resources of the Florentine treasury.[74] Constitutionally, the university was a corporation of foreigners; the rectorship and all major chairs went by university and communal decree to nonnatives of the city and countryside of Florence.[75] Many readers in medicine did not bother to matriculate in the guild; this state of affairs was initially tolerated and later condoned by the communal government, presumably to aid in the recruitment of lecturers.[76] Under these circumstances the guild physicians naturally saw the *studio* doctors as a threat to both their authority and their livelihood. This medical town-gown rivalry came to a head around 1390, probably as a result of the university's renewed vigor in this period. These years saw a continuing controversy over the teaching eligibility of Florentine citizens and a heated debate between university and guild over whether guild physicians could attend the public doctoral examination (*conventus*) of students in arts and medicine and vote on their degrees. This debate issued in the provision mentioned above concerning the participation of the doctors of the college in 1392.[77]

[74] Throughout this period the *studio* was a secondary university, well behind Bologna and Padua in size and prestige. For a general account see Brucker, "Florence and Its University." On the chronology of its openings and closings: Park, "Readers," 249-52, 268-71, and Novati, "Sul riordinamento." Although most of the *studio's* records from this period have been lost, Alessandro Gherardi has edited the statute of 1387/8, with a large number of related documents, in his *Statuti*.

[75] Alessandro Gherardi, *Statuti*, 149, and the deliberations of 1361, 1390, and 1404, on 137, 168-69, 182-83. This was frequently true of Italian universities in this period; a signal exception was the University of Bologna; see Rashdall, *Universities of Europe*, 1:213-15.

[76] Communal deliberation from 1413/4, in Alessandro Gherardi, *Statuti*, 190.

[77] See the deliberations of the university officials from 1388 and 1390 and the deliberation of the Signoria from 1391, in ibid., 166-70, 172-73; also Guild of Doctors, Apothecaries, and Grocers: amendment of 1388, III (Ciasca, *Statuti*, 330), amendment of 1389, II, III (334-35), amendment of 1392, IX (348). In various other towns physicians in the civic colleges also participated in the granting of degrees; see Palmer, "Physicians and the State," 50-51.

In the absence of university records there is no way to know whether the College of Doctors managed to make its presence felt in the matter of examinations, just as there is no way to know if disputations and dissections took place regularly as prescribed. The main piece of information concerning the functioning of the college appears in an entry in the guild's book of deliberations from 1473. Some guild members (presumably physicians) expressed concern about the competence and honesty of apothecaries in filling prescriptions; in response, the consuls ordered the College of Doctors to compose a book of recipes which was to be observed by all apothecaries and to elect two physicians to oversee its enforcement. The book was duly compiled, appearing in print in 1499, and served in the following century as a model for similar official pharmacopoeias in Mantua, Bologna, and other Italian cities.[78]

Thus the foundation of the College of Doctors in 1392 and the debate between guild and university over examination privileges represented a final effort to reform the medical profession under the auspices of the Guild of Doctors, Apothecaries, and Grocers following the plague of 1348. Doctors with influence in the guild were concerned both to buttress their public reputation and to reconfirm the authority of the established medical profession, embodied in the College of Doctors, over both apothecaries and irregular and foreign doctors, including readers at the University of Florence. On paper at least, their efforts in the second sphere seem to have been successful, not only in the case of the recipe book but also in the communal statute of 1415, which incorporated licensing privileges for doctors, alone among all the city's guilded occupations, in virtually the words of the guild statute of 1349.[79] But it would be a mistake to make too much of the foundation of the college; the laxity that had marked the licensing procedures of the fourteenth-century guild seems to have continued into the fifteenth century, as later complaints confirm.[80] And the

---

[78] AMS-49, fol. [84]. *Nuovo receptario*; on the influence of this work see Panebianco, "Contributo," 10.

[79] *Statuta populi et communis Florentiae*, IV, 53; 2:202-3: "Nullus medicus civis vel comitatinus possit, vel debeat admitti ad collegium dictae artis, vel civitatis, seu comitatus Florentiae medicare, nisi primo talis medicus examinatus in scientia medicinae fuerit per consules dictae artis, et eos, quos ipsi consules habere voluerint ad faciendum examinationem praedictam, et per ipsos pro sufficienti approbato in scientia medicinae, quam operari voluerit, sub poena librarum ducentarum f. p. cuilibet medico contrafacienti, et quod nullus spetiarius aliquem medicum, qui primo non fuerit approbatus modo praedicto in sua apotheca, teneat, vel tenere praesumat ultra decem dies, sub poena librarum centum f. p. eidem spetiario tenenti auferenda."

[80] For example amendment of 1422, V (Ciasca, *Statuti*, 422).

college could do nothing whatsoever to halt what was perhaps the most alarming change in the status of doctors traceable to the effects of the plague: their virtual disappearance from the power structure of the guild.

DOCTORS AND GUILD OFFICE

In order to understand this last development, we have to look beyond the plague and its effect on doctors to the upheavals which marked Florentine political life in the second half of the fourteenth century.[81] The tug of war between proponents of oligarchy and the supporters of a more democratic republican government based on the guild system had issued in the restoration of a slightly broadened form of oligarchy in the years after 1346. The "corporate revival" of the mid-1370s, which led to the revolt of the Ciompi in 1378 and the establishment of a broadly based guild regime, was of short duration. With its collapse and the gradual restriction of the power of the lower guilds and the lower ranks of the greater guilds, a new, more aristocratic regime emerged in which political power was ever more tightly concentrated in the hands of a small group of prominent families in the merchant guilds, including the Guild of Doctors, Apothecaries, and Grocers. The effect of these changes on the political status of doctors within the guild is clear. At the same time that political office was being restricted to a narrower elite of Florentine citizens and the barriers to officeholding for those outside this elite were being strengthened, the composition of the medical profession in Florence was changing, as immigrants and those outside the politically empowered class came to predominate in the branch of doctors. As a result, doctors found themselves gradually excluded from Florentine political life in general, and in particular from the power structure of their guild.

This process had begun as early as 1349. Whereas the guild's first surviving statute, from 1314, assigned a third of all offices to each of the three principal branches, the compilers of the statute of 1349 worked out a new apportionment, which decreased the number of positions assigned to doctors in the consulate, council, and various electoral bodies of the guild from a third to a quarter. This trend continued in the amendments of 1360 as well as in a comprehensive electoral reform

[81] On Florentine political life in this period see Najemy, *Corporatism and Consensus* and "*Audiant omnes artes*," from which I take the phrase "corporate revival"; also Brucker, *Florentine Politics and Society* and, for the decades following the revolt of the Ciompi, *Civic World*; and Becker, *Florence in Transition*, vol. 2.

after the revolt of the Ciompi in 1378, which further reduced the role of doctors in the governance of the guild.[82]

It would be a mistake to interpret this early set of reductions as the result of a political vendetta against the medical profession.[83] As the guild's matriculation lists show, the number of apothecaries and grocers had increased substantially relative to the number of doctors; thus the reforms between 1349 and 1382 appear as a reasonable attempt to bring the proportion of doctors in guild offices into line with the proportion of doctors in the total membership (see table 1-3).[84] The electoral reforms after 1382 are another matter. They were not meant to favor or disfranchise any particular occupational group within the

TABLE 1-3

Proportion of Consulships Held by Doctors

	Guild Matriculations			Guild Consuls		
Years	Total	Doctors	Doctors (%)	Total	Doctors	Doctors (%)
1320-53	2,006	170	8			33
1353-86	1,192	122	10	612	54	9
1386-1408	1,101	81	7	414	32	8
1409-44	1,445	91	6	648	35	5
1445-90				828	17	2

SOURCES: Ciasca, L'arte, 712-18 (to 1353); AMS-46 (from 1353); AMS-7, 9, 21. For details see note 84.

[82] Statute of 1349, I, 1; I, 2; I, 4 (Ciasca, Statuti, 94-105, 108-10); amendment of 1360, I and IV (255, 257); amendment of 1378, IV-VI (301-7). See Ciasca, L'arte, 91-99, 117-18, 131-35.

[83] Ciasca's discussion takes this tack, arguing that the doctors corresponded to a local aristocratic element in the social and political structure of the guild. After the plague, he claims, the guild was swamped by large numbers of gente nuova—parvenus and immigrants (specifically apothecaries and grocers)—who proceeded to disfranchise the doctors, the older ruling elite; thus with the oligarchical reaction after 1382 doctors reacquired a substantial part of their previous influence in guild politics. See Ciasca, L'arte, 116-17, 141-42; this interpretation was first advanced by Doren in Entwicklung, 59. It ignores the fact that the representation of doctors in the political hierarchy in the guild in fact decreased dramatically after 1382 and that doctors were the parvenus and immigrants, while grocers and especially apothecaries were often considerable merchants and part of Florence's oligarchical elite. The average wealth of apothecaries in the catasto of 1427 was high, only slightly below that of lawyers; see Herlihy and Klapisch-Zuber, Les toscans, 299.

[84] Sources for table 1-3 include the lists of consuls in Ciasca, L'arte, 712-18 (to 1353), and AMS-46 (from 1353); matriculation figures are calculated from the matriculation lists in AMS-7, AMS-9, and AMS-21. In the years before 1349 the proportion of doctors in the consulate was set by statute at 33%. No matriculation lists survive for the period from 1445 to 1490.

guild, but rather they reflect general communal efforts to tighten eligibility for office and to restrict it ever more closely to natives of the Florentine territories who were long-term inhabitants of the city and members of an increasingly narrow ruling elite.[85] The net result of these various changes after 1349 was a progressive erosion in the number of doctors holding positions of responsibility in the guild—an erosion which became acute in the fifteenth century. The decline in the number of consulships held by doctors illustrates the point dramatically. In the second half of the fourteenth century doctors were elected to 8 or 9 percent of the available consulships; by the second half of the fifteenth century, however, the figure was 2 percent—a drop out of proportion to their representation in the guild membership.

The reasons for this gradual exclusion of doctors have to do with their changing social and geographical origins in the century after the advent of plague. As a study of toponymics in the matriculation lists shows, doctors formed the most important immigrant element in the guild; apothecaries and grocers, in contrast, were overwhelmingly of Florentine origin, and many were part of the Florentine merchant oligarchy. (Apothecaries ranked high in average wealth in the *catasto* of 1427, standing only slightly below lawyers.)[86] As medical practitioners continued to immigrate and as Florentine citizens continued to flee the medical profession, doctors took on more and more the complexion of a group of newly arrived although often prosperous outsiders, who were not even technically eligible for communal office under the stricter birth and residence requirements passed in the early fifteenth century. Rather than corresponding to the most established and oligarchical elements of the guild, as Raffaele Ciasca and others have argued, they were the guild's most notable class of *gente nuova*.

This fact in turn explains the changing distribution of consulships within the medical profession charted in table 1-4.[87] As the immigrant

[85] Ciasca, *L'arte*, 137-46. The amendment of 1414 (Ciasca, *Statuti*, 402-5) barred from the consulship anyone who had not paid city taxes for a full thirty years or whose father or other male forebear had not met the same condition, in accordance with communal legislation from 1404. On the progressive exclusion of immigrants from public office in this period see Kirshner, "Paolo di Castro."

[86] See table 4-1. Ciasca's position in note 83 above. Bullough—in a clear projection of modern expectations—simply asserts that the apothecaries, and no doubt the grocers, were wholly subordinated to the branch of doctors, in the same way that the modern medical profession dominates auxiliary medical personnel like nurses and pharmacists; see his *Development of Medicine*, 88.

[87] See note 84 above. Ciasca's lists were compiled largely on the basis of records of the Mercanzia; they are often incomplete, particularly for the years before 1338, but the contents are no doubt typical. The average number of consulships per doctor-consul for the earlier period is calculated using those lists that do survive.

TABLE 1-4
Distribution of Consulships among Doctors

Years	Consulships Held by Doctors	Doctors Holding Consulship	Average Number of Consulships per Doctor
1320-53	70	42	1.7
1353-86	54	21	2.6
1386-1408	32	8	4.0
1409-44	35	9	3.9
1445-90	17	5	3.4

SOURCES: as in table 1-3. For details see notes 84 and 87.

doctors joined the guild and well-established Florentines left the medical profession, there was a progressive concentration of offices in the hands of the small group of doctors with ties to the ruling oligarchy. Of the 67 consulships held by doctors between 1386 and 1444, 51 went to only five individuals: Maestro Cristofano di Giorgio (21), Maestro Antonio di maestro Guccio da Scarperia (10), Maestro Galileo di Giovanni Galilei (8), Maestro Piero di Giovanni (7), and Maestro Giovanni di maestro Ambruogio (5). All but one of these doctor-consuls (Maestro Antonio) were natives of the city; all but one (Maestro Giovanni) were physicians; and three (Maestro Antonio, Maestro Galileo, and Maestro Giovanni) were wealthy, while Maestro Cristofano and Maestro Piero were at least comfortable.[88]

The effect of the plague and concomitant political developments on the position of doctors in the guild was therefore complex. As the proportion of immigrants and newcomers to the profession grew larger during the century after 1348, doctors as a group found themselves increasingly on the margins of the political community of the guild, barred from office by a series of stringent eligibility requirements and, perhaps more important, by their lack of an established family political tradition. But the group was not all of a piece. The few doctors who did come to occupy positions of influence in the guild were in general physicians from well-to-do citizen families or wealthy immigrants from the countryside, two groups which became less and less representative of the Florentine medical profession as a whole. The response of these and other Florentine physicians was a natural one: faced with popular skepticism regarding the competence of the profession and declining influence within the guild, they attempted first to impose stricter standards for admission and practice. When these failed, they founded

[88] On M⁰ Cristofano, the only doctor included by Brucker in his list of the *reggimento* (inner circle of the ruling elite) of 1411, see his *Civic World*, 269-71. The political status of individual doctors in this period is discussed below in Chapter Five.

their own corporation, the College of Doctors, in an attempt to assert their authority and distance themselves from their empirically trained colleagues by forming an exclusive community within the inclusive community of the guild's branch of doctors.

From all available evidence, however, the College of Doctors remained relatively uninfluential until the plague began to recede in severity over the course of the sixteenth century; only then did prominent Florentines begin again to elect medicine as a career, and only then did doctors begin to reappear in significant numbers in the guild's political hierarchy.[89] Throughout the period with which we will be concerned, however, most doctors—natives and immigrants, physicians and lower practitioners—participated in the guild community not as political leaders but as members of its rank and file. They matriculated and practiced, contracting ties with apothecaries and other guild members with whom their work or their social circumstances brought them in contact. Thus the guild served for most doctors as their point of entry into the medical profession of Renaissance Florence. But just as matriculation was only the first step in a doctor's career—a career shaped by many other institutions and circumstances—so to study the place of doctors in the guild gives only a preliminary picture of their practice and their profession. For more details we must turn to the doctors themselves.

[89] Only in the years after 1560 were doctors again elected to the consulate with any regularity, and only after 1580 were they elected in significant numbers; see the relevant years in AMS-46.

· II ·

The Doctors

THE COMPOSITION of the medical profession in Florence naturally reflected the policies of the Guild of Doctors, Apothecaries, and Grocers. The guild set standards for admission to medical practice in the city and countryside, but it defined those standards
broadly and applied them laxly. Thus the Florentine example confirms
for early Renaissance Italy what Danielle Jacquart has recently established for France and Margaret Pelling and Charles Webster for England; we can no longer think of the early medical profession as a small
group of university-trained and theoretically oriented doctors who catered to the rich, while the rest of society made do with a miscellaneous collection of folk healers and charlatans.[1] The reality is more
shaded and more complex. In Florence, as in many other Italian cities,
the organized profession opened its doors to those who could plausibly claim or demonstrate competence in some field of healing, including women, Jews, and others without access to a university degree [2]

In many ways the key to the nature of the Florentine medical profession is its stratification and specialization. Medical knowledge and
medical practice in the fourteenth and fifteenth centuries were not
monolithic but embraced a number of distinct and well-established
traditions, ranging from the sophisticated textual learning of the physician to the manual skill of the bone or hernia doctor. There was less
resentment or rivalry among these different kinds of practitioners than
might be expected; doctors and patients acknowledged in general that
each group was authoritative in its own area of practice and that each

[1] Jacquart, *Le milieu médical*; Pelling and Webster, "Medical Practitioners," esp. 232.
For the older view see, for example, Bullough, "Population and Medicine," and Freidson, *Profession of Medicine*, 12.

[2] On the practice elsewhere in Italy see, for example, Ruggiero, "Status of Physicians
and Surgeons," 169-71, and Marangon, "Professores," 30. The case of Padua is important: even in this university town, where the medical faculty dominated the guild in the
regulation of medical practice, we see the same broadly inclusive model.

had a legitimate place in the Florentine medical economy—a place determined less by the social class of its clientele than by the illnesses it treated and the methods it used. The expertise of the surgeon complemented rather than challenged the expertise of the physician. (The position of empirics was more ambiguous; in many cases, however, they too were accepted as legitimate practitioners by physicians and more formally trained surgeons.) The resultant profession was large and heterogeneous, embracing men and women who differed greatly in their social and geographical origins as well as in their training and practice.

It was also, as we have already seen, a profession under pressure in the years after 1348, and this pressure affected its composition. In this chapter we will study not only the basic outlines of the Florentine medical profession—how many doctors practiced in the city, how they were trained, what they did, where they came from—but also the way these patterns changed over the course of the later fourteenth and the fifteenth centuries.

DOCTORS AND OTHER HEALERS

Doctors did not enjoy a monopoly on the arts of healing in fourteenth- and fifteenth-century Florence. The inhabitants of the city could turn to other sources of therapeutic power: folk medicine, the vernacular or domestic medical tradition, and the Church. Each had its own character, and each resided in a different group of healers. Before we look at the medical profession in detail, we need to understand where it fit into this broader world of healing. How did the services offered by doctors differ from those offered by these other groups? When and with what expectations did Florentines choose to consult professional practitioners?

We know next to nothing about pure folk medicine in this period, since it remained an overwhelmingly oral tradition. The best information about popular or domestic medical practices comes from vernacular treatises put together from various Latin sources and translated into Italian for the use of literate heads of household and their wives (a relatively select group, even in Florence), the staffs of abbeys and convents, and similar readers. One example of this genre is the collection of remedies and recipes compiled in 1364 by an otherwise unknown Florentine named Ruberto di Guido Bernardi.[3] Bernardi's book

---

[3] Bernardi, *Una curiosa raccolta*. References to other similar works of Florentine origin on 6n.

is a miscellany; drawing on a long tradition of books of "secrets," it includes instructions for refining precious metals, making wine, and predicting the weather. Most of the collection, however, is devoted to domestic remedies for common conditions, such as constipation, diarrhea, warts, headaches, ringworm, scabies, minor burns, and nosebleeds. The recipes for the most part call for a few simple ingredients already on hand in a normal household or easily available from an apothecary. One of the several treatments for worms, for example, prescribes drinking milk followed by garlic crushed in vinegar, while others call for poultices made with crushed leeks or oil of almonds.[4] A smaller number of Bernardi's remedies involve appeals to the supernatural in the form of charms and prayers. The victim of toothache, for example, is advised to fast on the eve of the feast of Saint Apollonia (martyred by having her teeth extracted) and to petition her to remove the pain. Bleeding may be stanched by reciting three times a short incantation recalling the Passion: "Blood, blood, blood, stand fast in your vein as Christ stood in his pain. Stand so, blood, in your vein, as Christ stood in his pain. Stand even so, blood, firm in yourself as Jesus Christ stood firm in himself. Amen, amen, amen."[5]

Although Bernardi's treatise was not itself widely read, to judge by the lack of surviving manuscripts, it reflected common practices. Domestic medicine of this sort drew on traditional beliefs as well as simplified and antiquated versions of the theory taught to medical students.[6] At times these traditions conflicted with professional medical practice. Ser Lapo Mazzei maintained that an onion crushed in butter and applied to the buboes was a better remedy for plague than all the pills prescribed by all the doctors in the world, while the fifteenth-century physician Antonio Benivieni recalled laughing, "as the young do," at a patient who insisted on treating her toothache with paternosters and magical formulas. (He was less amused when her remedies worked where his had failed.)[7] For the most part, however, there was little sense of competition between domestic and professional medicine. Remedies like Bernardi's were not necessarily expected to substitute for a doctor's care; they were proposed as a first line of defense.

[4] Ibid., 31.

[5] Ibid., 43, 45: "Sangue sangue sangue, sta fermo inella tua vena, chome stete Gieso Cristo nella sua pena. Chosì sta, sangue, fermo nella vena tua, chome istete Gieso Cristo nella pena sua. Chosì ista tu, sangue, fermo in te, chome istete Gieso Cristo in se. Amen amen amen."

[6] See Paul Slack's discussion of these issues in his "Mirrors of Health," 237, 261; also Faye Getz, "Gilbertus Anglicus Anglicized."

[7] Mazzei, *Lettere*, 1:259. Benivieni, *De abditis*, unpublished sections, 638-39.

Only the rich could call in a physician for the minor or chronic illnesses which Bernardi professed to be able to treat. The very absence of instructions for acute conditions in his book suggests that these would have been confided to a doctor.[8]

The Church and the Christian religion served as another source of healing power complementary to that of the medical profession. Doctors themselves acknowledged that not all diseases were of natural origin and that some conditions resulted from direct divine or demonic intervention; this was one of the reasons that the Guild of Doctors, Apothecaries, and Grocers forbade doctors from attending a seriously ill patient before he had confessed his sins.[9] In these cases, of course, conventional medicine was impotent. Antonio Benivieni recorded a typical instance in his *Several Hidden and Wonderful Causes of Diseases and Cures*, a collection of notable observations taken mostly from his own practice. Called in to treat a young woman afflicted with intense pain and swelling of the belly, his first diagnosis was hysteria, a common and treatable physical condition. "Investigating this disorder," he wrote,

> I concluded that it arose from the ascent of the womb, harmful exhalations being thus carried upwards and attacking the heart and brain. I employed suitable medicines, but found them of no avail. Yet it did not occur to me to turn aside from the beaten track until she grew more frenzied and, glaring round with wild eyes, was at last violently sick and vomited up long bent nails and brass pins, together with wax and hair mixed in a ball. . . . As I saw her go through exactly the same procedure many times, I decided she was possessed by an evil spirit who blinded the eyes of the spectators while he was doing all this. She was handed over to the physicians of the soul and then gave proof of the matter by plainer signs and tokens. For I have often heard her soothsaying and seen her doing other things besides, which went further than any violent symptoms produced by disease and even passed human power.[10]

In this case even the clergy, the "physicians of the soul," could work no cure.

---

[8] The main exception is his discussion of epilepsy, which was probably included because it did not respond to conventional medical treatment; see Bernardi, *Una curiosa raccolta*, 42.

[9] Statute of 1349, II, 70 (Ciasca, *Statuti*, 186). See Diepgen, *Die Theologie*, 48-52.

[10] Benivieni, *De abditis*, tr. Singer, 37. Most of Benivieni's cases date from the 1480s and 1490s.

Benivieni cites several other instances, however, in which his patients successfully sought divine aid, not only for supernaturally caused illnesses but also for recognizable diseases and injuries grown too severe to respond to normal treatment: an arrowhead embedded in a rib, for example; an intractable abscess of the knee; a "flux of the bowels" which his relative Giovannina Bencio had allowed "to continue for so long that it could be stayed neither by drugs nor other remedies nor even by baths." The last two cases were cured by a Dominican friar from Pescia who had a reputation for miraculous cures. Benivieni himself was skeptical about Giovannina's recovery, but after she had lived three years without a relapse, he "frankly admitted and declared that this had been done by God's will alone, through the faith and prayer of that saintly man, to the praise and glory of His Name."[11]

As Benivieni's accounts show, clerical intervention was in general used only as a last resort in severe and hopeless cases where standard treatment had failed. In this sense the religious medicine of the Church, like the domestic medicine in Bernardi's treatise, acted not as a rival or alternative to professional medicine but as its supplement and complement. Mild and common illnesses, as both doctors and patients realized, could be treated at home through common remedies and simple prayers, while extraordinary cases might be confided to the clergy. The great range between was the proper domain of Florence's medical profession.

Unlike the traditions of domestic and Church healing, the medicine practiced by Florentine doctors was entirely naturalistic. Patients went to them for physical explanations and physical remedies. According to contemporary medical theory, diseases could spring from various causes. Fractures and wounds, for example, were classified as "dissolutions of continuity" (*solutiones continuitatis*). Other conditions were referred to an imbalance in the four primary qualities which characterized the human body (hot, cold, wet, and dry) or to an accumulation of harmful humors; these states could affect the whole body or a single member, producing a range of effects from fever to insanity, depending on the parts affected.[12] The doctor had three kinds of remedies at his disposal: diet, medication, and surgery. Diet was the treatment of choice;

[11] Ibid., 97; also 36-43. For the miraculous cure of Benivieni's own intestinal pains. Benivieni, *De abditis*, unpublished sections, 640-41.

[12] For a contemporary Florentine discussion of the three main categories of disease (*solutio continuitatis, morbus in complexione,* and *morbus in compositione*) see Falcucci, *Sermones medicinales,* I, 2, 13-16; vol. 1, fols. 28ra-30vb. For a general account of the techniques of medical practice and their relation to theory see Siraisi, *Taddeo Alderotti,* chap. 9.

defined as the manipulation of food, drink, air, sleep, exercise, and the emotions, it was considered less disruptive to the patient's physiology than drugs.[13] The action of internal and external medicines was considered to be similar but more violent; composed for the most part of herbal ingredients, some medicines altered complexional imbalance, while others evacuated humors or—like laxatives, soporifics, or purgatives—produced specific effects. Surgery, the doctor's third therapeutic tool, embraced the application of external remedies and the physical manipulation of the members; surgical techniques included cupping (with or without scarification), cautery, phlebotomy, and the use of leeches and plasters as well as more specialized operations such as setting fractures, repairing hernias, rectifying dislocations, and treating wounds, sores, and sprains. It is important to remember that various therapies which might appear to us supernatural or "magical"— the appeal to astrology or the use of precious gems, for example— were actually explained in naturalistic terms.[14]

This does not mean, however, that doctors as a group were anti-Christian or irreligious. There is little evidence that the philosophical biases of fourteenth-century physicians and their exposure to radical Aristotelian ideas led them into theological heterodoxy, as has been claimed.[15] The esoteric textual knowledge of the physician, his access to powerful and dangerous medicines, his claimed mastery of natural forces, even the prominence of Jewish doctors may well have encouraged associations between medicine and magic or demonism in the popular mind and made physicians a natural target for zealous inquisitors. This does not entail, however, that such doctors were actually guilty as charged. In 1350, for example, the head of the Florentine inquisition fully exonerated Maestro Francesco di ser Simone da Carmignano from charges that he had "trafficked in necromantic books and notebooks containing invocations of demons, magic characters, forbidden experiments, and heresy," on the grounds that he had confessed to those crimes through fear of torture.[16] The only documented

[13] Falcucci, *Sermones medicinales*, II, 1, 1; vol 1, fol. 2va of the second *sermo*: "melius est in quibus convenit dieta solum utendo adipisci finem in eis et abcedere pharmacos." See also II, 1, 9-24; II, 2, 1-15; vol. 1, fols. 25v-34rb of the second *sermo*.

[14] See Siraisi, *Taddeo Alderotti*, 139-45, 294-95. On medicine and natural magic, as codified later in the fifteenth century in Florence by Marsilio Ficino, see Walker, *Spiritual and Demonic Magic*, chaps. 1-2.

[15] See the classic statement in Bruno Nardi, "L'averroismo bolognese," and the comment by Siraisi in *Taddeo Alderotti*, 148-51.

[16] Diplomatico-Patrimonio ecclesiastico-27.iii.1350: "se habuisse et tenuisse, emisse et vendidisse et alteri commodasse libros et quaternos nigromanticos, invocationes demonum, caratteres et experimenta plurima vetita et heresiam continentes adhoc ut ipsis

case of a man who was both a doctor and a confirmed heretic was that of Maestro Giovanni di Bartolomeo da Montecatini, executed and burned in 1450.[17] But Maestro Giovanni was in many ways a marginal member of the medical profession; the poorest doctor in the *catasto* of 1427, he was the only physician to own no books, and the nature and extent of his medical practice is unclear.[18] His case was notorious because it was unique. To judge by their letters, diaries, and wills, Florentine doctors were responsible and orthodox Christians who joined religious confraternities and made religious bequests with the same devotion as other citizens. Many served in hospitals and monasteries for token salaries and treated the poor without charge. If they did not appeal to supernatural forces in their healing, it was not because they did not believe in such forces but because medicine itself was part of the physical realm: as both theoreticians and practitioners, doctors were expected to work within the established natural and social order.

This matter-of-fact attitude toward medicine appears everywhere in Florentine culture. The city's inhabitants had few religious or social taboos about their bodies. Autopsies, routinely used for teaching under the auspices of the university and the guild, were also common in private practice. Benivieni regularly performed dissections of patients who had died from mysterious causes, including three noblewomen and a nun, and considered it an aberration worth recording when relatives of one of the deceased refused permission "through I don't know what superstition."[19] Even patrician women had little reticence about being treated or examined by male doctors, before or after death. Consider, for example, the death of Bartolomea Rinieri in 1486, as described by her husband: "At 1:30 in the morning my wife Bartolomea died at the age of forty-two or thereabouts. She died of a diseased

---

libris uteretur, et quantum in eo fuit operatus est et operam dedit ut ipsis libris uteretur, licet operatus non fuerit, et dixisse se habere spiritum sub gemma anuli inclusum, licet verum non esset." M° Francesco had been convicted by the previous inquisitor, Pietro dell'Aquila, who was notorious for his abuses; see Stephens, "Heresy," 34, and Becker, "Florentine Politics and Heresy," 63-64.

[17] See Morçay, *Saint Antonin*, 167-68. Although M° Giovanni was also accused of necromancy, his main crime seems to have been to deny the immortality of the soul; see Pietro Pietribuoni, *Priorista*; BNF: Conventi soppressi MS C.4.895, fol. 152v: "fu acchusato allo inquisitore per hareticho perchè diceva che doppo alla morte nonn era nulla. Et sempre mai non volle nè confessarsi nè comunicharsi. Et sempre iste' fermo in suo [*sic*] oppinione."

[18] Catasto-76, fol. 307v.

[19] Benivieni, *De abditis*, tr. Singer, 80: "mortuo eo experimento comprobare volentes corpus incidere tentavimus. Sed nescio qua superstitione negantibus cognatis voti compotes fieri nequivimus." See also cases 3, 33-37, 61, 76, 79, 81, 83, 89, and 94. Another example in Thorndike, *Science and Thought*, 125-32.

womb; this caused a flux which had lasted about eighteen months and which no doctors could cure. She asked me to have her autopsied so that our daughter or others could be treated [should the need arise]. I had this done, and it was found that her womb was so calcified that it could not be cut with a razor."[20]

On the whole, Florentines had confidence in the medical profession, at least where diseases other than plague were concerned. There were of course always complaints. The *ricordanza* of Francesco di Tommaso Giovanni, for example, includes a long description of his wife's illness in 1452. Francesco was highly critical of the treatment ordered by Maestro Piero Toscanelli; her condition worsened under his care, and she began to make progress only after a second physician, Maestro Girolamo Brocardi da Imola, was called in. "After about ten days of delirium she began to improve and take food and recuperate," Giovanni wrote. "I attribute this first to God and then to Maestro Girolamo, while her danger I attribute to Maestro Piero alone."[21] But such episodes were comparatively rare, and they usually reflected criticism of a particular doctor rather than of the profession or medical art in general. A more typical sentiment is found in the will from 1411 of Michele di Donato Pianellari: one of his smaller legacies was a bequest of fl. 25 to Maestro Cristofano di Giorgio, "who for the past fourteen years had diligently treated Michele in his illness and never abandoned him, but was always there when needed."[22]

SIZE OF THE PROFESSION

In his description of Florence in 1338, Giovanni Villani estimated the number of inhabitants engaged in various of the city's more presti-

[20] CS-95, 212, fol. 171r (9.iv.1486): "circha a ore 1½ di notte morì la Bartolomea mia donna, ch'era d'età d'anni xlii in circha. . . . E morì di mal di matrice che gli fe' frusso di ventre che gli durò mesi 18 in circha, e mai i medici trovarono rimedio. . . . E perchè mi preghò la facessi sparare per vedere se'l mal suo fusse di tisicho per poter remediare alla figliuola o ad altri, e chosì fe', e si trovò esser male di matrice, ch'era la matrice inchallita in modo chon rasoio non si poteva taglare." A similar account appears in the diary of Filippo di Matteo Strozzi, CS-5, 22, fol. 97r (23-24.i.1477/8).

[21] Carte Strozziane-II, 16bis (8.vii.1452): "E così per Dio gratia avengha che stesse fuori della memoria x dì o circha. Cominciò poi a migliorare e a piglare il cibo e guarire, il che reputo primo da Dio e poi da M° Girolamo. E così il pericolo suo reputo solo da M° Piero ecc."

[22] Diplomatico–Santa Maria Nuova–25.iv.1411: "Egregius doctor magister Cristoferus Georgii medicus civis florentinus et de populo Santi Apollinaris de Florentia iam quatuordecim annis elapsis dictum Michaelem diligenter in infirmitatibus suis curavit et ipsum numquam in aliquo egritudinis casu dereliquit, sed fuit semper adsistens."

gious occupations: "The association of lawyers had some eighty members; the notaries, some six hundred; physicians and surgeons, some sixty; shops of apothecaries, some hundred."[23] Although later historians often dismissed many of Villani's figures as a figment of his evident civic pride, recent work on Florentine demography has tended to confirm the accuracy of many of his estimates. It is possible to check Villani's figures for physicians and surgeons against other contemporary archival sources; rather than discredit his estimate, these make it seem if anything conservative.

There are two obvious places to look for information on the number of doctors practicing in Florence in this period: the matriculation lists of the Guild of Doctors, Apothecaries, and Grocers and the communal tax records. The usefulness of the former is limited; without a good idea of the average professional lifetime of a doctor after matriculation, it is impossible to convert the number of matriculants per year into an estimate of the number of doctors practicing in the city at any one time. City tax records are a better point of departure. Assessed at frequent intervals in the fourteenth and fifteenth centuries, the *seghe* (hearth taxes), *prestanze* (forced loans), and *catasti* (wealth taxes) were recorded in large ledgers organized by quarter and *gonfalone*.[24] From these ledgers it is possible to reconstruct the city population of taxpayers (nonindigent heads of household) in any year for which complete records survive.

Of course an estimate of the size of the medical profession based on doctors appearing in tax records will be low. It will not include most doctors who were paupers, women, dependent members of households, or tax-exempt, nor will it include recent immigrants from the Florentine territories who were still taxed in their places of origin.[25] It will also miss the sizable number of transient practitioners—close to a quarter of all matriculants—who never established themselves firmly enough in the social and economic fabric of the city to be taxed at all.[26] Yet despite these limitations, the records of the *seghe* and *pre-*

[23] Giovanni Villani, *Cronica*, XI, 94; 3:325.

[24] See Appendix I for information on the various taxes and the geographical divisions of the city.

[25] There are records of doctors in all these categories: for example Mº Luca di Cecco, declared "miserabile" (indigent) and cancelled from the rolls of the *prestanza* of 1369/70 (Prestanze-156, fol. 23); Mº Piero and Mº Paolo di mº Domenico di Piero, listed under the name of their father in the *catasto* of 1427 (Catasto-65, fol. 96v); Mº Lionardo di mº Iacopo da Volterra, exempted in 1388 (PR-77, fols. 178r-79r); and Mº Antonio di Giannetto, who was allowed to pay taxes in his home town of Castelfranco (PR-85, fols. 122r-24r).

[26] This estimate is based on an examination of the *seghe* of 1352 and 1355; the *pre-*

stanze, levied in the later fourteenth and early fifteenth centuries, and of the *catasto*, assessed beginning in 1427, give good minimum figures for the number of doctors with established medical practices in Florence at any given time. Furthermore, these figures can be improved by adding the number of doctors known from communal records to be tax-exempt and by increasing the total by a calculated percentage to approximate the number of doctors who were not heads of household.[27]

We can confirm these results by looking at several years for which we have reliable figures for the size of the medical profession in Florence. The first is 1358, when the Guild of Doctors, Apothecaries, and Grocers compiled a list of all current members; this list included fifty-six doctors.[28] The second is 1427, the year of the first *catasto*; in this assessment, unlike some of the later ones, even residents with tax exemptions filed declarations, and dependents were listed for each household. Thus to the twenty-six doctors listed as taxable heads of household we can add six dependent sons or brothers who had already—according to guild matriculation lists—entered medical practice as well as two surgeons from Norcia with lifetime tax exemptions. With these we should certainly include two doctors who lived in the portions of the city parishes of San Frediano and San Piero in Gattolino, located just outside the city walls, and who therefore appeared in the *catasto* of the countryside. This yields a grand total of thirty-six doctors for the city of Florence—a figure which may not include one or two transients or recent immigrants but which is substantially reliable.[29] Finally, we can supplement these numbers with Villani's estimate for 1338, cited above, and with Benedetto Dei's list of the thirty-three

---

stanze of 1359, 1379, 1390, 1399, 1406, and 1414; and the *catasti* of 1427, 1451, and 1458; a study of each separate tax distribution between these years would no doubt have turned up more doctors, but not enough to alter the picture substantially. Note that a significant minority of the transients were readers at the University of Florence and thus exempt from taxation; see, for example, the documents concerning M° Iacopo della Torre da Forlì (1365) and M° Ugolino da Montecatini (1396) in Alessandro Gherardi, *Statuti*, 309-10, 366.

[27] Regarding the latter, I have arrived at the corrective figure of 20% using as a guide the *catasto* of 1427, where, in addition to the thirty doctors recorded as heads of household resident in Florence, the rolls list six doctors as dependents. This figure is almost certainly too low for the fourteenth century, when there was greater occupational inheritance within the profession, as will be discussed below. Tax exemptions appear throughout this period in the registers of provisions voted by the communal councils (PR).

[28] AMS-9, fols. 1r-39r.

[29] See Appendix III. I have not included in my calculations M° Niccolò Leonardi, who lived in Venice.

TABLE 2-1
Size of the Florentine Medical Profession

Year	Doctors	City Population	Doctors per 10,000
1338	60*	120,000	5
1352	50*	40,000	13
1358	56	42,000	13
1379	71*	50,000	14
1399	58*	55,000	11
1427	36	37,000	10
1451	26*	37,000	7
1470	33	40,000	8

SOURCES: Giovanni Villani, *Cronica*, XI, 94 (1338); Estimo-306, fols. 7-184 (1352); AMS-9, fols. 1-39 (1358); Prestanze-355, 367, 368, 369 (1379); Prestanze-1787, 1788, 1789, 1790 (1399); Catasto-65 to 83, and Catasto-Campioni del Monte-San Giovanni-1427 (1427); Catasto-687 to 722 (1451, cross-checked with *campioni*); Dei, *Memorie*, BLF: Ashburnham 644, fol. 31. Estimates of city population from Herlihy and Klapisch-Zuber, *Les toscans*, 176-83.

* Adjusted as in note 27.

doctors practicing in Florence in 1470.[30] The final results appear in table 2-1.

As the figures show, Florence, unlike many smaller cities, was well served with doctors in this period. At its height, in the second half of the fourteenth century, the profession numbered approximately seventy—more doctors per capita than in Rome three hundred years later—and it averaged a respectable eleven doctors per ten thousand inhabitants during the period between 1350 and 1450.[31] Nonetheless, the number of medical practitioners fluctuated significantly. As we have already seen, it dropped after the Black Death, provoking remarks on the "great shortage and small number of competent doctors" in the 1351 amendment to the statute of the Guild of Doctors, Apothecaries, and Grocers. The commune, sensitized by the recent epidemic, quickly responded to this lack. Not only did the government vote to refound the long-suspended University of Florence, including its medical school, but it also initiated a consistent policy of attracting immigrant doctors by granting them full citizenship and generous tax exemptions.[32] This

[30] Benedetto Dei, *Memorie*; BLF: Ashburnham 644, fol. 31v. Transcription in Uzielli, *Toscanelli*, 651. Dei almost certainly did not include empirics in his tally.

[31] Figures for Rome in Cipolla, *Before the Industrial Revolution*, 82.

[32] Amendment of 1351, IX (Ciasca, *Statuti*, 231). Examples of citizenship and tax grants to doctors in PR-36, fols. 62r, 73r; PR-39, fols. 163v, 164r; PR-47, fol. 138v; and PR-50, fol. 179v.

policy enjoyed notable success. The number of doctors practicing in Florence rose quickly in the decades following the plague of 1348. Doctors reestablished themselves much faster than the population as a whole, and soon the number of medical practitioners reached a much higher level, relative to the total population, than in the first half of the fourteenth century. This situation, however, was not to last; by 1400 the size of the profession had begun to decline again, and the decline, both in absolute numbers and per capita of the city population, continued through the middle of the fifteenth century. By 1468 the situation was alarming, and the government again felt it had to take action. Contrasting "the lack of doctors well versed in the art of medicine" with the needs of the expanding city, the legislative councils appropriated fl. 1,000 over three years to hire one or more communal doctors.[33]

If the drop in the number of Florentine doctors after the plague makes good sense, its later fluctuations are more puzzling. We must remember, however, that these figures are aggregates; the members of Florence's medical profession varied greatly both in level of training and practice and in geographical origin, and any analysis of the profession as a whole must take this variety into account. Thus in order to understand the increase in the number of Florentine doctors in the later fourteenth century and its decrease in the fifteenth, we must form an idea of the levels within the profession and of the origins of the doctors themselves.

CLASSES OF PRACTITIONERS

By statute, the guild's branch of doctors embraced a wide variety of practitioners, including "all persons in the city and countryside of Florence who practice physic or surgery, set bones, and treat mouths." In practice, contemporaries recognized three main groups of doctors: physicians, surgeons, and empirics.[34]

Physicians (*fisici* or *physici*) were doctors who had attended a university (*studium generale*) or other recognized medical school and had been examined and granted a degree which licensed them to teach

---

[33] Alessandro Gherardi, *Statuti*, 267-68. On the situation in Venice see Ruggiero, "Status of Physicians and Surgeons," 176-77.

[34] Statute of 1349, II, 23 (Ciasca, *Statuti*, 132). The three groups were formally distinguished in the matriculation lists of the guild beginning in the mid-sixteenth century; see Mannelli, "Il Collegio medico fiorentino."

medicine and to enroll in the guild without further examination.[35] Their studies included theoretical and practical work in both surgery and internal medicine. Physic—in Latin *physica*—referred originally to the entire field of natural philosophy; the homonymous medical discipline, which emerged at the end of the twelfth and beginning of the thirteenth centuries, justified its name by its interest in the speculative and philosophical (i.e., scientific) foundations of its theory. By 1300 both the discipline and the associated university curriculum had been consolidated in Italy, and Italian writers and teachers were using Aristotelian ideas as well as more recently developed logical and mathematical systems in their elaboration and interpretation of the work of classical and medieval authors.[36]

Most Florentine physicians seem to have studied at the universities of Bologna, Padua, and Florence, although Perugia and Siena were also popular.[37] Students moved from one *studio* to another with little difficulty, since the degree course was fairly standard.[38] Medicine could be studied alone or, more commonly, combined with one or more of the arts subjects—typically logic, philosophy, and astrology. At Bologna the standard course in medicine was four years, reducible to three for a student with a background in the arts; at Florence, Perugia, and a number of other universities the requirement was for seven years, reducible to five.[39]

[35] Nonuniversity medical schools granting degrees in this period included the school in Lucca; see Ceccarelli, *La tradizione chirurgica lucchese*, 17-18.

[36] The fundamental study is Siraisi, *Taddeo Alderotti*, which focuses on the University of Bologna; see also her *Arts and Sciences at Padua*, chap. 5, and Kristeller, "School of Salerno." For the contribution of Florentine writers to this tradition see below, Chapter Six.

[37] It is difficult to prove this assertion, given the lack of any systematic collection of matriculation lists and degrees in medicine for Bologna and Florence in the early period. (Degrees from the University of Padua appear in Gloria, *Monumenti*, and Zonta and Brotto, *Acta graduum*.) It is known that law students from Florence attended the *studio* of Bologna in preference to that of Florence, as did medical students from nearby towns like Pistoia; see Martines, *Lawyers*, 81, and Chiappelli, *Medici e chirurghi pistoiesi*, 162. Almost all the scattered instances of medical diplomas of Florentine doctors I have found, at least for the later fourteenth century, come from Bologna or Florence; see, for example, Diplomatico-Acquisto Polverini-12.iv.1367 and Diplomatico-Acquisto Mannelli-12.iv.1369.

[38] M⁰ Giovanni di m⁰ Dino di ser Martino da Firenze, for example, took his private exam in Florence but was *conventuatus* at the University of Padua (Gloria, *Monumenti*, 1:454); M⁰ Lorenzo d'Agnolo da Prato seems also to have studied at both Bologna and Padua (ASP: Datini CP-1102, letters of 2.ix.1400 and 8.ii.1400/1). Often the examination fees were lower at one *studio* than another, encouraging students to move for the purposes of being examined; sometimes they would leave to follow a particular lecturer.

[39] University of Medicine and Arts of Bologna: statute of 1405, 45 (Malagola, *Sta-*

From at least the second half of the fourteenth century the three principal subjects which made up the medical curriculum in physic were *theorica*, which included the study of physiology and the general principles of medicine; *practica*, the study of specific diseases, their symptoms, and their treatment; and surgery, the study of external abnormalities and the operations used to correct them. All three were taught through lectures on set texts, of which those by the Greek and Arabic writers Galen, Hippocrates, and Avicenna were the most important. These lectures typically included a section-by-section reading of the text with a commentary by the lecturer. (See Appendix II for the particular books prescribed at Bologna in 1405.) *Theorica* was the central subject; its lecturers enjoyed the highest salaries, and it had the most time devoted to it: two lectures in the morning and an additional class or review session (*repetitio*) by a less prestigious reader in the afternoon. *Practica* and surgery, in contrast, were each lectured on only once a day, in the evening and afternoon.[40] On Thursdays and feast days disputations were held on tricky or debated points. Students had to read publicly and to take part in several disputations as part of the requirements for the degree.[41]

The medical student's training was not, however, confined to the study of books. "Because," as the 1388 statute of the University of Florence noted, "no one can be a good or fully trained doctor unless he is familiar with the anatomy of the human body and because it is the custom and tradition at other universities," two human dissections were to be performed each year for the benefit of the more advanced

---

tuti, 255-56); University of Florence: statute of 1387/8, II, 69 (Alessandro Gherardi, *Statuti*, 77-78). These requirements had been set in 1321 by Pope John XXII in the bull *Dum sollicite* and confirmed in 1355 by Emperor Charles IV. The following synthesis of medical training in the fourteenth and early fifteenth century is based primarily on the statutes of the University (association of students) and College (association of teachers) of Medicine and Arts of the University of Bologna, edited in Malagola, *Statuti*. Both Florence and Padua tended to model their curricula and requirements on those of Bologna. The earliest surviving statutes for Florence are those of the university, compiled in 1387/8 and edited by Alessandro Gherardi in *Statuti*, 3-104. The earliest printed statutes in arts and medicine for Padua are those of 1465, revised in 1498, in *Statuta dominorum artistarum*. I will record the points on which the statutes of Florence differ from those of Bologna. On the Bolognese medical curriculum in general see also Bullough, "Medieval Bologna," and esp. Siraisi, *Taddeo Alderotti*, chap. 4.

[40] University of Florence: statute of 1387/8, I, 41 (Alessandro Gherardi, *Statuti*, 50). The rolls of the teaching faculty at Bologna are collected in Dallari, *Rotuli*, esp. vol. 4; and Park, "Readers," 260 (1366/7). Surgery was strictly speaking part of *practica* but was also taught separately; see Siraisi, *Taddeo Alderotti*, 109.

[41] University of Medicine and Arts of Bologna: statute of 1405, 45 and 54-55 (Malagola, *Statuti*, 255-56 and 260-61); University of Florence: statute of 1387/8, II, 69 (Alessandro Gherardi, *Statuti*, 78).

students—one of a male and one of a female cadaver. Attendance at both was mandatory for graduation.[42] (The body was supplied by the Florentine *podestà* from among the foreign criminals executed by the commune. The records of executions kept by the religious company of Santa Maria della Croce al Tempio testify to this practice; a typical entry from 1421 includes the notation: "Baldassare di Giovanni da Ferrara, locksmith, was hanged, anatomized by the doctors, and buried in Santa Maria in Campo on January 23.")[43]

Medical students also accompanied experienced doctors on visits to patients. At Pavia, for example, the university required each student to "practice for six months with one or more physicians."[44] Neither Bologna nor Florence specified a particular length of time for this stage of medical training, but it was clearly taken for granted. Gabriele Zerbi, professor of medicine at Bologna in the later fifteenth century, included in his treatise on medical conduct a section on how a doctor should behave toward students accompanying him on his rounds. The practice was also familiar in Florence, as a will from 1417 shows. Made on his deathbed by one Ricco di Niccolò, it included as one of the witnesses Ugolino di Piero da Siena, "a medical student assisting the testator."[45] Both doctors and patients valued experience highly, and no young doctor without clinical training would have found patients in a large city willing to entrust their lives to his care.

Once the student had fulfilled the requirements, he was allowed to present himself for examination by the university's College of Doctors, the association of lecturers with a medical degree.[46] There were in fact two examinations. The first, called "private," was a true examination.

[42] University of Florence: statute of 1387/8, II, 62 (Alessandro Gherardi, *Statuti*, 74); see also II, 63-67. Similar provisions appear for the University of Medicine and Arts of Bologna: statute of 1405, 96 (Malagola, *Statuti*, 289-90), and for the University of Padua. See Siraisi, *Taddeo Alderotti*, 110-14; Premuda and Ongaro, "Dissezione in Padova."

[43] BNF: MS II, I, 138, no. 25: "Baldassare di Giovanni da Ferrara, chiavaiouolo, fu appiccato, fecesene nutumia per i medici, sep[ellito] in Santa Maria in Campo, 23 gennaio." See also nos. 169 and 206.

[44] College of Arts and Medicine of Pavia: statute of 1409 (*Statuti e ordinamenti*, 124).

[45] Zerbi, *De cautelis*, 69-70; see also 22. Notarile-L.196, no. 1410, unpag. Medical students also appear as witnesses to deathbed wills in Padua; see, for example, Gloria, *Monumenti*, 1:504, and Marangon, "Professores," 17.

[46] Although in more established universities like Bologna only senior professors conducted these examinations, it was apparently common in Florence for city physicians without formal ties to the university to sit in on one or both of them; see, for example, the examination certificate of M° Piero di m° Duccio da Montevarchi (1364) in Alessandro Gherardi, *Statuti*, 299. At the time only one of the five examiners listed was a salaried lecturer at the *studio*. This practice became a matter of conflict between the guild and *studio* in the 1380s; cf. Chapter One.

The student was assigned passages selected from the most important medical texts he had heard in lecture, and he was asked to comment on them, responding to questions from the examining doctors. A vote was taken, and if the student passed he was declared *licentiatus*—licensed to teach.[47] The second, or "public" examination (*conventus*) was less an exam than a formal ceremony in the cathedral; there the bishop or his representative conferred on the candidate the beret, ring, and other doctoral insignia. Once *conventuatus* or *doctoratus*, the young physician could, and often did, matriculate immediately in the medical guild of the town in which he intended to practice.

Whereas physicians by and large practiced internal medicine, surgeons treated external conditions like sores, wounds, fractures, and dislocations.[48] In Italy surgery could be a university discipline, and the *studi* of Bologna, Padua, Florence, and elsewhere offered surgical degrees which required training in medical theory as well as surgical practice. (The situation was very different in northern Europe, where surgeons were considered artisans and associated with the lower craft of barbering.)[49] In 1361 Maestro Iacopo da Prato, reader in surgery at the University of Florence, composed a treatise for the use of his students called *On Manual Operation*. In it he emphasized that surgery, like physic, required both theoretical knowledge and practical skill:

> The science of manual medicine is made up of rules by which the doctor is guided to success in his work and acquires trust, honor, praise, and profit. All these things are contained in the books of earlier writers like Galen, Albucasis, and others. . . . The surgeon

[47] College of Medicine and Arts of Bologna: statute of 1378, 16 (Malagola, *Statuti*, 438-39); at this time the two set texts for the examination were Galen's *Tegni* and the *Aphorisms* of Hippocrates.

[48] Internal operations were extremely rare in this period, since without antisepsis the success rate was very low. Only military doctors, faced with dying patients on the battlefield, attempted them with any regularity. On the teaching of surgery in Italy in this period see Marangon, "Professores," 1-30, passim.

[49] See Jacquart, *Le milieu médical*, 1:57-59, on the French case. The difference in status between surgeons in Italy and France is well illustrated in a doctor's letter from the Datini archive in Prato. M° Naddino di Aldobrandino, a Pratese physician, had emigrated in the early 1380s to Avignon, where he found success as a court doctor to various bishops and cardinals and finally to the pope himself. In 1387, however, he wrote home to discourage his surgeon friend, M° Giovanni Banducci da Prato, from trying the same thing: "Al maestro Giovanni dirai per mia parte che qui ora per l'arte sua in guadangni son picholi, e'l più del'arte della cirugia se fa per barbieri. E acci alcuno cerusico bene sufficiente in scientia e in pratica, e non sanno niente, e quell'onore o pagamento si fa a llui che a uno barbiere. . . . Con questi singnori non vedo modo aconciarlo, inperochè que' che sono potenti son forniti, e apresso vogliono dottori in fisica" (ASP: Datini CP-1091₂, letter of 11.iv.1387).

must study the anatomy of the members with great diligence, so that he knows their composition, position, and function. . . . And let him not attempt a difficult operation unless he has performed it before or seen it performed successfully, because in many cases the art [of surgery] cannot be written down or understood completely except through manual operation. . . . For this reason students must frequent the places where experienced surgeons operate and observe their operations carefully.[50]

For surgery as for physic, the normal course of study seems to have been about four years, though students often stayed longer. At the university they read a variety of other medical topics in addition to surgery. The license conferred in 1391 on Maestro Niccolò di maestro Francesco da Serravalle, for example, specifies that the candidate had "attended the University of Padua from 8 March 1387 to the present, studying surgery and working with Iacopo Zanettini da Padova, ordinary lecturer in [theoretical] medicine; Antonio da Conegliano, doctor of arts and medicine, extraordinary lecturer in medicine; Benedetto Galmarelli da Padova, lecturer in surgery; Baldassare da Padova, extraordinary lecturer in medicine; and Girolamo Anzeleri da Venezia, doctor of arts and medicine, lecturer in *practica*."[51] Thus the surgery curriculum included a grounding in physiology and the principles of scientific medicine as well as specific training in the treatment of eyes, bones, sores, and other particular conditions. Lectures in surgery took the accustomed form of textual commentary, and surgical students also

---

[50] Iacopo da Prato, *Liber in medicina de operatione manuali*; BNF: Pal. 811, fol. 1r: "Scientia medicine manualis agregatur ex regulis quibus medicus dirigitur ad subcessionem laudabilem sui operis, unde exhibetur sibi fides, honor, laus et lucrum. Omnia hec sint comprehensa sufficienter in libris anthiquorum sicut Galieni, Albucasis et aliorum. . . . Cuius artifex cum s[umma] diligentia debet esse inspector anothomie membrorum, ut sciat compositionem, situm et iuvamentum ipsorum, quoniam ex anatomie ignorantia labitur in multos [erro]res, ut Albucasis in prohemio 13 particula Azerui: et nullam operationem difficilem faciat, nisi prius operatus fuerit vel viderit aliquem operari cum salute. Quoniam in multis casibus ars ista non potest scribi nec concipi ita complete quam descendendo ad operationem manualem, nisi prius visa operatione singulari, non sequatur magnum periculum. Et propter hoc debent scholares frequentare loca ubi periti cirugici operantur et eorum operationes diligenter insp[icere]. . . ." The beginning of the treatise and table of contents are transcribed in Sudhoff, *Geschichte der Chirurgie*, 2:426-28.

[51] Gloria, *Monumenti*, 2:252 (2.v. 1391). See College of Medicine and Arts of Bologna: statute of the early fifteenth century, 14 (Malagola, *Statuti*, 490); College of Arts and Medicine of Pavia: statute of 1409 (*Statuti e ordinamenti*, 127-28). The other surgical licenses printed in Gloria for the 1390s indicate periods of study from four to six years: Gloria, *Monumenti*, 2:261 (5.iv.1392), 261-62 (16.iv.1392), 277 (14.x.1393), and 289 (17.x.1394).

attended disputations and the annual anatomical dissections. In addition they apparently served a clinical apprenticeship; the statutes of the University of Pavia called for two of the student's four years to be spent in this kind of training, and practice was probably similar at Bologna and Florence.[52]

At the end of his formal education in surgery the student presented himself for a private examination which, like the physician's, consisted of reading and commenting on sections from two texts: the 1378 statute from Bologna prescribed Avicenna, *Canon*, IV, 3, and the first part of the *Surgery* of Bruno da Longoburgo.[53] If he passed he received universal license to "read, dispute, profess, gloss, practice, and perform other surgical functions." He was further granted most of the sumptuary privileges of the university graduate in medicine; he could wear the doctor's long gown, ring, gold ornaments, and "clothes lined with any lining except for miniver and ermine"—the last two items being the exclusive prerogative of the physician by virtue of his doctorate.[54] While the *conventus* or doctorate was the usual terminal degree in physic, it was much rarer among surgeons. The surgical student usually took only the private examination; this qualified him to teach as well as to practice, and it was functionally equivalent to the physician's doctorate except that the diploma was conferred by the prior of the university's College of Doctors rather than by the episcopal authorities.[55] At Bologna and apparently at other universities, readers in surgery, like readers in grammar, were permitted to lecture without a doctorate.[56]

[52] University of Medicine and Arts of Bologna: statute of 1405, 35 (Malagola, *Statuti*, 247-48). For the books assigned at Bologna in 1405, see Appendix II. College of Arts and Medicine of Pavia: statute of 1409 (*Statuti e ordinamenti*, 127-28).

[53] College of Medicine and Arts of Bologna: statute of 1378, 24 (Malagola, *Statuti*, 442-43). At Pavia the examination texts in surgery were the surgical writings of Galen and Avicenna; College of Arts and Medicine of Pavia: statute of 1409 (*Statuti e ordinamenti*, 128).

[54] Zonta and Brotto, *Acta graduum*, 2:239 (2.v.1442). Note that the surgeons of Pavia, in contrast, were allowed to wear miniver; see College of Arts and Medicine of Pavia: statute of 1409 (*Statuti e ordinamenti*, 128).

[55] Gloria, *Monumenti* 1:369; Sarti and Fattorini, *De claris archigymnasii*, 1:522. This is confirmed in the case of Bologna by the fact that each year one poor student in *physica* and one in surgery were to be examined free by the College of Medicine and Arts; the former was to be examined both privately and publicly whereas the latter was to be examined only in private and then placed immediately on the roster of surgeons. See College of Medicine and Arts of Bologna: statute of 1378, 14 (Malagola, *Statuti*, 438). It must have been possible to be *conventuatus* in surgery, at least in theory, because the university statutes of both Bologna and Florence give fees for the surgical *conventus*: see College of Medicine and Arts of Bologna: statute of 1378, 25 (Malagola, *Statuti*, 443).

[56] University of Medicine and Arts of Bologna: statute of 1405, 42 (Malagola, *Sta-*

The number of surgeons willing to invest the time and money in this full course of university study seems to have been quite small. The records of the University of Padua yield fewer than ten surgical diplomas for the entire period from the late fourteenth century through 1434, in contrast to hundreds of doctorates in physic. One student in surgery chose not to take the examination but received a certificate from the rector attesting that he had completed the regular course of study, while another, a Jew named Abraham, was licensed "in the vernacular," presumably because he knew no Latin; this authorized him to operate but not to prescribe any drug or medicine. There were in addition several men recorded as "students of surgery" for whom no certificate or diploma of any sort survives.[57] This evidence implies that university study in surgery was both less common than in physic and less standardized. Instruction was offered in both Latin and Italian, and it is likely that many surgical students enrolled for short periods—hence the one-year cycle of courses at Bologna shown in Appendix II. Because the degree was not necessary for practice in Florence, the student could leave when he felt prepared and enroll in the Guild of Doctors, Apothecaries, and Grocers on the basis of his university training alone or of the guild exam.[58] Furthermore, courses in surgery seem to have had a degree of independence from the other university medical courses. In Florence, for example, after the *studio* was temporarily closed in 1370, Maestro Lodovico di Bartolo da Gubbio continued to give lectures in surgery under the auspices of the communal government.[59]

As the lack of surviving diplomas suggests, however, most surgeons probably had no formal academic training at all. This impression is

---

tuti, 254). This appears to have been true at Florence as well. For example M° Lodovico di Bartolo da Gubbio, a lecturer on surgery, figures in the communal payment records for 1368 as "experienced in the art of medicine" (*artis medicine perito*) rather than as the more usual *artis medicine doctor* (CCCU-186, fol. [22v]). Later, in 1377, he is listed as a doctor of medicine (CCCU-228, fol. [6r]); he probably passed a further examination to earn the title; see Chapter Six.

[57] Marangon, "Professores," 8-10. The paucity of surgical diplomas might represent an accident of survival, given that they were issued by a different body. However, the relatively small number of surgeons on the teaching staff of the University of Bologna—two or three in the late fourteenth and fifteenth centuries—would argue that this kind of teaching was less in demand; see Dallari, *Rotuli*, vol. 4, passim.

[58] The colleges of medicine and arts of the various Italian *studi* attempted at times to require a university license for legal surgical practice, but such efforts seem to have been sporadic and ineffective. See College of Medicine and Arts of Bologna: statute of the early fifteenth century, 14 (Malagola, *Statuti*, 490); College of Arts and Medicine of Pavia: reform of 1433 (*Statuti e ordinamenti*, 129); and Marangon, "Professores," 30.

[59] See Park, "Readers," 264-67.

confirmed by the records of the *catasto* of 1427; whereas all but one of the fifteen physicians declared sizable personal libraries in their lists of assets, only one surgeon, Maestro Piero di Feo da Arencio, doctor to the city's prisons, owned any books at all, and his four volumes, worth fl. 10, were the smallest medical collection in the *catasto* (see Appendix III). Most surgeons in this period in fact learned their craft through regular apprenticeship to a recognized practitioner. A typical contract, drawn up in Verona in 1452 between Maestro Antonio di Nasimbeni, a surgeon from Treviso, and Bartolomeo di Tebaldi, the fifteen-year-old son of a Veronese dyer, provided for the boy to enter into an eight-year unpaid association with Maestro Antonio; in return Maestro Antonio agreed to "teach the said Bartholomeo, as much as he is able, his trade and craft."[60] At the end of his apprenticeship the young doctor would have petitioned for membership in his local guild. Once examined by the guild's commission of doctors, if such an examination was required, he would have matriculated as a qualified surgeon, permitted to perform the whole range of known operations but forbidden to prescribe internal medicines. Such doctors could not claim the sumptuary privileges of university-educated physicians and surgeons, but they used the honorific title maestro; they were often highly prized as practitioners, and some enjoyed both wealth and high social status.[61]

In addition to surgeons and physicians, contemporaries recognized a third class of doctors usually called empirics (*empirici*).[62] These were

[60] Text of the contract in Lecce, "Un maestro," 748-50. This kind of training was the rule for surgeons in northern Europe; see Bullough, "Training." On the private teaching of surgery in Bologna see Siraisi, *Taddeo Alderotti*, 14-15, and Zaccagnini, "L'insegnamento privato," 290-91.

[61] See below, Chapter Five; also, for Padua, Marangon, "Professores," 14-20; for Venice, Ruggiero, "Status of Physicians and Surgeons," 179-80, and Palmer, "Physicians and Surgeons." Because of the differences in their dress, such surgeons have been called surgeons of the "short robe" to distinguish them from university surgeons of the "long robe," with their special sumptuary privileges; MacKinney, *Medical Illustrations*, 65. On problems of enforcement see the deliberations of the Guild of Doctors, Apothecaries, and Grocers, AMS-49, fol. [19v].

[62] The titles used by empirics were somewhat flexible; a number matriculated in the guild without the honorific maestro but soon acquired it in nonguild records, perhaps because they appropriated it illegally, but probably because it was the title in general use for doctors. This was certainly the case, for example, for the man who matriculated under the name Andrea di Bartolo, doctor, but who appears in later communal records of payment for his services in the city army and prisons as M° Andrea (PR-38, fol. 57r-v; PR-48, fol. 42r). Marangon implies that in Padua empirics and barbers formed a single group ("Professores," 29-33); in Florence, however, they were seen as distinct, and barbers never enjoyed the title of maestro.

distinguished from the former two groups by their lack of formal training and the general knowledge it conferred. Like many surgeons, some empirics had doubtless learned by watching and assisting, while others seem to have been self-taught, as is implied by a reference in the guild's deliberations of 1475 to "those who begin to practice medicine on their own authority, based on simple and fallible experience."[63] Often illiterate, they were to a large extent specialists in treating a particular condition or performing a particular operation. Some moved regularly from town to town, while others owned or rented shops.[64] Some of the Florentine empirics practiced internal medicine; this was doubtless the case with Maestro Simone di Pacino, who identified himself in the *catasto* of 1427 as an "herbalist," or Piero di Bello, who matriculated as an apothecary but who appears in later records as a doctor. Most of the identifiable empirics, however, seem to have been surgical specialists and were identified as such when they matriculated in the guild.[65]

Matriculation lists, tax rolls, and government deliberations all testify to the importance and variety of empirical practice in fourteenth- and fifteenth-century Florence. Some empirics handled relatively routine and straightforward conditions. Of these, the most common were bone doctors (*medici ossium*), who treated fractures and dislocations. Both the commune and the rectors of various hospitals hired bone doctors to treat the poor without charge. Maestro Iacopo dell'Ossa da Roma, for example, as his name suggests, served as the city's bone doctor for many years; his position was filled after him by his three sons, Maestro Giovanni, Maestro Niccolò, and Maestro Stefano. Similarly, Maestro Giovanni di maestro Ciuccio da Orvieto appears as bone doctor to the hospital of Santa Maria Nuova in the early fifteenth century, where he was replaced on his death by his son Maestro Domenico, a bone doc-

[63] AMS 49, fol. [19v]. The guild was concerned to distinguish "tra quegli che di loro autorità per senplice e fallace experimento si mettano a medichare e quelli che ad tale uficio sarano stato o fieno legiptimamente."

[64] Wandering empirics were apparently a common feature in late medieval Italy. In 1346, for example, two surgeons from Parma arrived in Lucca and circulated an announcement that they would be available for a short period of time at a certain inn to treat fractures, hernias, stone, "or any other illness"; see Corsini, *Medici ciarlatani*, 56. Finding fertile ground for practice, however, such doctors might elect to settle down; this was probably the case for M° Niccolò di Bartolino "da Parma o da Pavia," who spent the rest of his life in Florence (PR-90, fols. 289r-91r). In his 1451 *catasto* declaration the hernia doctor M° Luca di m° Antonio noted the rent of a shop as one of his obligations (Catasto-711, fol. 582).

[65] Note that I say "identifiable." Doctors who appear as medical specialists in tax rolls, matriculation lists, or citizenship grants can be identified with fair certainty as empirics. It is likely that a number of others noted in similar documents as "doctor" or surgeon" were also empirics. On this topic see also Giovanni Sacino, "Primi albori."

tor also trained as a physician.[66] Other empirics specialized in teeth (*magistri dentium*), poultices (*medici de emplastris*), or wounds (*medici vulnerum*); the last were frequently hired by the city as military doctors.[67] Still others concentrated on particular diseases: Monna Neccia appears in the *estimo* of 1359 as a ringworm doctor (*medica di tigna*), and Betto di Tieri di Betto da Castelfranco, according to the guild's matriculation list for 1426, treated what was described as *cancro*.[68]

Most or all of these conditions were within the repertory of any higher surgeon,[69] and wealthier patients could certainly have gone to one of them for treatment. There were, however, several specialized and complex operations considered too dangerous and difficult for the regular surgeon. In the fourteenth century Lanfranco da Milano referred to surgery for bladder stones, for example, as a "fearful operation" and recommended that it be left to the (empirical) specialist.[70] Other similarly dangerous operations were those for cataracts, performed by lowering the crystalline lens behind the pupil with a needle, and for hernias; the celebrated fifteenth-century physician Bartolomeo da Montagnana gave up performing hernia operations after three of his patients died.[71] Florence was well equipped with empirical sur-

---

[66] PR-32, fol. 105; PR-36, fol. 30; PR-52, fol. 138. On M° Giovanni da Orvieto, SMN-4458, fol. 103v (1406); SMN-4477, fols. 39r, 103v, 113v (1426/7-28).

[67] Florentine dentists from this period included M° Domenico de dentibus, in the hearth tax of 1352 (Estimo-306, S. Maria Novella), and M° Simone di Pacino, in the *catasto* of 1427 (Catasto-307, fol. 74r-v). Among the Florentine poultice doctors were M° Lodovico di m° Francesco, matriculated between 1345/6 and 1353, and his son Stefano, matriculated somewhat later. There is also reference to a woman, Monna Iacopa, "che medicava d'impiastri nel tempo della mortalità del 74," in BNF: Magl. XXV, 113; quoted in Targioni-Tozzetti, *Notizie*, 155. On military and wound doctors see below, Chapter Three.

[68] For Monna Neccia, Prestanze-5, fol. 64v; for Betto da Castelfranco, AMS-21, *ad annum* 1426: "medet de morbo clancli." *Cancro* seems to have included a number of skin conditions, not all necessarily malignant; see the discussion in Iacopo di Bartolo da Prato, *Liber de operatione manuali*; BNF: Pal. 811, fol. 18r-v.

[69] Medical faculties offered instruction in these specialties, presumably for both those studying for a degree in surgery and occasional auditors. The rolls of the University of Bologna in this period, for example, contain the names of a M° Paolo da Rocca Contraria, "medicus ciroxie, specialiter ad malum capitis et oculorum provixionatus"; M° Giovanni da Genova, "deputatus ad lecturam Dislocationum et fracturarum ossium"; M° Medicolo da . . ., "deputatus ad lecturam Dislocatorum ossorum [*sic*]"; and M° Lorenzo de' Flagelli da Pieve di Cento, "deputatus ad lecturam predictam Cirogie et fracturarum ossium" (Dallari, *Rotuli*, 4:19, 53, 55, 57, 59, 63, 65).

[70] In Tabanelli, *Chirurgia italiana*, 2:997. The Hippocratic oath contains the same caution, cited also by Zerbi, *De cautelis*, 57. See Fabbri, "Litotomia," on this operation.

[71] Marangon, "Professores," 11-12. Details in Feigenbaum, "Cataract," and Jandolo, "Ernia inguinale."

geons in such specialties. There are references to several eye doctors (*medici oculorum*) in communal and guild records from the fourteenth and fifteenth centuries. One, Maestro Beltrame di maestro Neri da Cortona, was granted Florentine citizenship in 1354 on condition that he treat the poor free. Another, Maestro Benedetto di Francesco di Michele, listed himself on his *catasto* declaration as "shoemaker and eye doctor," implying that his needle did double duty.[72]

A number of hernia doctors also matriculated in the Florentine guild. Notable among these were the two brothers Maestro Antonio and Maestro Francesco di Giovanni da Norcia. Norcia, a modest town to the southeast of Perugia, was the seat of a remarkable lay tradition of empirical surgery specializing in operations on the urinary-genital tract and, to a lesser degree, on eyes—skills generally passed on within families.[73] Of obscure origin, this tradition was firmly established by the end of the fourteenth century, when Norcia began to export surgeons in large numbers to Rome and other cities in central Italy. Florence was no exception. Between 1386 and 1444 the guild enrolled twenty-six doctors from Norcia and its district—twice as many as from Arezzo, Prato, Pisa, and Bologna combined. The Norcini tended to immigrate to Florence by family. There is no information about most of them apart from their matriculation entry in the guild records, and it is difficult to say anything certain about their medical practice; it seems likely, however, that most of them were empirics and specialized in various surgical procedures. Certainly the best documented Florentine family of Norcini falls into that category. Maestro Antonio di Giovanni immigrated from Norcia and joined the guild sometime toward the end of the fourteenth century. In 1406 the city granted him and his brother Maestro Francesco, described as "doctors for those with problems of the genitals," a highly unusual lifetime tax exemption, with the express purpose of keeping them in Florence.[74] Maestro An-

---

[72] For M° Beltrame, PR-41, fol. 38r-v (matriculated 1355). For M° Benedetto, Catasto-78, fol. 242r. Other documented eye doctors included M° Falcone di m° Rinuccio da Montalbino, matriculated between 1320 and 1338, and M° Lionardo di m° Iacopo da Volterra, granted citizenship in 1388 (PR-77, fols. 178r-79r).

[73] On the Norcian tradition see Fabbi, "Lebbrosario" (with bibliography). It reached its peak in the sixteenth and seventeenth centuries but is traceable as early as the fourteenth century. Much of the literature on the subject of Norcian surgery is of little value, at least for the early period. Less inadequate than most, besides Fabbi, are Cristiano Dominici, "Scuola," and Pizzoni, "Litotomia."

[74] PR-95, fol. 3r-v: "medicorum eorum qui in membris generantibus infirmitates patiuntur." He and his brother had been granted a partial tax exemption in 1398; see PR-87, fol. 237r-v. Note that not all hernia doctors were from Norcia; for example, M° Bartolo di Bettino da Arezzo matriculated as such between 1353 and 1386.

tonio had four sons, Maestro Iacopo, Maestro Bartolomeo, Maestro Luca, and Maestro Giovanni, all of whom matriculated as doctors and apparently carried on their father's work in the hernia business.

Empirical surgeons seem to have occupied a somewhat paradoxical position within the larger medical profession. On the one hand, many were viewed with pronounced suspicion and disapproval by formally trained surgeons and physicians as at best ineffectual and at worst a public menace. Guglielmo da Saliceto described them in his *Surgery*, an influential thirteenth-century textbook, as a threat to the newly consolidated scientific status of surgery. Maestro Iacopo da Prato attacked them on several occasions in *On Manual Operation*, as did Maestro Niccolò Falcucci, the most important Florentine medical writer of the early fifteenth century. "A great host of lay and empirical practitioners flourishes at present," he lamented, refusing to acknowledge them as colleagues: "We should not call just any empiric or wisewoman a surgeon, even though he lances boils, stitches up wounds, and does similar work. We should rather bar them everywhere from this kind of operation and shun their treatments, since they practice wrongly. And if they perform successful cures, it is not thanks to their competence but to luck. . . ."[75] To a certain extent the profession as a whole sympathized with this view and considered the more questionable of the empirics to be dangerous and unfair competitors; many of the guild's attempts to tighten matriculation requirements in the decades after the plague of 1348 were in fact directed against this kind of practitioner.[76]

On the other hand, many of the empirics were well entrenched within the profession and the guild. Some, like the bone doctors, were obviously highly effective at routine medical tasks, as a number of illustrious medical writers acknowledged,[77] while others, like the eye doctors and hernia experts, took on cases which general practitioners

[75] Guglielmo in Tabanelli, *Chirurgia italiana*, 2:524-25. Iacopo da Prato, *De operatione manuali*; BNF: Pal. 811, fol. 1r. Falcucci, *Sermones medicinales*, VII, 3, 1; vol. 4, fol. 43: "Non enim quilibet operator ydiota vel muliercula, quamvis secet apostemata aut suat vulnera et similia faciat opera, debet vocari cirugicus, sed ab huiusmodi operationibus sunt ejiciendi ubique terrarum, et a curis egrorum fugandi sunt, cum erronee et indebite operentur. Et si aliquando effectum sospitatum consequantur, non est eorum benemeritis gestis sed fortune. . . . Et horum ydiotarum et empiricorum operatorum nostris diebus copia magna viget, . . . et maxime in curandis solutionibus continuitatis ossis vel ossium et dissolutionibus iuncturarum." Also Mᵒ Giovanni da Arezzo, *De medicinae et legum praestantia*; BLF: Laur. 77, 22, fols. 5r-27r. See in general Agrimi and Crisciani, "Medici e 'vetulae.' " 144-59.

[76] See Chapter One, notes 63 and 64.

[77] These included Bartolomeo da Montagnana and Michele Savonarola; Marangon, "Professores," 37.

considered too dangerous to accept. And outside the profession these specialists were often more highly prized than the surgical generalist. Maestro Gregorio da Pisa, exiled in 1361 from his own city, was put on the communal payroll and invited to stay by the Florentine government, "because the city of Florence needs good surgeons, especially those expert in the treatment of eyes, hernias, boils, and fractured and dislocated bones."[78] In the decades following, virtually all the doctors who received special tax exemptions to tempt them to settle in the city were empirics and surgical specialists.[79]

In addition to empirics two other, smaller groups played a more established and respected role in the Florentine medical profession than we would at first expect: these were women and Jews. In some respects they were regular members of the profession; they matriculated in the guild like other doctors and were subject to its statutes and regulations. In other respects they stood apart, both because of their relatively small numbers and because they were as a rule excluded from positions of responsibility within the guild.

Information concerning female doctors in Renaissance Florence is sparse. Four women matriculated as doctors in the later fourteenth or very early fifteenth century: Monna Franca di maestro Filippo di ser Bindo (between 1356 and 1353); Monna Tessa di Guido del Rosso (1363); Monna Lisa, wife of Iacopo da Carmignano (between 1353 and 1363) and Monna Antonia di maestro Daniele, a Jew (between 1386 and 1408). I have found two more listed as doctors in the contemporary tax records—Monna Alfania (in 1353 and 1355) and Monna Neccia, a "ringworm doctor" (in 1359)—and there were no doubt others appearing in other distributions.[80] As their names indicate, at least two of these women were daughters of doctors and, like many sons, almost certainly learned their trade from their fathers. (Monna

78 PR-48, fol. 149v: "quod civitas florentina valentibus viris cirusicis indiget, maxime expertis in curis oculorum, crepatorum, antracis sive malarum bullarum, et in curis restaurationis ossium fractorum et dislocatorum."

79 For example, M° Beltrame di m° Neri da Cortona, eye doctor, in 1359 (PR-41, fol. 38r); M° Lionardo di m° Iacopo da Volterra, eye doctor, in 1388 (PR-77, fols. 178r-79r, new numeration); M° Niccolò di Bartolino da Parma, bone doctor, in 1401 (PR-90, fols. 289r-91r); M° Antonio and M° Francesco di Giovanni da Norcia, hernia doctors, in 1406 (PR-95, fol. 3r-v). The provision granting a universal tax exemption to these last two states explicitly that "aliis fuit concessa immunitas medicis forensibus habentibus aliquid singulare in exercitio medicine, maxime medicis ossium." Furthermore, an automatic tax exemption was granted to the communal bone doctor, as provided for in the communal statutes from at least 1355 and in practice from at least 1336; Statuti-11, fol. 146v.

80 Estimo-306 and 307 (S. Giovanni/Vaio); Prestanze-5, fol. 64v.

enrolled

Franca in fact matriculated without charge, because her father was also
a member of the guild.) Although they could not claim to be physicians in the strict sense, lacking doctorates; they might well have practiced internal medicine. To judge by her specialty, on the other hand,
Monna Neccia was almost certainly an empiric; it is characteristic that
she was one of the few documented doctors not to appear in the records of the guild. It is also worth noting that no women seem to have
matriculated before 1353 or after 1408. This would confirm the
impression left by the guild statutes and by contemporary accounts
that the medical profession was relatively open in the decades immediately following the first epidemic of plague.

We know much more about Jewish doctors, who formed a small
but visible minority of the Florentine medical community throughout
the fourteenth and fifteenth centuries. Trained and licensed for the
most part outside the universities, they were often, like empirics, the
object of official criticism and restrictions while still highly prized by
the commune and the population at large.[81]

From the early Middle Ages a series of conciliar decrees had restricted the practice of Jewish doctors, prohibiting them from treating
Christians, as this was seen as a particularly intimate and dangerous
form of contact. At the same time the thirteenth and fourteenth centuries witnessed the growth of a deep respect for the Jewish medical
tradition, based on its close historical and linguistic ties with Arabic
medicine in Spain and the Near East. This respect was particularly
marked in Spain, southern France, and Italy, where with increasing
frequency popes and rulers granted special dispensations to Jewish
doctors and hired them as court physicians. A series of papal bulls in
the fifteenth century substantially weakened the previous prohibitions
and exempted medical practitioners from wearing the special signs required of Jews: a red tabard, yellow hat, or yellow cloth circle, depending on the city.[82] In general, papal and communal dispensations
were easy to come by; even in periods or regions where Christians
were prohibited from consulting Jews except in emergencies, the practice was widespread, though deplored by certain ecclesiastics.

The training and licensing of Jewish doctors, like that of surgeons
and empirics, varied according to circumstance and place. By the middle of the fourteenth century a few Jews were attending lectures at
some universities, although they were forbidden by civil and canon

[81] The principal study on Jewish medicine in Italy is Friedenwald, _Jews and Medicine_,
vol. 2, chap. 41. See also Roth, _Jews in the Renaissance_, 213-27.
[82] Friedenwald, _Jews and Medicine_, 2:556-72.

law from taking degrees. Again, exceptions seem to have been granted from the early fifteenth century, most notably at Padua, which emerged as a center of Jewish medical studies in the Renaissance. Elsewhere, Jews learned medicine by apprenticeship and from private teachers. Those without university degrees were examined and licensed to practice by the guilds in the usual way.[83] Though rarely allowed to teach in Christian universities, Jews engaged in a wide range of medical activities, practicing privately or acting as salaried doctors for popes, princes, communes, and even for monasteries.[84]

These general remarks apply to Jewish medical practice in Florence. The Guild of Doctors, Apothecaries, and Grocers placed no special restrictions on Jewish doctors, and their names appear in the matriculation lists from the early fourteenth century; their numbers increased significantly after a communal provision of 1396, which authorized Jewish moneylenders in Florence and led ultimately to the first establishment of a real Jewish community in the city.[85] At no time were there many Jewish doctors. Between 1320 and 1444 only ten (including one woman) matriculated in the guild, although we have information on several more from other fifteenth-century sources.[86] Almost

---

[83] See Toaff, *Ebrei*, 32 and 48-50, for an analysis of contemporary legal opinions regarding university study by Jews. The first known degree granted to a Jew was at Padua in 1409. Later in the fifteenth century it became a standard although infrequent practice; Jews were required to hold a special banquet for all comers on the occasion of their *conventus*, and the financial outlay must have been considerable: Roth, *Jews in the Renaissance*, 37. On other sorts of training see Roth, "Qualifications," 835-38.

[84] The rare exceptions included M° Musetto di Guglielmo, who appears in the list of the teaching faculty of Perugia in the early fifteenth century (Toaff, *Ebrei*, 82), and M° Elia del Medigo, who taught in the *studio* at Padua later in the century (Ciscato, *Ebrei*, 99). No Jews appear in the extant records of the teaching faculty of the University of Florence for this period. Cf. the general remarks on Jewish doctors in France, in Jacquart, *Le milieu médical*, 1:160-67.

[85] PR-85, fols. 224v-26r. This arrangement did not become permanent in Florence proper until 1431. For the background to communal policy concerning Jewish moneylending and immigration to Florence see Anthony Molho, "A Note on Jewish Moneylenders in Tuscany in the Late Trecento and Early Quattrocento," in Molho and Tedeschi, *Renaissance Studies*, 99-117. On Jewish doctors in Florence see Cassuto, *Ebrei*, 180-85, and Münster and Malavolti, "Documenti."

[86] The lists of Jewish doctors in Cassuto, *Ebrei*, 183-85, and Münster and Malavolti, "Documenti," 24-29, are incomplete for the period to 1450; they should also include the following: M° Giovanni di Gaio da Moroso di Maiolica (*fu giudeo*), matriculated between 1312 and 1320; M° Dateo di Vitale, matriculated between 1320 and 1338, probably the M° Datillo da Roma mentioned by Cassuto on 9; M° Abraham, surgeon, matriculated ca. 1350, appears on tax lists of 1352 (Estimo-306, S. Spirito), 1369 (Prestanze-143, fol. 136v, as a pauper), and 1379 (Prestanze-369, fol. 105v); M° Bonaventura, matriculated between 1353 and 1386; Monna Antonia di m° Daniele (*ebrea*

all were foreigners, often from Rome, Spain, or Provence, although Maestro Aliuccio di Salamone di Aliuccio, who was also a moneylender and opened a bank in Florence in 1439, came from Arezzo and paid the reduced fees of a native of the district.[87]

Some of Florence's Jewish doctors were men of considerable eminence. Maestro Salamone di Abraham Aviziri of Arles, for example, who matriculated in 1412 and who alone of all the fifteenth-century Jewish or Christian matriculants had the money to pay his foreigner's fee of fl. 12 in two lump sums, is known as a Hebrew translator of Latin medical and philosophical works. Maestro Giovanni Agnolo, a Spanish physician, was "learned in the law" and a friend of the humanist Giannozzo Manetti and the cardinal Giuliano Cesarini. He converted to Christianity in the middle of the fifteenth century and was baptized amid great ceremony, with Manetti, Cesarini, and Agnolo Acciaiuoli as his godparents.[88] Others, though less distinguished in the world of letters, were equally prized as doctors. In 1416, for example, the Florentine government granted citizenship and a full tax exemption to two brothers, Maestro Diamante and Maestro Luigi di Anori (from Provence via Rome), "because the said Maestro Diamante and Maestro Luigi are very learned in medicine—Maestro Diamante in the science or art called *physica* and Maestro Luigi in that called surgery, as well as in bones and hernias."[89] They were the last doctors of any sort in the fifteenth century to receive such a privilege.

In Florence, as elsewhere, there was some suspicion of Jewish doctors; this attitude must have been fueled by the trial of Maestro Iacopo, a Jewish doctor from Provence, who confessed to supplying a woman with poison to murder her husband and who was executed in 1404.[90] On the other hand, there is evidence from later in the century that certain Jewish doctors were highly esteemed, as shown by the records of the Otto di Guardia, the Florentine police body responsible

---

medicha), matriculated between 1386 and 1408; Mº Iacopo debelchadre (?), matriculated between 1386 and 1408, possibly identical with Mº Iacopo Astrughi da Arillo di Provenza, condemned for conspiracy to commit murder (see note 90 below).

[87] AMS-21, fol. 374r.

[88] On Mº Salomone, see Münster and Malavolti, "Documenti," 24-25; Roth, "Qualifications," 839-40; and AMS-21, fol. 35. On Mº Giovanni Agnolo, Vespasiano de Bisticci, *Vite*, 1:144-45.

[89] PR-105, fol. 358v: "Quoniam prefati magister Diamante et magister Loysius doctissimi sunt in arte medicine, videlicet magister Diamante in ea scientia sive arte que dicitur fisica et magister Loysius in ea que dicitur cerusica ac etiam ossium et in eo defectu qui dicitur de' crepati. . . ."

[90] Atti del podestà-3965, fols. 40r-42r; tr. in Brucker, *Society of Renaissance Florence*, 243-45. Also PR-93, fols. 23v-24r.

for Jewish affairs and other matters of internal security. In 1460, for example, Maestro Bonaventura di Bonaventura, famed for his many successful cures, was granted a universal license to practice surgery and physic on all inhabitants of the Florentine territories, both Jews and Christians. In 1476 the commune further authorized him to enter the convent of Santa Veridiana to treat the daughter of Giacomo Ghiberti and any other nuns who required it.[91]

One final question concerns the relative numbers of physicians, surgeons, and empirics practicing in Florence. A compilation from the most informative tax rolls of the later fourteenth and the fifteenth centuries gives the results shown in table 2-2.[92] The most striking feature of these figures is the steadily increasing proportion of physicians. In the first decades after the plague of 1348 they were clearly outnumbered by surgeons and empirics; a century later the pattern had reversed itself, and most of the city's doctors were physicians.

The reasons for this shift are complex. On the one hand, there seems to have been a substantial influx of healers into the profession immediately after the epidemic of 1348—healers who, according both to lay observers like Boccaccio and to the framers of the guild's amendments of 1351 and 1353, were drawn from the lower ranks of practitioners.[93] This situation prompted the guild, as we have already seen, to make sporadic efforts to tighten entrance requirements for doctors;

TABLE 2-2
Classes of Doctors in City Tax Rolls

Year	Physicians	Surgeons	Empirics	Unidentified	Total
1359	9 (35%)	8 (31%)	6 (23%)	3 (11%)	26
1399	16 (33%)	14 (29%)	10 (21%)	8 (17%)	48
1427	19 (53%)	7 (19%)	10 (28%)	—	36
1451	14 (64%)	2 (9%)	2 (9%)	4 (18%)	22

SOURCES: Prestanze-5 (1359); Prestanze-1787, 1788, 1789, 1790 (1399); Catasto-65 to 83 and Catasto-Campioni del Monte-San Giovanni-1427 (1427); Catasto-687 to 722 (1451, crosschecked with *campioni*).

[91] Privileges from OG-12, fols. 34r-v, 38r, 40r, and OG-41, fol. 44r; transcribed in Cassuto, *Ebrei*, docs. LV and LVI, and in Münster and Malavolti, "Documenti," 32-37.

[92] I have supplemented the tax rolls with information about tax-exempt doctors and collated them with details concerning their practice from other records. Note that the classes of empirics and surgeons were not completely distinct; their relative numbers are thus more uncertain.

[93] Boccaccio, *Decameron*, 7-8; Guild of Doctors, Apothecaries, and Grocers: amendments of 1351, IX, and 1353, I (Ciasca, *Statuti*, 231 and 242-43).

these efforts may have had some success in reducing the relative numbers of surgeons and empirics. On the other hand, the increase in the proportion of physicians may well have had less to do with guild policies than with changing social and economic conditions in the Florentine territories and in Italy as a whole. One clue lies in a letter from the bishop of Pistoia to Lorenzo de' Medici in 1477. In it the bishop complained about the dearth of competent physicians in Pistoia: "We have here four doctors who do not add up to even half a good one. The best of them—or let us say the least pathetic—is thought to be Maestro Niccolò da Siena, who does not practice in Italian or rely on experience alone, like the others."[94] Twenty-five years earlier Pistoia had had a number of respected physicians, but by the middle of the fifteenth century it and other smaller cities like Prato and Volterra were witnessing the exact opposite of the trend in Florence: they experienced a decline in the proportion of physicians just as that proportion was rising in the capital.[95] The implication is that doctors were being drained from secondary cities; as we shall see in Chapter Four, Florence, center of an expanding state and a flourishing culture, offered more to ambitious and well-educated physicians than the stagnating economy and society of the smaller towns. This interpretation fits well with the changing immigration figures for Florentine doctors.

IMMIGRATION AND THE PLAGUE

The composition of the Florentine medical profession underwent important changes over the course of the later fourteenth and the fifteenth centuries. As we have already seen, the number of doctors expanded rapidly after 1348, reaching a peak in the last decades of the fourteenth century, and declined thereafter; this decline coincided with a rise in the proportion of physicians and a decrease in that of surgeons and empirics. Even more striking, however, was the shift in geographical patterns of recruitment among medical practitioners. Whereas in the mid-fourteenth century most Florentine doctors were natives of

[94] MAP-XXXV, 924 (8.xii.1477): "Noi habiamo qui quatro medici che non vagliano per uno mezo buono. Il meglio di loro, o vogliamo dire il mancho tristo, si riputa Maestro Nicolò da Siena, che non medica in volgare nè per pratica, come gli altri. . . ." (The bishop meant that the other doctors did not read Latin.)

[95] See Chiappelli, *Medici e chirurghi pistoiesi*, 69-118. Enrico Fiumi noticed a decline in the proportion of all professionals in the city of Prato by the end of the fifteenth century, where "professionals" are defined as notaries, doctors, lawyers, and others with an academic title; see his *Demografia*, 69-70, 78-80, 139-40. Statistical studies are generally lacking for the smaller towns.

the city, a century later citizens were strongly outnumbered by recent immigrants. (This shift, as we saw in the previous chapter, accounted for the declining presence of doctors in the power structure of the guild.) It would be a mistake to attribute this change exclusively to the plague: even before 1348 doctors had a high rate of immigration compared to other occupational groups, and patterns of geographical mobility established in the early fourteenth century continued to hold after the first epidemics. Nonetheless, the coming of the Black Death complicated these patterns as it complicated the practice of medicine itself.

As table 2-3 shows, doctors differed strikingly in their geographical origins from the merchants, shopkeepers, and artisans who made up the other branches of the Guild of Doctors, Apothecaries, and Grocers, particularly if we are concerned to distinguish immigrants from the Florentine territory (countryside and district) from "foreigners" (those who came from other cities and states inside and outside Italy).[96] Among the nondoctors of the guild, the percentage of foreign

TABLE 2-3
Immigrants in the Guild Matriculation Lists

	From the Florentine Territory	Foreigners	Total Immigrants	Total Matriculants
Doctors				
1320-53	42 (25%)	19 (11%)	61 (36%)	170
1353-86	41 (34%)	31 (25%)	72 (59%)	122
1386-1408	30 (37%)	25 (31%)	55 (68%)	81
1409-44	27 (30%)	46 (50%)	73 (80%)	91
Nondoctors				
1320-53	49 (3%)	15 (1%)	64 (4%)	1,836
1353-86	124 (11%)	17 (2%)	141 (13%)	1,070
1386-1408	142 (14%)	13 (1%)	155 (15%)	1,018
1409-44	94 (7%)	34 (2%)	128 (9%)	1,361

SOURCES: AMS-7, 8, 9, 21.

[96] As before, I have based these figures on a collation of AMS-7, AMS-8, AMS-9, and AMS-21. The toponymic method is not foolproof, as Herlihy and Klapisch-Zuber have pointed out (*Les toscans*, 304-6), since families and individuals tended to shed their toponymics at different rates, depending on social class and family background. In my experience, however, the problem is not great. For doctors and other members of the guild, the use of toponymics is remarkably consistent: matriculants born elsewhere than in Florence have them, whereas matriculants born in the city—even the sons of immigrants—do not. Thus the main source of error in my statistics lies in the fact that the

immigrants remained roughly constant and almost negligible for the entire period between 1320 and 1444; the percentage of immigrants from the Florentine territory, however, rose significantly in the half-century following the plague, peaking around 1400 before beginning to drop in the fifteenth century. Thus the influx of immigrants increased noticeably if temporarily after 1348, an increase drawn almost entirely from the surrounding countryside.[97] Among the doctors, on the other hand, the proportion of immigrants from the Florentine territory was very high even before the plague. It rose only moderately after 1348 and declined again in the fifteenth century. Thus the soaring immigration rate of doctors in the fifteenth century stems largely from a dramatic increase in the number of foreigners coming to the city.

In fact, the matriculation lists give a somewhat skewed picture of the profession; some doctors joined the guild without settling permanently in the city, and this tends to inflate the figures on immigration. But if we exclude transient practitioners by looking only at those doctors who appeared in the city tax rolls, we see a similar, if less extreme, pattern: the proportion of native Florentine doctors dropped steadily during the century after 1348, until in the *catasto* of 1427 they represented only 30 percent of medical practitioners in the city; meanwhile the proportion of immigrants from the subject territories increased into the mid-fifteenth century, to be rivaled only by the growing number of foreign immigrants. By 1470, according to Benedetto Dei's list of doctors, over three-quarters were immigrants, and almost three-quarters of them were foreigners.[98]

---

guild notaries occasionally omitted toponymics in their summary lists because of lack of space. This means that my figures should be taken as reasonably accurate minima for nondoctor immigrants. The figures for doctors should be accurate, because I have been able to crosscheck them with other documents. Note that the boundaries of the Florentine territories expanded markedly in the course of the fourteenth and early fifteenth century. I have taken this expansion into account in my calculations; it only intensifies the significance of the trend in favor of foreigners described in the next paragraphs.

There is no detailed study of population movement in and outside Florence in this period, although Herlihy and Klapisch-Zuber have offered a preliminary sketch in *Les toscans*, chap. 11. See also, esp. for the years before the plague, Plesner, *L'émigration*; Luzzato, "L'inurbamento"; Fiumi, "Fioritura e decadenza," 116(1958): 497-504; and de la Roncière, *Florence*, 2:679-96.

[97] My figures agree well with those of Herlihy and Klapisch-Zuber, who calculate the proportion of foreign immigrants at 2.1% and local immigrants at 10.2% for the Florentine population as a whole in the years around 1427; see *Les toscans*, 310.

[98] Sources as in notes 26, 30, and table 2-2. If matriculation lists give an inflated picture of immigration, tax lists give a deflated one, since households with their principal holdings outside the city were often taxed there. This seems to have been particularly

These figures suggest a number of conclusions. In the first place, doctors had a high immigration rate well before the plague; during the first half of the fourteenth century something like 40 percent of them came from outside the city, most notably from the *contado*. This group also included a smaller number of foreign immigrants—natives for the most part of other Tuscan cities, like Siena, Montepulciano, Arezzo, and Volterra. Thus doctors fit the pattern described by Plesner for notaries in this period: they tended to come from the *castelli* (fortified towns) of the Florentine territory, and like Plesner's lawyers and notaries they participated in a wider professional culture which encouraged them to think beyond the confines of their native town. They also possessed skills for which there was a ready market in the city, and this further enhanced their mobility relative to other inhabitants of the countryside.[99] Even after transferring their households to Florence they usually maintained strong personal and economic ties to their place of origin, deriving rents and income from property there and returning to the family house for the hot summer. Assimilation was thereafter a gradual process.

This pattern held for doctors at least through the second half of the fourteenth century. Maestro Antonio di maestro Guccio da Scarperia, who settled in the city with his brothers in the late 1380s, and Maestro Antonio Chellini da San Miniato, who matriculated in the guild shortly before 1400, are good examples of this kind of immigrant from the *contado*. Both retained strong economic and emotional interests in their native towns, as their *catasto* declarations show.[100] At the same time, however, we see an increase in doctors from the district—Tuscan cities newly subject to Florence, like Prato, Pistoia, San Gimignano, Volterra, and Arezzo. Before the expansion of Florence's boundaries in the course of the fourteenth century these men would have been clas-

---

true of residents of the district in general and foreigners in the *catasti* from the middle of the fifteenth century on. Dei's list, on the other hand, may exaggerate the proportion of foreigners, since he probably does not include empirics.

[99] Plesner, *L'émigration*, 128-50. Plesner estimates the proportion of city notaries born in the *contado* before the plague to be between a third and a half—a figure which fits closely with my results for doctors; see 149. Martines, who observed much the same thing for lawyers, has emphasized the "instrumental quality" of their legal education; their special skills acted as a kind of easily transferable capital (*Lawyers*, 72). Note that more recent historians than Plesner have pointed out that Plesner may have underestimated the numbers of poorer and less visible immigrants from the countryside in his period; see, for example, Luzzato, "L'inurbamento," 197-98.

[100] On M° Antonio see Baccini, "Maestro Antonio di Guccio da Scarperia," 339ff.; Catasto-78, fols. 1r-10r. On M° Giovanni see Lightbown, "Giovanni Chellini"; Catasto-79, fols. 47r-49v.

sified as foreigners; nonetheless they followed much the same pattern as doctors native to the *contado*. Maestro Tommaso di Baccio da Arezzo, for example, kept a house for the use of his family in Arezzo, where two of his sons were in business.[101]

As the influx of doctors from the Florentine territory began to tail off toward the middle of the fifteenth century, the number of foreign immigrants from distant areas was increasing. The largest group of these were natives of Umbria—many empirics from Norcia, as we have already seen—and of the nearest university towns like Bologna and Siena. As the fifteenth century progressed, however, more and more came from farther away: the Marches, Pavia, Milan, Venice, Friuli, Sicily, and even Spain, Germany, France, and elsewhere. One of the doctors in Dei's list for 1470 was "Maestro Giorgio the Greek, eater of caviar."[102]

To what can we attribute these fifteenth-century developments—the decrease in the number of local immigrants and the rise in the number of foreign doctors? It may be that many of the local immigrants, at least among physicians, had first come to Florence to study medicine and that with the university's decline in the mid-fifteenth century this conduit ceased to function.[103] It may be also that the towns of the *contado* and the district found themselves progressively exhausted of talent, as generation after generation of their best-educated and most ambitious citizens left for the big city. This is consistent with the complaints of contemporaries about the scarcity of doctors in towns like Pistoia and Volterra as well as with the observations of recent historians that fifteenth-century immigrants to Florence from the countryside were mostly poor laborers and agricultural workers—a far cry from the doctors, lawyers, and notaries of the thirteenth and fourteenth centuries.[104] At the same time, however, Florence was becoming more and more of a cultural and political center; the capital of one of Italy's principal states, it was able to draw doctors from the farther reaches of Italy and of Europe.

[101] Catasto-83, fols. 213r-217r.

[102] Dei, *Memorie*; BLF: Ashburnham 644, fol. 31v: "El maestro Giorgio ghrecho, magnatore di chaviaro." This tendency of doctors to immigrate from farther away was part of a general phenomenon; see Cohn, *Laboring Classes*, 96-104.

[103] Given the loss of university records from this period, it is difficult to estimate exactly how important the *studio* was in attracting physicians to the city. My impression is that relatively few professors immigrated permanently to Florence but that many students remained after taking their degrees; for a discussion of the motivations behind this kind of decision see below, Chapter Four.

[104] See Chiappelli, *Medici e chirurghi pistoiesi*, 9-10; Battistini, *Medici in Volterra*, 24-25; Herlihy and Klapisch-Zuber, *Les toscans*, 318-20; de la Roncière, *Florence*, 2:726.

But none of this explains the most striking aspect of the situation: the dramatic drop in native Florentine doctors. Whereas in 1359 they formed roughly 60 percent of the medical profession appearing in the communal tax rolls, by 1427 they had declined to less than a third— and by 1470, according to Dei, to less than a quarter. This drop is even more impressive if we look at the absolute numbers involved. Between 1409 and 1444 only seventeen of the ninety-one doctors who matriculated in the guild were natives of Florence, and of these five were sons of immigrant fathers. Thus only twelve came from families established in Florence for more than a single generation and were, for the purposes of political representation, full-fledged Florentine citizens.

The causes of this movement among native Florentines away from the medical profession are clearly complex, and we can only guess at them here. Florence was a large and varied city with a large and varied economy; thus it offered a much wider range of alternatives for young people choosing a career than smaller towns like Scarperia, San Miniato, or even Prato.[105] One possible explanation for the decline in doctors of Florentine stock lies in the market for medical services. If there was in fact a significant rise in the number of doctors active in the city after the plague (see table 2-1), it may be that the supply of medical services began to outstrip the demand. This would have led to more competition and shrinking fees; citizens who would otherwise have gone into medicine might well have opted for careers in other kinds of businesses where the return on their investment of time and money was greater. This explanation would be more convincing if the government had not continued to make preferential citizenship grants to doctors while complaining about the shortage of medical practitioners. Furthermore, there is no evidence that medical fees dropped in this period; if anything, medicine was more lucrative in the fifteenth century than the fourteenth.[106]

[105] See, for example, the petition of Mº Iacopo di Francesco Chiarenti da S. Gimignano, who described himself as "ob prolem suam motus" in his request for citizenship (PR-89, fol. 28v).

[106] It is difficult to cite hard evidence in support of this statement, given the paucity of documents on doctors' income. One of the best sources is the account books of the hospital of Santa Maria Nuova, which employed at least two salaried doctors during the fourteenth century. In 1353, for example, the standard salary seems to have been fl. 12 a year (SMN-4408, fol. 28); by 1427 the two doctors were receiving fl. 14 and fl. 24 respectively (SMN-4477, fol. 39r). There was no corresponding general inflation in the salaries of other employees of the hospital. As another indication, doctors in the fifteenth century tended to be wealthier on the average than doctors in the mid-fourteenth (see

Another, more plausible explanation for the decline in native Florentine doctors is that some of the sons of the more established doctors and medical families did not in fact choose an alternative career but instead opted for a life of leisure supported by rents or, in a number of cases, by liquidation of the family patrimony. It seems likely that in these cases sons of doctors of a certain economic and social status tended to associate and identify with the patrician elite among which they and their fathers moved. They may well have mimicked the patrician class in its increasing flight from trade toward rentier (*scioperato*) status or the "leisure of letters" described by Alberti.[107] This explanation works well for a number of individual cases, but it fails to account for the majority of native doctors' sons, who went into business of some sort, usually in spices or cloth. Similarly, there is no evidence that Florentines emigrated in numbers large enough to account for the decline in native doctors.[108]

The decisive factor seems to have been the plague. It is surely no coincidence that the sharp drop in the number of Florentine citizens entering the medical profession occurred during the period in which the city was ravaged by repeated epidemics of the Black Death. Under such circumstances there was every reason for boys with other prospects and alternative sources of employment to avoid medicine. To begin with, plague was thought to be highly contagious; the doctor, like the notary and priest, who also frequented sickrooms during epidemics, was considered to be at great risk even in attending a plague patient, as contemporary plague tractates show. Fearing contagion, many doctors, like their more prosperous clients, fled the city at the first signs of plague or, as contemporary chroniclers complained, declined to visit patients with the disease or took elaborate prophylactic

---

below, Chapter Five), although this may be due to a variety of factors extrinsic to medical fees.

[107] Alberti, *Libri della famiglia*, 76. The pull toward *scioperato* status and toward the life of letters was obvious even among wealthy doctors. M° Giovanni Chellini was an example of the former; in his *catasto* declaration of 1451 he noted, "I earn nothing from my profession except the good will of the citizens" (Catasto-715/I, fol. 293r). An example of the latter was M° Paolo Toscanelli, who treated only friends and spent the rest of his time on philosophy, astronomy, math, and letters; see Vespasiano da Bisticci, *Vite*, 2:75. (For more information on the cultural activities of Florentine doctors and their families see Chapter Six.) A more typical case of a doctor's son living off his patrimony is Francesco di m° Francesco di Ridolfo: Catasto-699, fol. 553.

[108] Examples of émigré Florentine doctors include M° Giovanni di ser Francesco Paci dall'Arena, teaching in Padua ca. 1400 (Gloria, 1:432-33), and M° Niccolò di ser Niccolò Leonardi, living in Venice in the 1420s (PR-116, fols. 52-54). I have found only a handful of such cases.

measures against it.[109] Those doctors who did remain in the plague-stricken cities were explicit about the danger and sacrifice it involved. Maestro Iacopo di Coluccino da Lucca, for example, left a vivid account of his practice during the epidemic of 1373. Attending patient after patient at great personal risk, many of them relatives or close friends, he was rewarded by seeing them die one by one under his care. "When Filippa had the plague," he wrote, "I cared for her with the greatest devotion, constantly, both day and night, six or eight times a day. She died of the worst kind of plague, and the most contagious: that involving spitting blood. This went on for four entire days. I would never have treated her for money, but for love alone."[110]

The frustations of Maestro Iacopo and other plague doctors were lost on their clients. As we have seen, the image of the profession also suffered, as the population at large began to view doctors as ignorant and powerless in the face of the disease, and grasping and unscrupulous in their willingness to demand fees for services unrendered. It is not hard to understand why Florentines, in such conditions, were attracted by other occupations. To many citizens a medical career must have appeared tantamount to suicide; if in addition medical theory was vacuous and medical practice futile, at least with respect to the disease which killed more Florentines than any other, the flight from medicine seems only reasonable. Young men in a large city would have had many alternatives to entering the medical profession.

Using our information concerning the geographical origins of Florentine doctors, then, we can take another, more analytical look at the significant decline in the size of the medical profession described in the beginning of this chapter. This decline masks two contrary trends. On the one hand, fewer and fewer sons and daughters of Florentine families were choosing medicine as a career. On the other, more and more doctors were deciding to immigrate to Florence, first from the countryside and district and then from increasingly far away. These immigrants filled the vacuum to a certain extent, but they could not fully compensate for the wholesale defection of Florentine citizens—both the scions of old city families and the sons of naturalized immigrants—from the medical profession. Nonetheless, Florence, unlike many

---

[109] See Tommaso Del Garbo's special advice to doctors in *Consiglio contro a pistolenza*, 22-23; also Chiappelli, "Studi," 799-800, and Amundsen, "Medical Deontology."

[110] ASL: Ospedale di San Luca-180, fol. 1: "Filippa quando moriò, medicaila con grandissima sollicitudine di dì e di notte, tutto il più tempo, e sei e viii volte il dì. Moriò dello pigiore modo di pestilentia che sia, e quello male che è più contagioso, cioè dello sputo del sangue, et questo fu iiii dì continui, chè per denari no'll'arei medicata se non fusse per amore."

of its smaller subject towns, continued to find itself relatively well supplied with medical practitioners of all levels—physicians, surgeons, and
empirics. Perhaps because of the high degree of specialization among
these different groups, conflict was at a minimum, at least between
groups. In a city as important and wealthy as Florence the market for
medical services was large enough, and the overlap of skills small enough,
to ensure that the established medical profession—in the form of the
branch of doctors in the Guild of Doctors, Apothecaries, and Grocers—could accommodate practitioners with a wide variety of education and skills. In many ways, therefore, the market for medical services is the key to the shape and vitality of the Florentine profession.

III

The Medical Marketplace

THE LATE medieval Italian cities, as is well known, were central in the development of capitalist forms of economic organization. This does not mean, however, that the economy of a large and prosperous town like Florence functioned as a free and impersonal market of goods and services. It is better visualized as a cluster of marketplaces—like Florence's many *piazze*, dominated by their churches and lined with shops and houses, where the inhabitants came together not only to buy and sell but also to make contacts, close deals, exchange news and gossip, and in general to see and be seen. In other words, Florentine economic life was organized by many concerns that we would identify as noneconomic, including social and political ties of patronage, friendship, and kinship, as well as more abstract ideas of honor, loyalty, and religious obligation.[1]

This environment shaped the economic life of Florentine doctors. They practiced in a marketplace defined largely in personal and social terms. This meant, for example, that even a physician of citywide repute would treat the humbler inhabitants of his own neighborhood in addition to his more far-flung patrician clientele. It also meant that doctors welcomed salaried positions and actively sought long-term contracts which guaranteed not only a stable income but also a continuing personal relationship with an employer. Furthermore, the market for medical services in Florence was dominated to a large extent by collectivities. The doctor did not approach his clients as an autonomous practitioner but as a member of a guild and, in the case of the physician, as the associate of an apothecary. His clients were often not individual citizens or even their families but corporations and institutions: a confraternity, a hospital, the state.[2] Finally, a doctor usually

[1] See the discussion of economic and social relations in Weissman, *Ritual Brotherhood*, chap. 2, esp. 35-41, and, on the importance of the *piazza*, 9.

[2] Martines emphasizes the importance of corporate clients for lawyers in his *Lawyers*, 97-104.

governed his practice by more than simply economic considerations; recall, for example, the personal loyalty which kept Maestro Iacopo da Lucca at the side of his patients during the plague. Doctors were also moved by Christian ideas of charity and penance to offer free medical care to the poor or to contract themselves to hospitals and other religious institutions at salaries much lower than those they could have commanded from other clients. This is not to idealize the Florentine medical practitioner, who could be, ample evidence shows, as ambitious, competitive, and greedy as the next man; it is merely to say that he lived and worked in a society where economic relations could not be easily separated from other basic aspects of Florentine culture.

For all these reasons, the medical marketplace in this period, like the profession itself, was larger and more complex than is usually portrayed. Doctors were hired for a wide variety of purposes by a myriad of private and institutional clients. On closer examination it is possible to identify three distinct sectors of medical practice: public, ecclesiastical, and private. In the first, the state commissioned doctors to perform services which ranged from emergency care for tortured criminals to highly paid consulting in forensic pathology and public health. In the second, religious institutions—primarily hospitals, monasteries, convents, and confraternities—employed doctors to attend to their members or those in their care. Even the third sector, private practice, was far more varied than standard histories indicate. The economic relationship between a bone doctor and an artisan who came to his shop with a fractured arm had little in common with that between a physician and the aristocratic patron he attended daily.

As we explore each of these sectors of medical practice, we must free ourselves from anachronistic assumptions about their structure and operation, and about who did or did not have access to professional medical services. Historians and sociologists of medicine have frequently claimed that only the urban patriciate, a very small fraction of the population of preindustrial Europe, was served by the organized profession, while the inhabitants of the countryside and the middle and lower orders of the cities fended for themselves or went to lay healers. Cipolla has challenged this view for later Renaissance Italy, and it seems equally misguided for the fourteenth and fifteenth centuries.[3] The tradition of public, ecclesiastical, and lay patronage of professional medicine was well established in Italy by 1348. The com-

---

[3] Cipolla, *Public Health*, 80-85. For the earlier view see for example Freidson, *Profession of Medicine*, 12, and Bullough, "Population and Medicine," 63.

ing of plague made great demands on this system but ultimately served only to root it more deeply in Florentine society.

THE STATE AS CLIENT

It was the public sector of the medical marketplace which embraced the most varied kinds of professional services. The Florentine government's earliest concern had been to provide medical care for high officials and the military. The first known reference to this practice dates from the twelfth century, when the city hired a doctor to attend consuls traveling on public business; soon thereafter it became common practice in Italy to send doctors into the field to look after the army.[4] By the early fourteenth century the commune's sense of responsibility had widened to include the lay and civilian population, particularly the poor, who lacked the resources to hire their own doctors. From this time on the city paid doctors of all sorts not only to treat particular classes of citizens but also to teach both inside and outside the university, as well as to provide expert medical opinions on matters ranging from natural resources to cause of death.[5]

The first extended description of doctors in the hire of the Florentine commune relates to military medicine and appears in the *Book of Montaperti*, an official contemporary account of the 1260 campaign between Florence and Siena. According to this document, the Florentine army was composed of a large number of citizens in addition to an unspecified number of professional soldiers, *contadini*, and allies. Among the citizens were several doctors, at least one of whom performed some medical services in the field.[6] The principal responsibility for such things, however, fell on a physician, Maestro Ruggiero di messer Beni da Obriaco, and two surgeons, Messer Gianni and one Berardo—all three chosen by the Florentine captains and "commissioned in the army on behalf of the commune to treat the wounded

[4] Ciasca, *L'arte*, 298. The practice of hiring army doctors was current in Bologna by 1220, in Siena by 1230, and in Cremona by 1240, as noted in Sarti and Fattorini, *De claris archigymnasii*, 2:214-15; Casarini, *Medicina militare*, 125-26; and Nutton, "City Physician," 25-27. Thus Fielding Garrison is mistaken in awarding priority to the Swiss in 1339; cf. his *Military Medicine*, 100.

[5] For brief surveys of this subject see Nutton, "City Physician," 26-34, and Ciasca, *L'arte*, 298-308.

[6] *Libro di Montaperti*, 309, 320; a wounded knight from the *sesto* of San Pancrazio was excused from fighting on the oath of a doctor named Apostolo, who appears among the foot soldiers supplied by the same *sesto*. See in general Cappellini, "Medici fiorentini."

and, in the case of Maestro Ruggiero, to attend those afflicted by other illness." One month after the first mention of their elections, payment was authorized to all three: £3 to Maestro Ruggiero and s. 40 to each surgeon.[7] Although the *Book of Montaperti* mentions only doctors who attended the army in the field, it is clear that the commune also provided for the medical care of its soldiers in other ways. The sick and wounded were often transported to the nearest town for treatment or carried home to their native city. In that case they were cared for by local practitioners; the government then either reimbursed the soldiers for their expenses or paid the doctors directly.[8]

Military doctors salaried by the commune were expected to see to all the medical needs of the army. The physicians, like Maestro Ruggiero, were charged with treating the various diseases ("fever and other illness," as it said in his commission) which could reach epidemic proportions in the camps.[9] The surgeons dealt with wounds and broken bones suffered by the combatants; this branch of medicine was highly developed in late medieval Italy, and all the standard surgical texts of the period discussed the techniques of treating wounds from swords, lances, and arrows in various parts of the body.[10]

As we have seen in the previous chapter, many of the surgeons most skilled in this kind of work (notably bone doctors and wound doctors) were in fact empirics. Thus it is not surprising to find that most of the army doctors hired by the commune in the years after the Black Death appear in guild and communal records as such. For example, there are a number of entries of payment to empirical doctors hired to accompany the Florentine army during the war with Pisa in the early 1360s. In September 1360 the legislative councils of the city authorized payment of up to £96 s. 5 to "Maestro Andrea di Bartolo, surgeon, for the thirty-five days which he spent with the army of the Florentine commune in the region of the Val di Nievole, on the order of the priors and the standard-bearer of justice of the people and the commune of Florence." A month later the communal treasurer registered

[7] Ibid., 53, 85. On money and salaries in Florence see Appendix I.

[8] This procedure was formalized in the statutes of Siena from the second half of the thirteenth century, although it was common practice earlier; see Garosi, "Organizzazione sanitaria," 233-34.

[9] *Libro di Montaperti*, 75. Garrison has referred to the epidemics which racked the French army in the fourteenth century during the Hundred Years' War; see his *Military Medicine*, 89. The principal diseases seem to have been plague, fevers like typhus and malaria, and dysentery.

[10] Note that although artillery was being used in battle by the earlier fourteenth century, no specific discussion of gunshot wounds appears until the second half of the fifteenth century; see Singer, "Early Treatment," esp. 452-58.

a further payment of £17 s. 10 to Maestro Andrea, who had been equipped by the government with a horse and sent to the "army of Monte Vinagni . . . to treat the wounded."[11] The war continued for several years, and with it sporadic references to military doctors. In June 1363 Maestro Stefano dell'Ossa, a Florentine resident and bone doctor, as his name implies, was paid fl. 7 for the seven days he "stayed with the army to treat the sick." The commune also made use of local practitioners. In particular it contracted with Maestro Michele di Coluccino, a wound doctor from the town of Barga, north of Lucca, to look after the Florentine wounded in that area; his contract ran for four months from May 1363, and his salary was fixed at £10 per month.[12]

The most striking thing about these entries is the size of the payments. They are typical of the public sector in medical practice, which was in general well remunerated. The monthly salary of Maestro Michele, who presumably remained in Barga and treated the injured as they were brought to him, was the same as that normally paid to the Florentine communal poor-doctors—respectable but not exorbitant. Maestro Andrea and Maestro Stefano, however, were compensated for the danger and inconvenience of their work in the field as well as for their medical services; the former received £2 s. 15 per diem, and the latter a princely fl. 1—a sum which, if calculated on a yearly basis, would have put him among the highest-salaried government officials.

It is also worth noting that Maestro Andrea and Maestro Stefano were both on the communal payroll back in Florence, the first as the prison doctor and the second as a doctor to the poor, so that the remuneration for their military services was added to their regular salaries. Maestro Andrea had at one time treated prisoners in the hospital of the communal prison (the Stinche) out of charity. In 1350 the legislative councils officially named him "doctor of the poor prisoners and of those who have a member amputated or removed at the Porta della Giustizia" (the public execution site outside the city's eastern gate) and assigned him a yearly salary of £50.[13] Maestro Andrea's

---

[11] PR-48, fol. 42r: "Magistro Andree Bartholi medico cerusico pro trigintacinque diebus quibus mandato offitii dominorum priorum artium et vexilliferi iustitie populi et comunis Florentie stetisse in exercitu comunis Florentie misso ad partes Valli Nebule." CCCU-147, fol. 132r: "in exercitu Monte Vinagni . . . ad medendum vulneratos."

[12] CCCU-161, fol. 29r; CCCU-165, fol. [7r].

[13] PR-38, fol. 57v: "medicus pauperum captivorum ac etiam illorum quibus amputatum seu extractum fuerit aut erit ad Iustitiam aliquod membrum. Et quidem Magister Andreas quando aliquod membrum incideretur vel extraretur alicui ad ipsam Iustitiam teneatur et debeat ire et esse ad curandum et medicandum illos. . . ." The previous

duties were threefold. He treated prisoners too poor to afford the services of a private doctor. He provided emergency care to any prisoner who had been sentenced to lose a "member"—the Florentine statutes specified crimes for which the penalty was an eye, foot or hand, or castration—at the hands of an executioner. And although his commission does not specifically mention it, we can assume by analogy with other Italian cities that the third of his principal tasks was to certify the suitability of prisoners for torture and to treat them afterward.[14] Maestro Andrea served the prison for many years until his exile in September 1378, in the aftermath of the revolt of the Ciompi. His successors are duly recorded in the treasury records and communal provisions relating to the Stinche.[15] Like the military doctors, who were often drawn from their ranks, these prison doctors were in general surgeons and empirics. They too received stipends considerably higher than those offered by most regular hospitals, stipends which they could augment by private practice. The same was true of the third type of doctor hired by the Florentine state: the communal doctor.

By the mid-fourteenth century the communal doctor (*medico condotto*) had become a standard institution in many Italian cities and towns as well as in some areas of the countryside, where various local authorities would salary one or more doctors to treat the local population. Such measures had two goals: the first was to ensure that adequate medical services were available to those who could afford them; the second was to subsidize the medical care of the nonhospitalized poor. Thus many communal doctors were hired on the stipulation that they remain in the city, provide free treatment for the poor, and charge wealthier patients according to a moderate scale of fees.[16] Smaller towns,

---

appointee, in 1347, had been Filippo di ser Bindo, who died shortly after; see BNF: Magl. XXVI, 116, fol. 290r.

[14] This was the case, for example, in Venice and Milan (Cecchetti, *Medicina in Venezia*, 41-44) as well as in Siena (Garosi, *Siena*, 301). The crimes for which torture was permitted included night thefts, arson, rape of an "honest woman," and assault and homicide; see statute of the podestà of 1325, III, 66, in Caggese, *Statuti*, 2:227-28.

[15] In 1378 M° Andrea was replaced by M° Niccolò di Valore, who had matriculated as a "barber or doctor" in 1372 but who appears in later documents as a surgeon (PR-67, fols. 45v-46r), and later by M° Bartolo di Chele, who was doctor of the Stinche at his death in 1390 (Prestanze-1264, fol. 169r). In 1402 the stipend of the prison doctor was raised to £60 (PR-91, fol. 180v), and in 1413—in favor of the incumbent, M° Nello di Berto—to fl. 3 per month (PR-102, fols. 80v-81v). In 1415 the position of doctor of the Stinche was incorporated into the communal statute. The next appointee was M° Piero di Feo da Arencio di Mugello, in 1416 (PR-106, fol. 181r).

[16] Some towns specified an elaborate sliding scale based on how far away the patient lived, how poor he was, and long his illness lasted. See Battistini, *Medici in Volterra*, 24-26, and Chiappelli, *Medici e chirurghi pistoiesi*, 11-12. On the institution of the *medico*

like Pescia or Volterra, required only a single *medico condotto*, while the most populous cities might support a large staff of doctors. In 1324, for example, Venice, with a population of close to a hundred thousand, had thirty-one doctors on the government payroll—thirteen physicians and eighteen surgeons. In towns with no scarcity of local doctors—particularly those like Parma, Pisa, Como, Urbino, or Naples, where free treatment of the poor was required of all practitioners, or at least of those with tax exemptions—the presence of a communal doctor was less urgent, and *medici condotti* appear only sporadically in local records; a town like Lucca, on the other hand, with few or no doctors of its own, might salary two or three.[17] Under special circumstances towns would hire doctors to meet a specific, temporary need; thus Volterra voted a special subsidy for a barber and a surgeon during the plague of 1467.[18]

Communal doctors were usually foreigners. A number of them, especially physicians, were at the top of their profession. Some doctors served a single town for the rest of their lives, while others moved from place to place on a series of one- or two-year contracts. In order to attract competent practitioners, given the high level of demand for medical services of this sort, towns offered yearly salaries which ranged as high as fl. 200 and sometimes included sweeteners like free lodging, the use of a horse, attendants, citizenship, or a tax exemption.[19]

Florence found itself in a peculiar position with regard to communal doctors. Because, as we saw in the previous chapter, the city had a plethora of medical practitioners in the later fourteenth century, the commune was concerned less with the general problem of attracting doctors than with the particular problem of providing medical treatment for the poor, in accordance with the ethic of charity which characterized the private and public spirituality of the period. The poor-doctors hired by the Florentine government tended to be surgical specialists, usually bone doctors, presumably because dislocations and fractures were both common and easy to treat. There are records of a communal bone doctor in Florence as early as 1336, when Maestro

---

condotto see Cipolla, *Public Health*, 88-91; Nutton, "City Physician," 28-34; and Palmer, "Physicians and the State," 47-49.

[17] Even after 1348 the number of communal doctors in Venice averaged about eighteen; Cecchetti, *Medicina in Venezia*, 22, 67-73. On Pisa and Lucca see Brugaro, "Contributo," 223; on Como, Naples, and Urbino, Chiappelli, "Studi," 629; on Parma, Nutton, "City Physician," n. 172.

[18] Battistini, *Medici in Volterra*, 27-28.

[19] See, for example, Battistini, *Medici in Volterra*, 24-26; Chiappelli, *Medici e chirurghi pistoiesi*, 11-12; and Brugaro, "Contributo," 233.

Iacopo da Roma, "commonly called 'dell'Ossa,' " was appointed by the commune to "attend and treat the people of the city and countryside of Florence, . . . particularly the needy and poor, without receiving any fee from them." For these services he was to receive £5 a month and—"considering that Maestro Iacopo is often required to go to treat the said needy and poor in the countryside and district of Florence and that he cannot conveniently go to them on foot"—the use of a horse owned by the commune and an additional £5 a month to keep it.[20] (This is not to imply that the commune put an equal value on doctor and horse; Maestro Iacopo also had a private practice.)

In 1344 Maestro Iacopo's salary was raised to £10 a month, and it was specified that he "be understood to be the doctor of the commune of Florence . . . with the immunities and privileges contained in the statute of the commune under the rubric 'On the immunity of doctors.' " The rubric in question appears in the Statute of the Captain from 1355 and exempted bone doctors hired by the commune to treat the poor from all taxes and forced loans.[21] Maestro Iacopo died during the plague of 1348 and was succeeded in the following decades by his three sons, Maestro Niccolò, Maestro Giovanni, and finally Maestro Stefano, who had previously served as an army doctor in the war against Pisa. Maestro Stefano died in 1374, and no more payments to communal bone doctors were recorded after that time.[22]

Besides its bone doctors, Florence supported two other poor-doctors in the decades after 1348, both surgical specialists. The first, Maestro Beltrame di maestro Neri da Cortona, an eye doctor, was granted citizenship in 1354 and hired on a series of two-year contracts between that year and 1362 to "treat all the infirm of the city, countryside, or

[20] PR-27, fol. 98r: "Magister Jacobus natus dudum de civitate romana, qui Magister dell'ossa vulgariter appellatur, fuit electus pro comuni Florentie in officium ad medicandum et curandum homines et personas civitatis et comitatus Florentie cum requisitus fuerit, et precipue impotentes et pauperes absque aliquo salario ab ipsis pauperibus et impotentibus percipiendo. . . . Considerantes quod Magister Jacobus sepe sepius requiritur ad eundum ad curandum in comitatu et districtu Florentie dictos impotentes et pauperes, et quod ad eos commode ire non possit pedes, etc." Mº Iacopo is also mentioned in a provision from 1326, in which he is described as "bone doctor and ambassador," but no specific mention is made of any public medical duties (PR-23, fol. 12v).

[21] PR-32, fol. 105r: "Magister Jacobus sit et esse debeat et intelligatur medicus comunis Florentie ad predicta faciendum cum immunitatibus, benefficio et privillegio contentis in statutis comunis Florentie positis sub rubrica De immunitate medicorum." Cf. statute of the captain of the people of 1355, IV, 74 (Statuti-11, fol. 146v). This rubric does not appear in the statute of the captain of the people of 1325 and must have been added between then and 1336.

[22] PR-36, fol. 30r; PR-52, fol. 138r. On the date of Mº Stefano's death see SMN-60, fols. 336r-338v.

district of Florence who are suffering any eye disease, without charge if they are poor, and if not, for a reasonable fee."[23] By 1359 his annual salary was a respectable fl. 50. The second, Maestro Gregorio da Pisa, was a surgeon "expert in the treatment of eyes, hernias, and boils, and in the care of fractures and dislocated bones." Noting that he was an exile, a man of good condition, and that he had been treating the poor free already, the commune hired him for a year in 1361, at £70, to continue his good work.[24]

By 1375, however, only one poor-doctor appeared on the payroll, and after 1380 there was none. Furthermore, the rubric concerning the immunities of bone doctors was dropped in the communal statutes of 1415, although the city did, as in the cases of Maestro Niccolino da Pavia and Maestro Antonio and Maestro Francesco di Giovanni da Norcia, offer individual tax exemptions to surgical practitioners in specialized areas. Other large Italian cities were moving away from subsidizing medical care for the poor in this period, but Florence seems to have done so earlier and more completely than most.[25] This change reflected in part the city's continuing fiscal crisis in the later fourteenth and early fifteenth centuries, which also made the university's life precarious, and it may also be that the revolt of the Ciompi in 1378 had taken the edge off the government's preoccupation with the plight of the poor. The main cause, however, was the great expansion in the Florentine medical profession in the last decades of the fourteenth century. The city was now well supplied, if not oversupplied, with doctors of all sorts, many of whom regularly treated the poor for free or worked at least part-time in Florence's numerous hospitals.[26] If the Church and the doctors themselves were willing to accept responsibility for the care of the city's poorer citizens, the commune saw no reason to spend scarce public moneys for the same service. Thus it was only in the mid-fifteenth century that the Florentine councils, worried

[23] PR-41, fol. 38r; PR-48, fols. 136v, 212r; PR-47, fol. 33r: "Ipse quoque Magister Beltramus teneatur omnes infirmos de civitate, comitatu vel districtu Florentie qui paterentur passionem aliquam oculorum medicare absque aliquo salario vel mercede si pauperes essent, et aliquos cum salario competenti." Mᵒ Beltrame had previously been employed for ten years as a communal surgeon in Perugia.

[24] PR-48, fol. 149v: "quod civitas florentina valentibus viris cirusicis indiget, maxime expertis in curis oculorum, crepatorum, antracis sive malarum bullarum, et in curis restaurationis ossium fractorum et dislocatorum. . . ." Mᵒ Gregorio was paid in April 1362; see CCCU-155, fol. 401v.

[25] See Nutton, "City Physician," 33-34; Palmer, "Physicians and the State," 47-48.

[26] The expansion in the number and size of Florence's hospitals is described below, in the next section. Doctors known to have treated the poor out of charity include Mᵒ Andrea di Bartolo and Mᵒ Gregorio da Pisa; see above, notes 13 and 24.

by the declining number of doctors in the city, appropriated an attractive fl. 225 for the salary of Maestro Giovanni di maestro Luca da Camerino, a physician and reader at the *studio*, in hopes of persuading him not only to continue his lectures in medicine but also to establish a permanent practice in Florence. The commune's renewed concern for public health was reflected even more clearly in an act passed during the epidemic year of 1448 which provided for the construction of a public hospital outside the walls of the city, where the sick could be isolated in times of plague. It was to be staffed by four doctors, four barbers, and sixty servants.[27]

It was not only doctors for the poor who were hired by the commune; the Florentine government on occasion also subsidized treatment for the rich. A rather special case of this involved the practice of sending illustrious physicians to treat allies or potential allies of the Florentine state. In 1431, for example, the newly elected Pope Eugenius IV fell ill and poison was suspected. Florence, anxious to cement her relations with the Papal See, decided to offer the services of one of her most respected physicians. According to an administrative memo from that year, "Maestro Lorenzo d'Agnolo da Prato was chosen to treat the pope, and fl. 200 were appropriated for a month's salary. He left Florence on 19 October 1431 and returned on 24 November 1431. At fl. 6⅔ per day, his fee amounts to fl. 240." Three years before, Maestro Lorenzo had been sent on a similar mission to assist Francesco Carmagnola, a Florentine ally against the Visconti, at the baths of Petriolo and San Filippo, near Siena.[28]

Besides treating special classes of patients, notably soldiers, prisoners, the poor, and diplomatic friends or allies, doctors also served the city as teachers and consultants. It is not known when and in what form the first official classes in medicine were given in Florence. By the mid-thirteenth century aspiring doctors could study medicine in a number of other Tuscan cities—at the cathedral school in Siena, at the town school in Arezzo, and with private teachers in Pisa.[29] In Florence, however, no evidence for the public teaching of medicine appears before 1320, when the city voted to hire the physician Maestro Bartolomeo da Varignana "to teach the art of *physica* to those wishing

[27] On Mᵒ Luca, PR-137, fol. 173r-v; there is no indication that he was invited to serve specifically as a poor-doctor. On the communal plague hospital of San Bastiano, which was not built until the late 1470s, Coturri, "Più antichi provvedimenti."

[28] Ricordanze dei Dieci di Balìa (15.vi.1431): "Maestro Lorenzo d'Agnolo da Prato fu eletto per medicare el papa, e diliberorògli fiorini 200 per uno mese. Partì di Firenze il dì 19 d'ottobre 1431; tornò a dì 24 di novembre 1431. Monta il suo servito a fiorini 6⅔ il dì, fiorini 240." (Quoted in Guasti, *Intorno alla vita*, 6.)

[29] See Coturri, "Vi furono," 341-44.

to learn and to practice that art in the city and the countryside."[30] Maestro Bartolomeo does not seem to have remained at his post very long, if indeed he taught in Florence at all; the next word on the subject is from 1348, when the commune, anxious to repopulate the city after the devastations of the plague, voted to establish a "permanent university (*studium generale*) in civil and canon law, medicine, philosophy, and the other disciplines," and to appropriate up to fl. 2,500 from state revenues to support it.[31] Among other professors, the city chose as its first regular lecturer on *physica* Maestro Tommaso Del Garbo, a doctor of Florentine origin who had been teaching at Perugia and Bologna. The University of Florence enjoyed a somewhat precarious existence for the next century and a quarter, but except for periodic vacations because of plague or lack of funds, it operated in Florence until transferred to Pisa in 1472.[32]

In its most prosperous period the university supported a teaching staff in medicine of five or six, including full-time professors and occasional lecturers in *theorica*, surgery, and *practica*. Their salaries, as was customary, depended on their fields, experience, and reputations. The highest-paid readers were those who gave the ordinary lectures in theory; the most famous, like Maestro Ugo Benzi da Siena, received salaries of up to fl. 600, although the usual sum was between a third and half that amount. Readers in lesser fields, like surgery, as well as "concurrent" or supplementary lecturers, were rarely paid more than fl. 50.[33] Most of the city's formal instruction in medicine took place in its university, but there is evidence that the state supported occasional medical lecturers while the *studio* was suspended. The most notable case was that of Maestro Lodovico di Bartolo da Gubbio, who had been lecturing on surgery since 1364. When the university closed in 1370 for financial reasons, the city governors, feeling that a supply of surgeons was essential to Florence's public health and well-being, hired Maestro Lodovico to teach surgery, first *in studio* and then, from 1376 to 1380, *in civitate*.[34]

[30] Alessandro Gherardi, *Statuti*, 278. It is unclear that Mᵒ Bartolomeo actually took up this position; see Münster, "Alcuni episodi." The town had already hired Mᵒ Guicciardo da Bologna several months earlier to teach grammar, and presumably logic and philosophy. He was paid for teaching those subjects at least through 1323; Alessandro Gherardi, *Statuti*, 277-79.

[31] Alessandro Gherardi, *Statuti*, 113-14.

[32] For a brief summary of the early history of the *studio* see Brucker, "Florence and Its University. On Tommaso Del Garbo see Chapter Six, below.

[33] On the teaching staff of the university and their salaries in this period see Park, "Readers." For many of these years the higher-paying appointments were closed to Florentine citizens.

[34] Ibid., 264-67.

Finally, the Florentine state hired doctors as experts—consultants whose specialized knowledge was required for decisions having to do with medicine and related fields. The most common context was judicial; throughout northern Italy the courts admitted medical testimony in a wide range of civil and criminal cases. In Venice, doctors were required to report to the authorities all wounds of suspicious origin and any cases of unusual or unexplained death.[35] In Florence, however, as in many other cities, doctors examined victims of assault or homicide only at the request of the podestà and his magistrates and in cooperation with the Guild of Doctors, Apothecaries, and Grocers, as specified in both its statute of 1349 and an amendment of 1351. According to the latter, "it often happens that the advice, judgment, and deliberation of doctors and experienced medical practitioners is needed in the courts of the rectors of the city of Florence, on the occasion of cases prosecuted every day against assailants and people who have seriously wounded others, injuring their faces, harming their members, and the like." The guild was to draw up a list of trustworthy city physicians and surgeons who could be called on to testify for a fee of up to fl. 2.[36] Among the issues they were expected to determine were the extent of injury (presumably to determine punishment or compensation); the cause of death; the number of assailants; and the number, nature, and location of minor, mortal, and postmortal wounds.[37] The guild was apparently justified in trying to supervise and control this process, given the opportunities for deception; in 1427, for example, Maestro Francesco di ser Conte Mini confessed to fraud in a case involving a head wound.[38]

Other kinds of cases required other kinds of medical judgments. Doctors were commonly called before courts of canon law to determine impotence and virginity where marriage or annulment was involved. Some decisions also concerned inheritances, as, for example, in a dispute over the will of a notary from Pistoia. Ser Francesco Camaggiori had died without issue in 1373, leaving his property to the

[35] See Ruggiero, "Cooperation," and Dall'Osso, *L'organizzazione medico-legale*, chap. 3. Also Amundsen and Ferngren, "Forensic Role."

[36] Amendment of 1351, IX (Ciasca, *Statuti*, 231-32). This represents the regularization of a practice already described in the statute of 1314, III, 58 (Ciasca, *Statuti*, 50); the main thrust of the amendment was to restrict this privilege to native Florentines and to exclude immigrant doctors attracted to the city in the aftermath of the plague.

[37] For a detailed discussion of the way this system worked in Bologna see Dall'Osso, *L'organizzazione medico-legale*, 18-38, including notarial records of doctors' testimony, and 75-77. The fifteenth-century Florentine physician Mº Antonio Benivieni recorded a typical case in his *De abditis*, tr. Singer, 206.

[38] Diplomatico-Camera fiscale-4.iv.1427.

Opera di San Iacopo (a pious foundation) in the event that his wife did not produce a posthumous heir. Three months later the widow declared she was pregnant. At the request of the Opera, a commission of two doctors and three midwives was appointed to examine her condition. (The commission tentatively announced her pregnancy real, but the woman was later caught when she tried to smuggle a poor woman's baby into her house for a staged "birth.")[39]

The state also hired doctors to give medical opinions in the area of public health. In June 1348, for example, when the plague epidemic was approaching its peak, the city paid doctors to perform autopsies on several victims, "in order to know more clearly the illnesses of the bodies."[40] In general, however, the medical profession played a relatively minor part in the Italian cities' attempts to defend themselves against the plague. Although the disease was immediately recognized as a new medical condition, the main line of defense adopted by public authorities, at least through the middle of the fifteenth century, was the conventional regulation of public hygiene—restrictions on the slaughter of animals in the city, the dumping of garbage, the emptying of privies, and so forth. Similar measures had appeared in the Florentine statutes at least as early as 1325.[41] The problem was treated as an administrative one, to be handled by the city's executive and other seasoned administrators; it is significant that the special Florentine commission of eight citizens formed in 1348 to implement plague measures included not one doctor.[42]

The commune, finally, used doctors as consultants on a host of miscellaneous issues touching on medical matters. In 1361, for example, when Florence annexed the territory of Volterra, it acquired a group of medicinal springs, called Bagno a Morbo, to the south of the city. The government saw the baths as a valuable asset, and soon afterward

[39] On this case see Chiappelli, "Singolare procedimento."

[40] They were paid on 30.vi.1348, as appears in the communal treasury records; see del Badia, *Miscellanea fiorentina*, 1:158: "per dare a' medici che spararono più corpi per potere più chiaramente conosciere le malattie de' corpi."

[41] During the worst of the first epidemic of plague special regulations were put into effect prohibiting the harboring of infected foreigners, the sale of clothing from the bodies of the dead, and similar actions; see Carabellese, *La peste del 1348*, esp. 41-66. A detailed list of sanitary ordinances from 1348 exists for Pistoia; see Chiappelli, "Ordinamenti sanitari." For the measures taken by Venice, which included a ban on foreigners entering the city (with the signal exception of merchants and ambassadors), see Brunetti, "Venezia durante la peste," 290-99, and Palmer, "Control of Plague," chaps. 1-2.

[42] PR-35, fols. 133v-34r. This was characteristic also of later commissions in Florence and elsewhere; it was not until well into the sixteenth century, for example, that a doctor served on the Venetian health board; see Palmer, "Control of Plague," 74-75.

sent one of the commune's most promising young doctors to the site to analyze the waters and to recommend how the area might best be developed. Maestro Ugolino da Montecatini visited the place some years later in the company of Salutati, the Florentine chancellor, and commented on the springs in his monograph *On Baths*: "These baths have been extremely well set up by the magnificent Signoria of Florence, following the advice and orders of the outstanding doctor Maestro Cristofano di Giorgio, a Florentine doctor and my dear colleague, who was delegated by the magnificent commune to refurbish them and who tried hard to make them famous."[43]

In the same way the commune also occasionally called on doctors to make judgments in areas related to medicine. One of the most common was astrology, which, although also practiced separately, was often taught as an ancillary discipline to *physica*. Usually the astrological opinions requested by the commune concerned auspicious times for engaging in some military operation, like the assault on Pisa in 1404, or for conferring the symbols of military authority (the rod, or *bastone*, and the banner) on the new captain-general of the Florentine army.[44] In 1453, for example, the Signoria, frightened by a recent earthquake, asked the Florentine physician Maestro Paolo di maestro Domenico Toscanelli to determine a propitious day to give the *bastone* to the newly elected commander, Sigismondo Malatesta. They relayed his reply to their officials in the field:

> We are writing to notify you that this morning when Maestro Paolo and others were informed of your commission to confer the *bastone* on the magnificent lord and knight Sigismondo, they reminded us that between now and the tenth of October there is no auspicious time to do it, for all the times are inauspicious. They encouraged us to delay the giving of the *bastone* until that time. We are content to do so. . . . We advise you that last night after the fifth hour there began most terrible and terrifying earthquakes, such as were never felt by any man, which destroyed many houses and buildings. This is the reason we were reminded of the evil disposition of the heavens that obtains at present and will continue to obtain for some days.[45]

[43] Ugolino da Montecatini, *De balneis*, 107. Cf. PR-84, fol. 100r; 85, fol. 104v. Bagno a Morbo became one of the favorite baths of the Medici in the later fifteenth century; Lorenzo rented it from the commune in 1477 and took over its administration in 1478. See Pieraccini, *Stirpe de' Medici*, 1:66-68.

[44] Casanova, "Astrologia."

[45] Riformagioni-Signori-Carteggio: Missive, Registri, I Cancelleria, no. 38, fol. 147v

Thus, between consulting on various matters of public health and security, teaching, and caring for groups with special claims on the commune's attentions like soldiers, prisoners, and the poor, there was a considerable public market for doctors' services in Florence. In general the state paid well; salaries were as high as or higher than the doctor would have received in normal private practice. This was not true of the other principal institutional clients in this period—the Church and the city's religious associations.

RELIGIOUS INSTITUTIONS AS CLIENTS

Florentine doctors in the employ of the ecclesiastical or pious foundations of the city viewed their services to those institutions at least partly as works of charity. Thus they were willing to treat patients at somewhat lower salaries than we find in either the public or the private sector. In other respects, however, such foundations acted like any other regular institutional client, contracting with individual doctors to provide specified medical services over a certain period of time (most often a year) for a fixed salary. The three most important kinds of religious corporations which hired doctors in late medieval and Renaissance Florence were convents or monasteries, hospitals, and confraternities.

Of the many monasteries and convents in the city of Florence at that time, virtually all the larger ones retained doctors to attend to the medical needs of their residents. There is ample evidence of this practice in the account books of the various religious houses and in their early fifteenth-century *catasto* declarations; the latter list doctors and their salaries among deductible obligations (*incarichi*), along with other regular staff: cooks, gardeners, factors, procurators, lawyers, and so forth.[46] Most of the medium-sized foundations (those with thirty to fifty residents) had one doctor, while the largest, like the Badia or the monastery of San Pier Maggiore, supported two or three. The duties of monastery doctors varied little from institution to institution. The diary of the abbot of the Badia in 1466 includes a typical job description: "We have hired Maestro Giovambatista, a former Jew, to treat our brothers in the Badia. . . . He must come at whatever hour and

---

(transcribed in ibid., 143). The letter was sent on September 29. On M° Paolo's interest and work in astrology and astronomy see below, Chapter six.

[46] Catasto-184, 185, 190, 194, 195. These volumes date from the late 1420s and 1430s. For evidence of similar practices in England see Hammond, "Westminster Abbey Infirmarers' Rolls" and "Physicians in Religious Houses."

time he is sent for to look after all the brothers and treat them for any and all illnesses—both in *physica* and in surgery. And we must give him for his services £40 a year, as was agreed by our prior; . . . he is to receive his salary at the beginning of each year."[47] In some cases it was specified that the doctor was also to treat the paid staff and dependents of the monastery, often for an additional fee.[48]

Maestro Giovambatista's salary of £40 (slightly less than fl. 10) was relatively high, as one would expect of an institution as large and rich as the Badia. The salaries paid by other monasteries and convents ranged from fl. 3 to fl. 10 a year, depending on their size. (It was also common for doctors to accept payment in kind, usually in grain or wax, or in the form of free rent.)[49] Thus a small convent like Santa Maria Maddalena, which housed twenty-two dependents, paid fl. 3 in 1429, while the convent of Santa Maria de' Servi (fifty residents) and the monastery of San Domenico (thirty-four) paid fl. 6, and the monastery of San Pier Maggiore fl. 10 to each of its two doctors.[50] These salaries were markedly lower than those of the full-time staff, and this suggests that the required services took only a fraction of the doctor's professional time. Because the lists of the foundations' employees include the names of the richest and most illustrious physicians in Florence, the fl. 5 or 6 in question can have been little more than a token payment.[51] Although this market was not particularly lucrative, it was large and—among the fifty-odd religious houses in the city—involved a good many

[47] CS-78, 261, fol. 135r: "abbiamo tolto a medicare li nostri frati della Badìa . . . Maestro Giovambatista che fu ebreo, . . . el quale debba venire a churare et medichare tutti li nostri frati d'ogni e qualunche male, così di morbo di fisicho e cerusicho, ed a qualunche hora e tempo si manderà per lui. Et noi li dobbiamo dare per sua faticha e provisione £ quaranta piccoli per ciaschuno anno, chome fu d'achordo col nostro priore, . . . e quali denari si li debbano dare in chapo di ciaschuno anno." M° Giovambatista may be the same converted Jew referred to by Vespasiano da Bisticci; see Chapter Two, note 88.

[48] Some employees had such a provision written into their contracts; see, for example, the documents relating to the Flemish singers associated with the monastery and church of Santissima Annunziata (CS-119, 49, fol. 33v).

[49] For an example of the latter see the *ricordanza* of M° Antonio Benivieni, in Notarile-B.1324, fol. 193r: "Facemo acordo le monache di sancto Nicholò ed io che loro mi donessino . . . l'abitazione d'una loro chamera [?] sopra el forno a lato a me, e . . . io l'avessi a medichare sanza altro salario, e questo per anni .v. a venire."

[50] For Santa Maria Maddalena, Catasto-185, fol. 502v; for comparison, note that the gardener was paid fl. 12. For Santa Maria de' Servi and San Domenico, Catasto-184, fol. 184r, and Catasto-194/II, fol. 673v. For San Pier Maggiore, Catasto-194/II, fol. 131r.

[51] This was especially true of the most important foundations. Thus the Badia had in its employ doctors like M° Lorenzo Sassoli da Prato, M° Tommaso di Baccio da Arezzo, and M° Simone di Cinozzo; see CS-78, 261, fol. 24r; CS-78, 77, passim.

doctors. The ecclesiastical sector assumes even greater importance in this period when we add to these institutions the more than thirty Florentine hospitals which took in pilgrims or travelers, the old, the sick, and the poor.[52]

The late Middle Ages saw an enormous growth in the number and size of hospitals and other charitable foundations in Tuscany and elsewhere in Italy. This growth corresponded to a significant change in spirituality, at least as reflected in foundations and bequests. (In the secular realm this change was manifest in the growing sense of social responsibility which prompted the commune to hire doctors for the poor in the years after 1300 and, especially, after 1348.) Using records of taxes levied on ecclesiastical institutions in Pistoia, Herlihy has found that at the end of the thirteenth century the richest religious institutions in the city were the corporation of cathedral canons, the bishopric of Pistoia, and three large Benedictine monasteries. By the early fifteenth century, however, the situation had changed dramatically: two hospitals and a foundation for charitable works had displaced the canons and all but one of the monasteries. This change, Herlihy argues, marks an important shift from an earlier form of piety—one emphasizing contemplation, retreat, or the ascetic veneration of God, and expressed in its highest form in the great monastic foundations of the Middle Ages—to a peculiarly late medieval and Renaissance form with a distinctly social emphasis on the exercise of charity. The new "civic" piety was embodied most perfectly in the charitable foundations and great hospitals of the period. One manifestation of this change in spiritual orientation was that by 1428 Pistoia, a modest town of 4,500 inhabitants, supported 200 hospital beds.[53]

Florence apparently experienced the same change. Beginning in the mid-thirteenth century the volume of lay bequests to pious foundations increased greatly; this increase was further accelerated by the advent of plague in 1348, as Matteo Villani testified in his *Chronicle*:

> In our city of Florence, during the year of the said plague, a surprising thing happened. People were dying, and the citizens of

---

[52] Using fourteenth-century wills, Saverio La Sorsa identified fifty-one Florentine convents and monasteries and thirty-four hospitals; see his *Compagnia di Or San Michele*, 172-74. By 1480, according to Cristoforo Landino, in his commentary on the *Divine Comedy*, there were seventy-four and thirty-six respectively; see his *Scritti*, 1:116. The most comprehensive account of Florentine hospitals in this period appears in Passerini, *Storia degli stabilimenti*.

[53] Herlihy, *Medieval and Renaissance Pistoia*, 241-58. See also Becker, "Aspects of Lay Piety," 177-81. Historians are not fully agreed on the importance of this trend, which requires further study.

Florence had faith in the organization and experience of the famous, good, and orderly charity which had long been administered and was being administered by the captains of the Company of the Madonna of Or San Michele. It was found that during the epidemic the citizens of Florence had willed . . . more than fl. 350,000 to be distributed to the poor by the captains of the company. When people saw themselves and their children and relatives dying, they made their wills. If they had living heirs they left their possessions to those heirs, and if the heirs died they wished to make the company their heir. . . . In the same way, more than fl. 25,000 in property and possessions was left to a new company called the Company of the Misericordia, which distributed it poorly through the negligence of its captains, and fl. 25,000 to the hospital of Santa Maria Nuova. The bequests to the hospital were well made, because the hospital gives much alms and is always full of sick men and women, who are cared for and treated with great diligence and abundance of food and medicines, and is administered by men and women of holy life.[54]

Perhaps even more important than the increase in the number and size of hospitals during this period was the change in their character. In the early Middle Ages the hospital had been above all a rural phenomenon; the typical "hospital" was in fact a simple hospice set up outside the city, often associated with a monastic foundation, to offer food and lodging to pilgrims and travelers. With the growth of cities in the later medieval period the spectrum of hospitals' activities widened, as urban institutions were founded to serve the old, the poor, and special occupational groups as well as those far from home. The next step in this evolution came in the second half of the thirteenth century, with the foundation of the first large city hospitals established specifically to serve the sick poor. Many other kinds continued to exist and flourish, but it is in the two centuries after 1300 that we see the emergence to preeminence of hospitals dedicated largely or exclusively to caring for the sick, and thus of hospitals with a large and growing demand for medical services.[55]

[54] Matteo Villani, *Cronica*, I, 7; 1:15-16.

[55] The only previous hospitals dedicated specifically to helping the sick were the leprosaria, like Florence's Ospedale di San Iacopo a Sant'Eusebio, probably founded in the twelfth century. In the fifteenth century its inmates were served by a nurse (*infermiere*), but there is no indication of any attached doctor (Catasto-190, fol. 32r). This was probably typical of the administration of such institutions, which were established largely to isolate lepers rather than to treat them. For contemporary English developments see Bullough, "Medical Care in English Hospitals"; for France, Wickersheimer, "Médecins et chirurgiens."

The first hospital of this kind in Florence, and indeed the city's largest hospital by the mid-fourteenth century, was the hospital of Santa Maria Nuova mentioned by Villani. Founded in the 1280s by the merchant Folco Portinari, it was supplemented in 1345 by the hospital of San Paolo, which had been established by Franciscan tertiaries in the thirteenth century to serve pilgrims and the homeless but which had shifted its attention to the sick by the middle of the fourteenth century. A similar foundation, the hospital of San Giovanni Batista—often called "di Bonifazio" after its founder and patron Bonifazio Lupi, an immigrant mercenary captain from Parma—was established in 1377; It was followed eight years later by the hospital of San Matteo (or "di Lemmo"), founded by Guglielmo Balducci, a banker from Montecatini, in atonement for usurious practices.[56] By the first half of the fifteenth century these four hospitals, all dedicated to the sick poor, accommodated close to four hundred beds, and the total number of beds in Florentine hospitals would have been more than double that, if we add the facilities of the other thirty hospitals in the city.[57] For the most part these hospitals housed travelers or the indigent; more prosperous citizens were cared for at home.

By 1428, then, there were some thirty-five hospitals in Florence serving various needy groups: foundlings (for example, Santa Maria della Scala and the much smaller San Gallo); the poor (many examples, including the four main hospitals mentioned above and other smaller foundations, like San Bartolomeo); specific occupational groups (for example, Sant'Onofrio, for old or poor dyers, or the Spedale de' Preti, for poor priests); sufferers from specific diseases (San Iacopo a Sant'Eusebio for lepers, Sant'Antonio for those with St. Anthony's fire); and pilgrims (for example, San Giuliano). These institutions were supported by funds from a wide range of sources, including the commune, guilds or other occupational associations, religious orders, lay religious companies, chivalric orders, and, above all, private bequests from Florentines of all classes and conditions.[58]

[56] Passerini, *Storia degli stabilimenti*, 149-60, 169-70, 216-84; Mannelli, "Lo spedale di San Paolo," 241-43; Coturri, "L'ospedale 'di Bonifazio' "; Mannelli, "Istituzione," 175-76; Mannelli, "L'ospedale di San Matteo."

[57] The hospital of Lemmo had 60 beds in 1410 and that of San Paolo 34 in 1404 (Passerini, *Storia degli stabilimenti*, 152, 169-70). Santa Maria Nuova had between 200 and 250 in 1400, according to Pampaloni, *Lo spedale di Santa Maria Nuova*, 12, while the hospital of Messer Bonifazio accomodated 31 invalids in 1428. Using the records in Catasto-184, 185, and 190 for the other hospitals, we can arrive at an average figure of roughly 16 beds per hospital in the late 1420s. On these other foundations see Passerini, *Storia degli stabilimenti*, passim, and Mannelli, "Istituzione." Most were listed in the *catasto* records as intended for the poor or, in a few cases, for pilgrims.

[58] On the issue of patronage and support see Passerini's discussions of individual

Doctors were associated with many of these hospitals from at least the early fourteenth century. Furthermore, hospital medicine, like plasters or bones, was a recognized specialty; thus a certain Francesco di Vanni matriculated in the guild around 1350 as a "hospital doctor" (*medicus hospitalarius*) employed at Santa Lucia de' Magnoli, and Maestro Agnolo di Cristofano, who worked at Santa Maria Nuova, appears with the same notation in the *catasto* of 1427.[59] All such institutions had to submit *catasto* declarations in 1428; these show that the hospitals employing the largest number of doctors were those catering to foundlings and, as we would expect, the sick poor. Most had two doctors on their payrolls, usually a physician and a surgeon, and paid them annual salaries ranging from fl. 2 (for the hospital of San Gallo, with its thirty beds for the poor) to fl. 24 (for the hospital of Santa Maria Nuova, which could accommodate 250 invalids).[60] Like the monasteries, hospitals often paid their doctors only token amounts, often in kind, and assumed that their fees would be supplemented by income from other forms of practice.[61]

The fiscal documents from the early Renaissance give no details about how patients were treated in Florentine hospitals. We can, however, get a good idea of contemporary hospital practice in Florence from a somewhat later document, a comprehensive description of the organization and administration of the hospital of Santa Maria Nuova prepared shortly after 1500 at the request of Henry VII of England.[62] By

---

hospitals and d'Addario, *Contrariforma*, 60-73. St. Anthony's Fire referred specifically to ergotism and in general to various skin diseases.

[59] AMS-8, fol. 8r; Catasto-81, fol. 171r. Note that Francesco's lack of an honorific implies that he was an empiric.

[60] San Gallo employed a physician and a surgeon with combined salaries of fl. 4 (Catasto-194/II, fol. 389r-v). Santa Maria Nuova employed the same with salaries of fl. 24 and fl. 14 respectively (SMN-4477, fol. 48v, and SMN-4479, fol. 43v). San Matteo paid its two doctors fl. 15 in all (Catasto-185, fol. 606v), while the hospital of Messer Bonifazio gave its two doctors fl. 24 together (Catasto-190, fol. 52r). The foundling hospital of Santa Maria della Scala, on the other hand, which housed mainly orphans and homeless boys and girls, had only one doctor on its payroll for twelve *staia* of grain (worth fl. 3) a year (Catasto-185, fol. 581r). Doctors were also sometimes called in especially to treat staff members or particular patients and were paid at rates equivalent to those in private practice for this kind of work; see, for example, SMN-4479, fol. 111r; 4408, fol. 44r; 4453, fol. 108v; 4456, fol. 94v.

[61] Thus a number of doctors appear on the payroll of both a monastery and a hospital, or of several hospitals. This is the case, for example, with the physician M° Cristofano di Giorgio, who at his death in 1425 was employed by both the hospital of Messer Bonifazio and that of San Paolo; see his will in Notarile-F.299 (1422-23), fol. 38v. Several decades earlier M° Cristofano had been on the staff of the hospital of San Gallo; see Pinto, "Personale," 133.

[62] For a transcription of the document see Passerini, *Storia degli stabilimenti*, 851-61;

that year the number of patients housed by the hospital had increased significantly, and with it the size of the medical staff. In other respects, however, the medical organization of the hospital was probably similar to that in the mid-fifteenth century.[63]

By 1480 Santa Maria Nouva was famous for the quality of its medical care. The humanist Cristoforo Landino praised it in the proemium of his commentary on Dante as "the first hospital among Christians":

> In it they care continuously for more than three hundred invalids. Difficult as it is to arrange, the beds are always clean, and there is always someone to look after the patient and see to his needs. Food and medicine are not distributed indiscriminately, but to each individual according to his disease. Both physicians and surgeons are always on hand and give individual directions for all. As a result, many noble and rich foreigners, afflicted with some illness during a voyage, have chosen to be treated in this institution.[64]

The early sixteenth-century description confirms Landino's claim. The general staff of the hospital—the male and female "oblates"—lived on the premises under their own rule. From them were chosen a man and a woman (*infirmarius* and *infirmaria*) with full responsibility for the day-to-day administration of the two sick wards, which were segregated by sex. The male ward alone housed a hundred bunk beds; these were made up with mattresses, bolsters, pillows, linens, and covers, and numbered to identify individual patients. On admission the patient was examined by the *infirmarius*, his clothes removed and stored under his name in alphabetically arranged cabinets, and standard clothing issued; finally he was registered in the book of admissions, also kept in alphabetical order.[65]

The actual medical care was the responsibility of a staff of nine doctors. Of these, the three youngest (called *adstantes* or "assistants") lived in the hospital. In return for their services they received room, board, and the valuable opportunity to study a wide variety of diseases: "while

---

Passerini's dating of the text is wrong; Henry VII died in 1509. (John Henderson and I are preparing a translation for publication.)

[63] Santa Maria Nuova had employed two doctors throughout the later fourteenth and early fifteenth centuries. By 1450 their number had risen to four (SMN-4495, fols. 52v, 87r); the four doctors in question were M° Bandino Banducci, M° Agnolo di Cristofano, M° Domenico di m° Giovanni, and M° Antonio di Francesco da Cagli. See also Chiappelli and Corsini, "Antico inventario."

[64] Landino, *Scritti*, 1:116.

[65] Passerini, *Storia degli stabilimenti*, 856-58, 865.

they are treating different illnesses in different ways," the document states, "they become more skillful and more prudent, for experience is the mistress of things." Together with the *infirmarius*, the three resident doctors divided the beds among them, each attending the patients assigned to him. They practiced under the supervision of six salaried senior doctors, "the most illustrious in the entire city," who came every morning to examine the sick, listen to the reports of the *infirmarii* and *adstantes*, and issue prescriptions for the treatment of each patient. The prescriptions were then made up by the hospital's resident apothecary and his assistants, registered in a book under the bed number of the sick person, and administered by the *infirmarii* and *adstantes*. Special classes of patients—"nobles," the wounded, priests and clerics, those mentally ill "from physical causes," and victims of diseases involving skin lesions—were isolated from the general wards and from one another. Of these, the wounded and the patients with skin conditions were treated by a seventh senior doctor, a surgeon, who came to the hospital for two hours each morning and evening.[66]

Thus the principal function of the hospital was to treat and house the sick poor, which it apparently did to good effect. (There is no evidence that it functioned either as a holding pen for the terminally ill or as a deathtrap; according to the hospital's records, of the 2,252 men admitted in 1524, for example, only 335 died, while the rest were discharged as improved or cured.)[67] In addition Santa Maria Nuova offered other medical services to the city at large, housing plague victims during major epidemics, furnishing medical advice and medicines for those who could not afford to call a doctor to their own houses, and occasionally sending members of its staff to the homes of gravely ill citizens, including "nobles and patricians."[68] Thus Santa Maria Nuova seems to have supplied medical care of a high quality to a wide cross-section of Florence's population, while concentrating on the needs of the poor. Other hospitals catering primarily to the sick may not have been as large or as well organized as Santa Maria Nuova, but it is clear that they and the more specialized small hospitals formed a large and varied market for doctors' services.

Associated with many of the Florentine hospitals, either as their patrons and founders or because they met on hospital premises, was yet a third kind of religious foundation which hired significant numbers of doctors: the confraternities. These were religious companies

---

[66] Ibid., 859-60.

[67] SMN-733, passim; this volume is one of the "books of the dead" meticulously kept by the hospital.

[68] Passerini, *Storia degli stabilimenti*, 860-61; Coturri, "Più antichi provvedimenti," 73.

composed for the most part of lay citizens, although they were frequently under the protection and supervision of established religious orders.[69] They varied considerably in size, membership, and function. Some were drawn largely or entirely from particular social groups—boys (like the company of San Giovanni Evangelista); women (like the company of women of San Lorenzo); or members of a particular occupation (like the company of Sant'Eligio of the goldsmiths)—while others embraced people of all ages and social origins. Their members met regularly to pray and sing together, hear sermons, and attend masses. Some had more specific purposes, including the various companies of flagellants (*disciplinati*) or the Company of Santa Maria della Croce al Tempio, which took as its particular task the physical and spiritual comfort of criminals slated for execution. Most, however, filled the three general functions of promoting collective devotion, dispensing charity, and providing a framework for fellowship and mutual aid among their members.

It was in the last two capacities that most confraternities required the services of Florence's doctors. A few of the larger and more important ones, and those with a strong charitable orientation, employed doctors to attend to the medical needs of the groups they chose to serve. Thus the Company of Or San Michele in the fourteenth century hired doctors to visit the sick poor at home, and the Company of Santa Maria della Croce al Tempio salaried a doctor and a barber to care for prisoners and condemned criminals.[70] Over the course of the fifteenth century, however, Florentine confraternities began increasingly to provide social benefits of various kinds to their members as part of the move toward civic piety described above, and one of the most important of these was medical care. By the middle of the fifteenth century many companies retained a doctor with a regular salary and specified his duties in their statutes.

The Company of San Lorenzo in Piano, a flagellant confraternity associated with the church of Santa Maria Novella, is typical. Its statute provided for a *correttore* to be sent by day or by night as necessary to sick members, to administer confession and spiritual comfort. "And in addition," it read, "just as we have a doctor for the soul, so we have a doctor for the body. Thus we ordain that our company always have a competent doctor for our sick, to be appointed and confirmed in the same way as the *correttore*. This doctor must treat with care and without cost to the patient all the sick members of our company, visiting

[69] On Florentine confraternities in the fourteenth and fifteenth centuries see Monti, *Confraternite medievali*, vol. 1, chap. 7, and Weissman, *Ritual Brotherhood*.

[70] Passerini, *Storia degli stabilimenti*, 488.

them day and night as needed." In return, the doctor was to receive a salary of £12, payable every four months, as well as £1 s. 8 for a goat at Easter, £1 s. 10 for a goose at All Saints', and a wax candle at Candlemas.[71] If the member was found to be seriously ill—"if the doctor finds fever," in the words of the statute of the Company of San Giovanni Scalzo—he was given a weekly allowance of up to s. 30; if he died in poverty, the confraternity would pay for both his funeral and a number of penitential psalms and masses.[72]

The importance of this kind of practice for the history of medicine and the medical profession lies above all in its scale. During the late Middle Ages and Renaissance, Florence supported between fifty and a hundred confraternities, each averaging on the order of a hundred members. About half of these companies offered medical benefits of the kind outlined above to members and (often) their immediate families. This means that at any given time roughly fifteen thousand people—about a third of the Florentine population—could have received their medical care in this way. Furthermore, these people consisted primarily of artisans and members of the city's middle classes; they thus represent a completely different pool of patients from those served by the hospitals or the more expensive varieties of private practice. It is even possible that many Florentines in fact joined confraternities, most of which set annual dues at about fl. 2, in order to enjoy these medical benefits, along with benefits concerning burial or dowries. In this way the confraternities would have been offering and doctors would have been participating in what corresponds to an early form of pre-paid health insurance.[73]

[71] BLF: Ashburnham 970, fol. 33r-v: "Et più vogliamo che come habbiamo el medicho dell'anima, habbiamo el medicho del corpo. Et però ordiniamo che sempre la nostra compagnia habbia uno medicho sufficiente pe' nostri infermi, da farsi e eleggersi e raffermarsi nel modo . . . del correctore. Et che detto medicho sia tenuto con sollecitudine curare tutti i nostri malati e infermi di nostra compagnia sanza costo e premio alcuno dello 'nfermo, et quegli visitare di dì e di nocte et anchora, come fusse di bisogno." The original statute dated from the 1360s; it was recopied in the early sixteenth century. For similar provisions see also Compagnie religiose soppresse-2170, filza statuti, fol. 57v (statute of the confraternity of San Zanobi from 1427, amended 1480); Compagnie religiose soppresse, Capitoli-606, chap. 6 (statute of the confraternity of Santa Maria della Neve in Sant'Ambrogio from 1447); BRF: Ricc. 2535, fol. 32r (statute of the confraternity of the Vergine Maria delle Laudesi di Santa Croce from 1470). The last two specified that the confraternity doctor must have a doctorate in medicine. I owe these references to John Henderson of the Cambridge Group for the History of Population and Social Structure.

[72] BRF: Ricc. 2535, fols. 6v-7v.

[73] I am indebted for the figures in this paragraph to Ronald Weissman of the University of Maryland (College Park).

The public and religious sectors of the medical marketplace in fourteenth- and fifteenth-century Florence, then, were important for several reasons. In the first place, they were comparatively extensive and may have provided the bulk of many doctors' practices. In the second place, they represented a market for a special type of medical practice—one in which the doctor was salaried by a third party or an institutional intermediary, a form of practice usually identified as a comparatively recent development. Finally, they catered overwhelmingly to the poor and the middle orders, those classes of Renaissance society which have traditionally been seen as cut off from the established medical profession and its services, and in many respects the care they provided—as even a cursory examination of the names of the doctors concerned shows—was the best that money could buy.

PRIVATE PRACTICE

Even in the private sector of the medical marketplace there was a great range of levels and types of practice, depending on the specialty of the doctor, the nature of the complaint, and the social standing of the patient. Private patients could be treated as outpatients in shops (*botteghe*) or visited at home. Many empirical surgeons worked out of regular shops which they owned or rented. This is true, for example, of the hernia doctor Maestro Luca di maestro Antonio da Norcia, whose specialized operations would presumably have required appropriate furnishings and a number of surgical instruments.[74] Similarly, the notary and author Ser Giovanni di Gherardo da Prato, after slipping on a cucumber peel in the Via Calimala and breaking his arm, went immediately to the bone doctor, where, he recounted, "he set it for me with excruciating pain."[75]

Physicians had less need to rent shops, both because their practices were more mobile and because most apothecaries employed a physician to staff a walk-in clinic on the premises for a certain number of hours every week. In return for a yearly salary the physician would write prescriptions for those who came to consult him, to be filled by his employer.[76] This form of practice was widespread in Florence, as

[74] Catasto-711, fol. 582r: "Iᵃ bottegha tengho a pigione del socio di Lorenzo."

[75] ASP: Datini CP-1093 (24.viii.1392): "andato subito al medicho, con grandissimo dolore e instimabile pena me rraconcia."

[76] For a typical example of a contract establishing this kind of practice see the *ricordanza* of Mᵒ Polidoro Bracali; ASPist: Archivio dell'orfanotrofio Puccini, Sala C, 2ᵒ piano, scaff. 237-38, fol. 6r (23.i.1459): "m'acconciai a bottega di Lorenzo di ser Cortese

elsewhere in Italy. In 1470 Benedetto Dei listed thirty-two large spice and drug companies in the city, noting the presence of doctors in each. He recorded only thirty-three doctors in the same year, at least one of whom was a surgeon; the implication is that virtually every physician was employed by at least one apothecary.[77] Furthermore, as the account books of physicians show, this was usually the first kind of contractual employment a young doctor enjoyed, and it was lucrative as well as a common practice; in 1385 Maestro Iacopo di Coluccino da Lucca received fl. 40 from his apothecary out of total annual earnings of fl. 182.[78] Thus even physicians at the peak of a successful career chose to retain both the professional contacts and the regular income and pool of patients generated by this kind of contract. The patient too stood to gain, since the cost to him was lower than a private visit; in fact it seems likely that the majority of private individuals who were not very sick received their medical care in apothecaries' shops.

Nonetheless, the practice of making house calls was apparently widespread on all levels of the profession. (Virtually all doctors included in their *catasto* declarations a horse or donkey to carry them to visit patients in the more far-flung parts of the city, and above all in the *contado*.)[79] Perhaps the most vivid and detailed contemporary Italian description of such home visits appears not in a diary or account book but in a treatise by Maestro Gabriele Zerbi. Zerbi never practiced in Florence, but his *On Precautions to Be Taken by Doctors (De cautelis medicorum)* relied heavily on the Florentine writer Niccolò Falcucci's *Practica*, among other classical, Arabic, and contemporary sources. Though part of a long medieval tradition of deontological writing, it nonetheless gives a fair picture of medical practice in the urban centers

---

spetiale, con patto dovessi ordinare le medicine a bottega sua et live pratichare secondo la consuetudine delli medici physici da Pistoia, et lui me debbe dare per anno fiorini octo larghi di Firenze. Acconciami per due anni, et debbe incominciare l'anno a dì a dì [*sic*] primo di febraio anno soprascritto."

[77] BRF: Ricc. 1853, fols. 42v-43v. See also Zerbi, *De cautelis*, 70, for advice on how a physician should behave toward his apothecary.

[78] See his *ricordanza*, in ASL: Ospedale di S. Luca-180, verso of first, unnumb. fol., and 41v; also the *ricordanza* of Mº Polidoro d'Antonio Bracali da Pistoia, esp. fols. 3r, 6r, 10v. For transcriptions of some relevant passages in the first see Chiapelli, "Maestro Jacopo di Coluccino da Lucca." As these entries show, doctors did not always stay with a single apothecary but typically moved from one shop to another two or three times in the course of a career.

[79] The fourteenth-century communal bone doctors received from the Florentine treasury, along with their regular salaries, the use of a horse and a stipend to maintain it; see above, note 20. See also Catasto-688, fol. 644r (Mº Piero and Mº Paolo di mº Domenico): "Faciamo esercitio di medichare; tegniamo due chavagli"; and Catasto-307, fol. 74r-v (Mº Simone di Pacino): "Truovasi lº asino il quale adopera a suo asercizio [*sic*]."

of fifteenth-century Italy.[80] In his fourth and fifth chapters Zerbi described how doctors should behave toward the patient and others present at the sickbed of a private client; his discussion included both ethical and practical considerations as well as a long description of the course of a standard medical visit.

To begin with, Zerbi recommended that the doctor call on his patient twice daily, morning and evening, except in cases of acute or life-threatening disease, when he should not leave the bedside.[81] (Letters and account books show that this was indeed standard practice.) It is clear from Zerbi's discussion as well as from contemporary *ricordanze* that the doctor supervised the treatment of the patient but that he did so in close cooperation with the sick person's family and friends, servants, and attendants, and that he was expected to keep the family informed at all times of the patient's condition and needs.[82] The doctor relied on members of the household not only to administer the more mechanical parts of the treatment but also as an important source of information about the course of the illness.

Zerbi emphasized that the doctor should proceed to examine and question the patient after having ascertained from those around him his case history, his symptoms, and the remedies previously administered, and after having formed, on the the basis of this information, a preliminary idea of the condition and its causes. Only then was the doctor ready to see the patient and—after ensuring that he had confessed recently and after engaging in some obligatory small talk—to undertake the examination itself. The examination was to consist of a careful look at the patient's face (a good indicator of his condition), followed by taking his pulse, palpating his members, and looking at his urine. Having assured the patient of his curability, the doctor was supposed to take the relatives and friends apart and inform them of the real state of affairs: the cause and nature of the disease and, if pressed, its prognosis. He could then proceed to the actual "curative act," the prescription of measures for treatment.[83]

At the end of this section Zerbi took up the sensitive question of

---

[80] On Zerbi and *De cautelis* see Lind, *Pre-Vesalian Anatomy*, 141-47, 151-54, as well as Lind, "Deontologia medica," 60-83. On the broader tradition see the discussion and references in Lind's article, Amundsen, "Medical Deontology," and Wellborn, "Long Tradition."

[81] Zerbi, *De cautelis*, 38; Latin text in Zerbi, *Opus perutile*.

[82] Zerbi, *De cautelis*, 40, 46; see also the *ricordo* of 1452 of Francesco di Tommaso Giovanni, where he describes the illness of his wife, Bartolomea (Carte Strozziane-2, 16bis, fol. 11r).

[83] Zerbi, *De cautelis*, 40-53.

the doctor's fee. One should not hesitate on this matter, he warned his readers; the fee itself is a powerful therapeutic tool for discouraging malingering and spurring the patient and his attendants toward a rapid cure. "Thus the doctor acquires more authority, is better respected, and will be treated humanely and correctly. All those involved will make an effort to obey him in order not to waste the money paid, and the patient will heal more quickly. As the saying goes, 'Medicine bought dear is of great efficacy; given free it is of little use.' "[84] Exceptions to this rule might be made for relatives of the doctor or for charity cases, but in general, unless the patient was a noble or known to be generous, the fee was best fixed at the beginning of the treatment. Zerbi's recommendations imply that the doctor was to be paid per visit, although not necessarily at each of his twice-daily calls. The ideal was to arrange daily payment, although payment every other day was also acceptable; if the client fell off this schedule, however, the doctor was to consider omitting either the morning or the evening visit as a gentle reminder of financial obligations.[85] Zerbi did not specify the amount to be charged per visit, and it is difficult to ascertain the size of the doctor's standard fee from contemporary account books, since the entries usually specify the money disbursed during the entire course of an illness.[86] Occasionally, however, the length of the illness is recorded, and in these cases the fee seems to have ranged from s. 5 to fl. 1 per visit (s. 10 to fl. 2 per day), depending on the patient's wealth and status.[87]

It is clear both from Zerbi's account and from other documents that Italian doctors treated a wide variety of patients, even within the arena of private practice, and that it is wrong to assume that empirics catered only to the lower orders while physicians restricted their attention to the elite. An ordinary bone doctor, as we saw in the case of Ser Giovanni di Gherardo da Prato's broken arm, might treat a notary and future professor of literature at the University of Florence, while a physician of high repute might care for many humbler citizens, either as part of his duties in the apothecary's shop or on a strictly private

[84] Ibid., 58; *Opus perutile*, fol. 69r: "Sic enim medicus maioris apud illum efficietur auctoritatis; illum excellentiorem iudicat ipsum sibi ad humanam communicat pollitiam. Illi omnes obtemperare conantur ne amittantur expense; sicque demum citius sanatur. Iuxta illud: Empta solet care multis medicina iuvare; si data sit gratis nihil confert utilitas."

[85] Zerbi, *De cautelis*, 58-61.

[86] See, for example, Carte Strozziane-5, 5, fol. 45r (1411): "A Mo Lorenzo da Prato medico per lla malattia d'Antonio, fl. 1 s. 5."

[87] See SMN-4456, fol. 94v (1404), for the lower figure; Origo, *Merchant of Prato*, 254, for the higher.

basis; Maestro Antonio Benivieni, for example, a man of letters and one of the most important physicians in later fifteenth-century Florence, included among his patients not only the families of Lorenzo de' Medici and other notable patricians but also, as we know from his collection of case histories, a carpenter, the son of a butcher, and a woman he identified as "my baker's wife."[88]

It is through physicians like Benivieni that we can get some sense of a very restricted kind of private practice—that which catered to the small group of aristocratic and princely patrons characterized by Zerbi in *On Precautions* as "generous and courtly."[89] Such clients were willing to pay for medical care on a scale inaccessible to most Florentine citizens. When Giovanni Rucellai's daughter-in-law Caterina fell gravely ill in 1464, for example, six doctors were called in; an even more extravagant patient, the wealthy fourteenth-century banker Bonifazio Peruzzi, had a certain Maestro Alberto travel to Florence from Bologna for a fee of fl. 60 to cure his sore throat.[90] Illustrious doctors were paid even to deliver expert written opinions *in absentia*, on the basis of a description of the case.[91] And if mere patricians like Rucellai and Peruzzi could command such treatment, princes and popes frequently paid prized physicians regular salaries amounting to hundreds of florins in order to enjoy their exclusive, or nearly exclusive, attention.[92]

Even in this rarefied environment, however, physicians did not regularly command fees for specific services rendered; there is a good deal of evidence that here, as in their dealings with the state, with apothecaries, or with religious corporations, they appreciated the security of a contract and a salary. Furthermore, they often neither expected nor wished to be paid in cash. When Maestro Antonio Benivieni contracted with Francesco di Tolosino de' Medici to attend to his medical needs and those of his family, he did so in exchange for a two-hundred pound pig. Maestro Polidoro d'Antonio Bracali da Pistoia, who had attended Cardinal Carlo Forteguerri during an illness of seventy-five

[88] Benivieni, *De abditis*, tr. Singer, 20, 164, 76.

[89] Zerbi, *De cautelis*, 58.

[90] On Caterina see MAP-XVI, 157; on Bonifazio Peruzzi, Peruzzi, *Storia del commercio*, 414.

[91] These opinions were known as *consilia*; see the discussions in Siraisi, *Taddeo Alderotti*, chap. 9, and Lockwood, *Ugo Benzi*, 44-78 and chap. 6.

[92] M° Ugolino da Montecatini was appointed court doctor to the lord of Pesaro for a salary of fl. 500 a year; see his *De balneis*, 105. M° Naddino di Aldobrandino da Prato received similar amounts from one of the cardinals in Avignon; see ASP: Archivio Datini-Carteggio privato-1091₂ (?.vii.1387). Doctors appointed in this capacity acted as much as courtiers as medical practitioners.

days, received a silver cloth with figures woven in gold and twelve silver spoons: "He said," wrote Maestro Polidoro, "that he was not giving them to me in payment, because he knew that I would not have accepted them, but in memory of our long, firm friendship."[93] The Medici often enjoyed doctors' services in return for promises of patronage. Thus they made a practice of rewarding the service of esteemed doctors with coveted teaching positions at the universities of Florence and Pisa, and physicians frequently approached them for this kind of favor. Maestro Luca di messer Antonio da Foligno, for example, sent Piero di Cosimo a sample of ointment and pills for his gout. "Piero, because I wish always to please you and be near you," he concluded the accompanying letter, "I pray you dearly to arrange that I come to read medicine in your University of Florence with a reasonable salary, and you will see that I do honor to you and to myself. . . ."[94]

On this highest level of private practice, the financial and social rewards of patronage and employment were substantial enough to generate a certain amount of friction among doctors. This competition could take on a personal tone. In *On Baths*, Maestro Ugolino da Montecatini described several episodes from what seems to have been a prolonged rivalry between himself and Maestro Giovanni Baldi over the care of patients like Giovanni di Bicci de' Medici and Raimondo degli Albizzi. The papal court in Avignon half a century earlier generated the same kind of rivalries when physicians like Maestro Naddino di Aldobrandino da Prato, for example, jockeyed for positions as

[93] *Ricordanza* of M° Antonio Benivieni, Notarile-B.1324, fol. 193r (entry of 1.xi.1485); *ricordanza* of M° Polidoro, as in note 76 above, fol. 14r (entry of 10.xi.1473): "dicendomi non melo dava per pagamento, perchè sapia non lo harei tolto, ma per memoria della buona amicitia anticha et al."

[94] MAP-XVI, 348: "Piero, perchè io desideravo sempre fare cosa che ve piaccia et d'essere ad presso de vui, io ve pregaria caramente ve volessate operare che io venga a llegere una lectione de medicina nellu studio vostro di Firenze con uno salario rasionevele, et vidrate io farò honore ad vui et ad me, prima quanto alli facti dellu studio et poy quanto allo facto del medicare, advisando che quando m'avirite provato uno anno, non me vorite lassare partire più, et io ve prometto mantenerve sensa dogle." There are many such letters in the archives of Medici correspondence; see also the series from M° Iacopo da Pistoia (MAP-XXVIII, 550; XXIII, 545; XXXIII, 359; XXIII, 694, 689) and from M° Giovanni da Arezzo (MAP-XXV, 291 and 249) as well as the letter from M° Francesco di ser Niccolò da San Miniato (MAP-XXX, 446). The Medici had a regular household doctor, M° Mariotto di Niccolò, but frequently called in consultants from Florence and other Italian cities for particular advice or in cases of serious illness. For more information on the health problems of the Medici and their doctors see Pieraccini, *Stirpe de' Medici*, 1:29-33, 57-68, 87-92, 128-33; Ross, *Lives of the Early Medici*, passim; and Maguire, *Women of the Medici*, passim.

doctor to the pope, cardinals, and other high Church officials.[95] At this level, however, the competition was often as intense among patients as among doctors. Clients who could afford the services of the few physicians with stellar reputations were forced to vie with one another for those services, often to the distinct discomfort of the doctor in question. Thus Maestro Benedetto Reguardati da Norcia found himself in the middle of a tug of war between Francesco Sforza, duke of Milan, whose wife he had cured of infertility, and Cosimo de' Medici, both of whom strove to monopolize his attention.[96]

In general, however, collaboration among doctors seems to have been the rule far more often than strenuous competition, even in private practice. As Zerbi pointed out in *On Precautions*, there were strong practical benefits to be gained from consultation, as long as the number of practitioners involved was not excessive, for while "collegiality does not jeopardize the doctor's reward, practicing alone [when the patient is critically ill] commonly leads to disgrace. Thus the doctor should press the friends and relatives of the patient to call in a colleague as a condition of his treatment.[97] (Zerbi's only exception to this rule involved collaboration with empirics; he considered this beneath the dignity of the more qualified surgeon or physician.) As always, however, he warned that the doctor must have an eye to appearances. He should seek as colleagues only those of his own rank who would not act as overt rivals or critics. Collaborating doctors might engage in a certain amount of personal promotion, but they should always present a united front to the client, reserving their disagreements for private discussion in order to avoid "scandalizing the layman and reflecting badly on the profession."[98]

Zerbi's discussion of cooperation among doctors tends to confirm the image of the profession which emerges from the statutes of the Guild of Doctors, Apothecaries, and Grocers. Like the guild statutes, Zerbi's treatise shows a certain tension between empirics and the higher levels of the profession, although no strong animosity. Greater em-

---

[95] Ugolino da Montecatini, *De balneis*, 46, 48; on M° Ugolino and M° Giovanni see below, Chapter Six. ASP: Datini CP-1091₂ (letters of M° Naddino di Aldobrandino da Prato); esp. letters of 7.i.1386/7, 21.i.1386/7, 21.iii.1388/9. See Brun, "Quelques italiens."

[96] Reguardati, *Benedetto de' Reguardati*, 112-28, 170-93.

[97] Zerbi, *De cautelis*, 65; *Opus perutile*, fol. 70v: "Non presumas solus curare egritudinem de qua rationabiliter mors cognoscitur, sed socium vel plures petas. Societas enim non aufert premium, sed singularitas plerumque infamiam parit; immo affinibus et amicis qui patientis sunt astringat ad dandum sibi socium alias se curaturum nequaquam."

[98] Zerbi, *De cautelis*, 66. Benivieni includes many accounts of such collaboration and consultation in his *De abditis*.

phasis was placed on professional unity and on avoiding direct competition. That this was the case in reality as well as the ideal seems clear from letters in which Florentine doctors described their relationships to their clients and to other doctors. In 1408, for example, Maestro Lorenzo Sassoli da Prato, fresh out of medical school, was approached by the prior of the Servite convent about an illness previously treated by one of the most prominent Florentine physicians, Maestro Cristofano di Giorgio. Rather than jumping at the opportunity, Maestro Lorenzo informed the prior that, as he related, "I did not want to [take the case], for the sake of his honor and mine, before talking it over with Maestro Cristofano."[99] In a later letter he referred to a similar incident:

> I wanted several times to talk with Maestro Cristofano, but this was never possible. Thus the case remained his alone as was fitting, and I did not know what remedies he prescribed or what the patient's condition was, or how his nature and accidents reacted [to treatment]. For our nature can change not just over two months but in a day, as you see all the time. I have often told you, both in person and by letter, that it is shameful for a doctor, and dangerous to his salvation, to prescribe or administer a remedy without knowing why. . . .[100]

Maestro Lorenzo may have been exceptionally scrupulous in his professional ethics; he was certainly unwilling to offend an influential senior colleague. It is nonetheless clear that the guidelines for conduct in private practice that we find in the guild statutes and Zerbi's *On Precautions* were not merely pious hopes. The impression created by these and other documents is that the doctor's main concern was not competition for patients. Florence seems to have supplied an adequate pool of institutional and private clients to support the medical profes-

[99] ASP: Datini CP-1102, busta (12.i.1407/8): "voleva che io il cominciassi a curare; rispuosegli che questo io non voleva per suo onore e per mio, se prima io non mi abochassi chon m° Cristofano."

[100] Ibid. (letter of 13.iii.1407/8): "Poi, passati alcuni dì, el priore mandò per me e vidilo due volte, e per quello che allora mi parve, parvemi il caso suo esere di gran pericolo e piutosto da pensare la morte che lla salute. . . . Io mi volli più volte abocare con m° Cristofano, e mai non ci fu modo, onde la cura rimase a llui solo come si convenia, per la qu[ale] cosa io non sepi che remedi s'egli facesse o in che dispositione remanesse o come poi la sua natura o suoi acidenti sieno seguitati, chè non che in due mesi si varii la nostra natura ma in un dì si può mutare, e voi tuto il dì lo potrete vedere. Per tanto come a boche e per letera molte volte v'ò detto, egli è grande vergongnia a un medico e danno all'anima a ordinare o dare niuno rimedio se non vede perchè lo dà. . . ."

sion, particularly at its shrunken fifteenth-century level. Rather, he looked to ensure his practice by seeking out long-term contracts and by cultivating a professional reputation based on cures achieved and (perhaps even more important) disasters avoided. Maestro Ugolino da Montecatini doubtless spoke for many doctors when he acknowledged, "our art is one that often depends on luck."[101]

In part this defensiveness was the product of a particular view of physiology and disease. Health and illness in Renaissance medical theory were not seen as distinct conditions but as constantly shifting points on an infinitely divisible continuum, which altered according to the complexion of the patient as well as his age, sex, and external circumstances; thus the doctor often relied as much on guesswork as on knowledge.[102] In part it was also the result of the relatively undeveloped state of medical knowledge. In the absence of antisepsis, anesthesia, and other more advanced techniques, both surgeons and physicians understood clearly that except in extreme cases the path of least intervention was usually the safest.[103] Both considerations urged a policy of caution and restraint on the doctor, a policy doubtless made more urgent by the intractability of the plague. But it is also true that the doctor did not see his practice in heroic or individualistic terms, because that was not the nature either of his society or of the market for medical services it supported. Like the artisan or the merchant, he worked in a world of communities. His practice was organized and regulated by one corporation, the guild, and it constantly brought him into contact with other collectivities, from private households to drug companies to hospitals and confraternities to the state itself. The themes of profit, ambition, and competition were by no means absent in this period, as the next chapter will show, but they were modulated by the corporate world of contract and mutual obligation in which the doctor's practice was embedded.

[101] Carte Del Bene, Busta 49, no. 201 (5.vi.[1381]); transcribed below, Chapter Four, note 90.

[102] For some sense of this aspect of contemporary medical learning see Siraisi, *Taddeo Alderotti*, chap. 4 and 286-90.

[103] Zerbi makes this point with great emphasis; see *De cautelis*, 37, 68. In particular he recommends that the doctor first attempt a cure using the mild action of what was called "diet"—the manipulation of air, food, drink, sleep and waking, exercise and rest, and the emotions. If such measures fail he might look to medication, but even then he should prescribe natural and nutritive medicines before strong ones, and external remedies before internal ones. Only as a last resort, or in very serious illnesses, should he turn to phlebotomy, "solutive" medicines (emetics and laxatives), or opiates; ibid., 51-54.

IV

Medical Careers

IN ORDER to understand the world of medicine and medical practice in fourteenth- and fifteenth-century Florence, it is not enough
to consider only the profession as a whole and the corporate groups
which shaped that world; we must also study the practitioners as individuals. Each doctor made his way among the competing demands
and possibilities of guild and family, Church and state to shape a career
in keeping with his abilities, ambitions, and opportunities. At various
points he was faced with important decisions: which occupation to
choose, how to train for it, whether to teach or practice, where to
establish his practice. And once the decisions had been made, both the
doctor and his family, friends, and associates had to carry them through.
The kinds of considerations which went into these decisions and actions contribute at least as much to our understanding of the medical
profession as the more cut-and-dried information of who paid which
doctors how much to do what.

One of the themes of the previous chapters has been the relative
complexity and sophistication of medicine in this period. Despite differences in medical theory and therapeutic technique, we can see in
early Renaissance Florence the outlines of a system of medical organization which is in important respects the ancestor of the one we know
today. The sense of familiarity becomes even stronger when we look
at medical careers. In part this is because doctors were moved by basic
impulses toward a life that was personally rewarding and materially
secure. In part it is because the social topography of fourteenth- and
fifteenth-century Tuscany is in itself familiar—highly urbanized and
organized through a network of primary and secondary towns, which
served as the centers of an active culture and a well-developed commercial economy. In many respects, however, the sense of familiarity
springs from the particular character of the doctors around whom this
chapter is constructed. The best sources for doctors' attitudes and motivations are letters and personal account books or diaries. These doc-

uments are rare, and they tend to survive only for relatively wealthy and well-educated physicians and for geographically mobile immigrants who corresponded regularly with absent family and friends. Living to some extent on the margins of a tightly organized corporate society, these men articulated desires and feelings which have a strong contemporary ring.

In their literary and intellectual ambitions, such physicians stood apart from the ranks of surgeons and empirics who filled out the rest of the profession. As immigrants to Florence, however, their experience was broadly typical. The settled Florentine doctor—one who trained in the city and practiced there for the rest of his life—did exist, but we have seen that he was in the minority, particularly by the middle of the fifteenth century, when 80 percent of the practitioners matriculating in the guild came from beyond the city walls. What was the city's attraction? What were the advantages and disadvantages, both real and perceived, of living and practicing there? At what point did doctors decide to immigrate, and how did they establish a practice and clientele? What ties did they retain with their place of origin? Were their decisions temporary or permanent? Taking these questions as a point of departure, we can begin to understand many of the decisions and episodes which marked the medical career of the Italian Renaissance doctor.

Choosing a Career: Education and Training

The first step in the doctor's career was the choice of medicine as an occupation. Because the training involved was long, such decisions were generally made when the child was quite young—usually by the time he was in his early teens—and were as much the work of the parents as of the son in question.[1] A number of Florentine moralists, including Paolo di ser Pace da Certaldo and the influential friar Giovanni Dominici, touched on the subject in the fourteenth and fifteenth centuries; their works advised that a number of considerations be kept in mind, including the spread of occupations already represented in the family and the particular talents and inclinations of the child. Leon Battista Alberti took a somewhat broader view in his own treatise on the family, recommending that parents also take into account the entire social, economic, and cultural environment. He wrote of "the great

---

[1] This was not invariably the case. M° Ugo Benzi, for example, chose to go into medicine as an adult; see Lockwood, *Ugo Benzi*, 25.

care fathers must exercise in choosing what art, what profession, what way of life is more suitable for the child, keeping in mind the child's nature, the family's honor, the country's traditions, present fortunes, time, conditions, opportunities available, and the citizens' expectations."[2]

The works of Alberti and his contemporaries were at best idealized prescriptions for enlightened action; they did not necessarily speak to the more pragmatic concerns which faced the fathers of adolescent boys. Alberti's implicit denigration of the profit motive, and Dominici's smiling assurance that all trades, even the most menial, were necessary and honorable, would have met with little sympathy from the more prosperous and respectable families which sent their sons to study medicine. But the more practical points made by Paolo da Certaldo and the others—the importance of occupational diversity within the family, of a fully mastered trade, and of the child's own talents and inclinations—certainly influenced many parents. This mix of anxieties and ambition appears clearly in the correspondence between Maestro Marco di maestro Antonio, a physician in Pistoia, and his young son Antonio, whom he had packed off in 1458 to study medicine at the University of Florence.[3]

The letters received by Antonio during his two years in Florence returned again and again to two arguments intended to spur his studies and lighten his homesickness: *utile* and *onore; denari* and *fama*; money and reputation. Many of the epistles from Maestro Marco and the boy's other correspondents were merely elaborate variations on that double theme:

> Marshal your strength to prepare yourself and to study. You can't do anything more pleasing to me and more productive of money and reputation.[4]

> You know that I have never asked anything else from you than that you attend to your studies, so that you won't be too old when you graduate. For a man who graduates when he is old is

[2] Paolo da Certaldo, *Libro di buoni costumi*, 104 and 193-94. Dominici, *Regola*, 141-42. Alberti, *Books on the Family*, I, in Guarino, tr., *The Albertis of Florence*, 61; original in Alberti, *Libri della famiglia*, 36.

[3] On the background of this prominent Pistoiese medical family see Chiappelli, *Medici e chirurghi pistoiesi*, 89-118; Chiti, "Marco Carafantoni"; and Verde, *Studio Fiorentino*, 3/1:356-57. A full index to these and other letters cited in this chapter is included in Appendix IV.

[4] Letter of M⁰ Marco to Antonio (17.iii or v.1459): "tue forze a pparare e a studiare. Non mi puoi fare chosa più grata e a risultare utile e onore."

like a man who buys only to sell at a loss; thus a man who graduates when he is old has wasted his time and his money in study, and his age doesn't allow him to earn either reputation or money.[5]

When you see things in the market which please you, close your eyes and shut your purse; otherwise you would reap loss and shame.[6]

If you do well, you will acquire reputation and money.[7]

Antonio's friends and relatives were not the only ones to navigate by those twin stars. Often linked, sometimes opposed, the terms reappear with tedious frequency in many other letters and treatises of the period.[8]

From the point of view of money and reputation, the career of a physician was attractive. Particularly in the period of the plague, medicine could be highly profitable, as chroniclers complained and doctors' accounts show. According to the Florentine *catasto* of 1427, the medical profession was the third richest occupational group in the city, in

TABLE 4-1
Wealth of Doctors and Other Occupational Groups (1427)

Occupation	Mean Net Wealth (fl.)
Bankers	8,748
Merchants and wool dealers	3,301
Physicians	3,063
All doctors	1,856
Other textile dealers	1,696
Lawyers (and notaries?)	1,079
Apothecaries	1,019
Stationers	599

SOURCES: Herlihy and Klapisch-Zuber, *Les toscans*, 229; Catasto 65 to 83 and Catasto-Campioni del Monte-San Giovanni-1427.

[5] Letter of Mº Marco to Antonio (22.xii.1458): "Tu ssai ch'io non t'ò preghato d'altro se non che tu attend'a studiare acciò che ttu non abbi a uscire vechio di studio, chè chi escie vechio di studio è chome chi chonpera una merchantantia per perdere; choxì chi escie vechio di studio à perduto el tenpo a studiare e chonsummati e denare, e ll'età non patiscie ghuadagnare nè fama nè denari ecc."

[6] Letter of Mº Marco to Antonio (7.x.1458): "E quando tu vedi delle chose in merchato che tti piaccino, chiudi gli ochi e sserra la borsa, chè non facciendo chosì tene risulterebbe danno e verghognia."

[7] Letter of Talento di Simone to Antonio (17.?.[1460]): "riusciendo tu valente tene risulterà onore e utile."

[8] See, for example, the letters from Mº Lorenzo Sassoli da Prato to Francesco Datini of 7.x.1402, 20.vii.1403, and 15.iii.1403/4.

the classification used by Herlihy and Klapisch-Zuber. The mean net wealth of households headed by doctors (surgeons and empirics as well as physicians) came to fl. 1,856, and that of physicians alone to fl. 3,063 (see table 4-1).[9]

The *onore* of the physician was also well established in Florence. In the city's sumptuary laws, as we saw in Chapter Two, doctors of medicine, including university-trained surgeons, were one of three privileged groups (lawyers or knights, doctors, and notaries) with special dispensation from the regulations against unnecessary display. The doctor's bier could be decorated with gold brocade and fur, his corpse dressed in a miniver-lined cloak, his funeral procession accompanied by a horse bearing a book (the symbol of his learning) and eight wax torches instead of the usual four.[10] In life, special laws also allowed the physician to wear a silver or gold belt buckle, a long robe, and a cloak lined with miniver.[11] Legally these privileges depended on the physician's university degree and were conferred as part of the ceremony of the *conventus*. But they were also considered symbols of the peculiar moral dignity of the medical profession, as Bernardino da Siena emphasized in one of his sermons: "What does the gentleman's coat of arms signify? That he is a gentleman in his speech, his heart, and his deeds; and if he acts otherwise, the coat of arms is not truly his. And what does it mean that the doctor wears miniver? It means that he must treat each person with charity and faith, in his speech, his heart and his deeds."[12] In this period, then, medicine was a prestigious occupation. It did not, perhaps, have the cachet in Italy that it enjoyed in northern Europe and other, less commercially developed parts of Italy, where it and the other "liberal" professions of law, the notariate, and the priesthood ranked above all forms of trade in dignity and honor. Nonetheless, even in Florence, where large-scale commerce

[9] See Herlihy and Klapisch-Zuber, *Les toscans*, 299. Their results depend on a rather quirky grouping of occupations. Thus they have amalgamated doctors and barbers, lowering the average wealth of this group to fl. 461. The same thing seems to have been done for lawyers and notaries; lawyers alone would probably have ended up considerably higher on the list. For the wealth of individual doctors in the *catasto* of 1427 see Appendix III.

[10] Communal statute of 1415, IV, 13-16, *Statuta populi et communis Florentiae*, 2:374-76. See also statute of the captain of the people of 1355, IV, 78 (Statuti-11, fols. 150r-153r), and statute of the captain of the people of 1321, V, 7, in Caggese, *Statuti*, 1:222.

[11] On the laws dealing with doctors' dress see Corsini, *Il costume*, 3-7, and Ciasca, *L'arte*, 291-92. Doctors' wives also had special privileges. As in the case of all such sumptuary laws in Florence, it is unlikely that these were effectively enforced.

[12] Bernardino da Siena, *Le prediche volgari*, 335. Bernardino makes a similar point about the special attire of the lawyer.

was accorded great respect, the physician was considered of equal occupational status with the international merchant or banker.[13]

Moved by such considerations, parents usually decided on a child's career as a physician quite early in order to provide him with the appropriate education. After primary school the boy would probably have gone to one of the more advanced city schools, along with other university hopefuls, for the basics of logic and grammar.[14] The next step was to choose a university. The letters from Maestro Marco to Antonio during his years at the Florentine *studio* illuminate the factors involved in this decision. One of the most important was academic reputation. Not all universities were of equal quality. In the mid-fourteenth century Bologna apparently had the faculty of choice for medical studies, although it seems to have been surpassed by Padua during the course of the fifteenth century. Florence was not in the front rank but grouped with a cluster of smaller and less illustrious universities, including Perugia, Siena, Ferrara, and Pavia.[15] Antonio, like his compatriots, was attracted by the reputations of Padua and Bologna. His father at first encouraged his hopes of transferring from Florence to one of those two universities. "Content yourself," he wrote, "to stay there for two or three years so as to master the fundamentals, and in the meantime I will arrange to place you at Padua or at Bologna with what money you require, wherever seems more appropriate to me, so that you will reach the goal if it please God."[16] By the end of Antonio's second year, however, financial considerations had come to the fore, and Maestro Marco had other plans: "And where you say that you

[13] Herlihy and Klapisch-Zuber, *Les toscans*, 574-75.

[14] There were three types of school in Florence in this period: one in which reading and writing were taught, one in which future merchants learned practical mathematics, and one which prepared prospective university entrants in Latin grammar and logic. On elementary education in Renaissance Florence see Bec, *Les marchands écrivains*, 384-91.

[15] The question of the relative reputations of Bologna and Padua in this period requires further research. Bologna had been the first university for medical studies in Italy in the first half of the fourteenth century, but by the beginning of the fifteenth century that position had apparently been taken over by Padua—"the most famous university that we have in Italy," according to a letter of Mº Lorenzo Sassoli da Prato to Francesco Datini (1.vi.1401). Padua maintained its primacy in medical studies throughout the fifteenth and sixteenth centuries; nonetheless, at least in the beginning of our period, Bologna retained much of its glory and seems to have been the most popular university for Florentine citizens. On the relative standing of the University of Florence see Park, "Readers," 251-52, 271.

[16] Letter from Mº Marco to Antonio (19.xi.1459): "Sie chontento volere istare due o tre anni chostì, tanto sia un pocho introdotto, ed io in questo mezo ordinerò metterti in Padova chol bisognio tuo o in Bolognia, dove io vedrò più attitudine, tanto che ttu giungha al palio, se ffia piacere d'Idio."

would be happier at Bologna than at Siena, I would like to do your will, but . . . we will choose the most promising and profitable alternative."[17] Antonio's future income, he reminded his son, would not depend on where he took his medical degree.[18]

As Maestro Marco's later letters show, reputation was not the only factor in choosing a university; expense also figured. It cost a good deal merely to maintain a son at the university, counting room, board, and masters' fees. Maestro Marco estimated that it would run him fl. 30 a year to send Antonio to Bologna, as opposed to lesser sums for Florence, where he could live with friends of the family, or for Siena, which had a residential college, the Sapienza.[19] A related issue was the emotional and moral environment of the university. Like many fathers, Maestro Marco worried about sending a fifteen-year-old away alone to a large city, partly for fear that the child would be homesick and partly "because it seems very dangerous to send young sons away from paternal authority, to live and associate with other, misguided youths and with foreign and unfamiliar people. This is responsible for the fall of many promising minds."[20] In fact, Maestro Marco eventually determined that Antonio would go first to Florence, where, as he reminded him, the family had so many friends and relatives that "it is as if you had never left home," and then to the Sapienza, where his brother had ecclesiastical connections and students lived under the watchful eyes of university authorities.[21]

Once at the university, the future doctor followed a well-defined course of study, progressing from Latin grammar, if he still needed it, to more strictly professional training, first in logic, then in philosophy, and finally in medicine. The timetable for university studies in arts and medicine was flexible. As a rule, boys were sent off at about fifteen (Antonio's age). Most finished the arts course in their early or mid-twenties and then began their medical studies; this was a somewhat shorter course which seems to have taken four or five years to com-

[17] Letter from M° Marco to Antonio (6.vii.1460): "E dove di' che ti chontenteresti più tosto in Bolognia che'n Siena, io farei della volontà tua, ma . . . dove vedremo che stia più utile e vantagio, quivi ci apicheremo."
[18] Letter of M° Marco to Antonio (19.vii.1460).
[19] Letter of M° Marco to Antonio (19.xi.1459).
[20] Florentine provision of 1428/9, in Alessandro Gherardi, *Statuti*, 211. This was given as an argument for supporting an adequate local *studio* with a residential college.
[21] Letter of M° Marco to Antonio (26.ix.1458): "A me non pare essendo chostì che tu sia fuori di chasa tua, e massime avendi tu chostì Messer Tommaso, Ser Giovanni e Buonachorso e Iacopo di ser Antonio, che sono quello medessimo che siamo noi." On the general growth of residential colleges in fifteenth-century European universities see Ariès, *Centuries of Childhood*, 155-57.

plete, so that the doctor received his final medical degree in his late twenties.[22] Some students chose to remain in the same place for their entire university career, while others, like Antonio, were more peripatetic, changing schools (sometimes several times) in the course of their studies.[23]

A fact which constantly shines through Maestro Marco's letters as well as through many of the other documents concerning university life in this period is that a medical education demanded a great investment of time and money on the part of the aspiring doctor and his family, particularly compared with other, nonprofessional careers. Crafts and commerce or banking were learned in a period of apprenticeship, which lasted roughly six years, depending on the occupation. Boys entered this apprenticeship earlier—usually in their very early teens or even younger, because the necessary primary education was less elaborate—and stayed in it for less time than their counterparts at the university. Thus their economically productive life began about ten years earlier than a doctor's, and their living expenses were generally paid during apprenticeship, so that from the moment they began to train for their careers they were no longer a burden on the family finances.[24] The opposite was true of medical education. Not only was the cost to the family and the individual great in terms of income lost during the long years of study, but university costs were also high. Although Maestro Marco's estimate of fl. 30 a year may have been inflated for rhetorical purposes, it was not unrealistic; a piece of Florentine legislation from 1429 put the annual expense of maintaining a

[22] There was a good deal of variation within this pattern as to when one took the four exams (private and public, in arts and medicine). One could, as Antonio's father wished him to do, take both exams in arts and receive the A.D. before beginning medical school (letter from M° Antonio, 1.xi.1459); or one could take the private exam in arts but wait to be *conventuatus* in arts and medicine simultaneously (like M° Piero Toscanelli of Florence, who was licensed in arts at Padua in 1420, at the age of about 24, but who received his A.D. and M.D. together in 1424; see Zonta and Brotto, *Acta graduum*, vol. 1, nos. 544 and 603); or one could postpone all four exams until near the end of one's university career, like M° Iacopo di Coluccino da Lucca, who passed his private exam in arts in April 1364 and his private exam in medicine in October of the same year and who was *conventuatus* in both in January 1365 (see his diary, ASL: Ospedale di S.-Luca 180, verso of first, unnumb. fol.).

[23] Examples of more mobile students include M° Ugo Benzi, who studied first at Florence and then at Bologna (Lockwood, *Ugo Benzi*, 23-24); M° Lorenzo Sassoli da Prato, who went from Bologna to Padua (Origo, *Merchant of Prato*, 339-40; note that M° Lorenzo did not, as Origo claims, study at Ferrara); and M° Giovanni di m° Dino da Firenze, who petitioned in 1374 to take his public exam at Bologna even though he had done all his work at the University of Florence (Gloria, *Monumenti*, 2:105).

[24] See Herlihy and Klapisch-Zuber, *Les toscans*, 574-75.

son at a foreign university at fl. 20.[25] Additional, occasional costs raised the total even higher. Books, for example, were expensive; the average medical library in the *catasto* of 1427 was declared at fl. 52—one very practical argument in favor of occupational inheritance among doctors, since students like Antonio relied heavily on borrowing books from relatives.[26] The *conventus* itself, including examination fees, new clothes, the procession, and the celebratory dinner, cost even more: Maestro Lorenzo Sassoli da Prato, who received his doctorate from Padua in 1402, projected his expenses for the entire proceedings at 70 ducats (roughly fl. 70).[27] Students often contributed to their upkeep by teaching—Antonio, for example, conducted *repetizioni*, or review tutorials, for less advanced students during his second year at Florence[28]— but the fees were small. If we accept recent estimates of the yearly salary of a day laborer as about fl. 40 (see Appendix I), we can understand what a drain the expenses of a medical education would have been, even for a relatively prosperous family like Antonio's.[29]

Most doctors' families must have found the investment worthwhile. They knew that the career of a physician could be both lucrative and honorable, and they thought that the university provided not only a professional education but also a cultural and moral one. For many small-town students the university was the first taste of city life, and the cities of fourteenth- and fifteenth-century Italy were the centers of its civilization. This was true for Antonio, moving as he did from Pistoia (a provincial town of some five thousand inhabitants in this period) to Florence, capital of the entire region and a flourishing cultural center. Maestro Marco had a strong sense of the value of an urban education, and he encouraged his son during the initial home-

[25] See Alessandro Gherardi, *Statuti*, 211: "avendo noi di questo danno investigato, troviamo fuori della città e provincia vostra circa ducento cinquanta scolari continuamente vivere, i quali traggono del nostro distrecto circa cinquemilia fiorini per anno. . . ." This financial drain was one of the reasons given for attempting to reform the Florentine *studio* in order to prevent Florentine students from going abroad; see Molho, *Florentine Public Finances*, 134-35.

[26] *Catasto* figures are given in Appendix III. Many letters between Antonio and his father and uncle involve the loan of books. See, for example, the letters of Mᵒ Marco to Antonio (?.i.1459, 8.v.1459, 19.xi.1459, 13.xii.1459).

[27] Letter of Mᵒ Lorenzo to Datini (30.viii.1402). Cf. Le Goff, "Academic Expenses," esp. appendix I.

[28] See letter of Mᵒ Marco to Antonio (19.xi.1459) and letter of Mᵒ Bartolomeo to Antonio (1.ii.1460). Antonio probably taught grammar or basic logic.

[29] Mᵒ Marco frequently reminded Antonio of the family's sacrifices; see, for example, his letter of 15.xii.1458: "aresti da mme tutte quelle chose mi fusse possibile, e patirei per te, io e lla familia mia, ogni disagio."

sickness with a proverb also quoted by Paolo da Certaldo: "the country breeds strong animals and the city valiant men."[30]

And indeed urban life did begin to seduce Antonio. The letters from his first autumn in Florence are full of complaints about loneliness, homesickness, poverty, and discomfort. Maestro Marco replied again and again with encouragement: "You must swallow these pills if you want to perfect your character [virtù]," he wrote in September, "because as soon as you are competent to take your doctorate, you can see patients in the comfort of your own home."[31] By December, however, Antonio had settled in well to city life, and the encouragement in his father's letters yielded to scolding.

> I am informed that you spend the lesser part of your time studying and the greater part in the Piazza and in the Mercato Vecchio. The reason I sent you [to Florence] was so that you would study and make an effort to become capable, and not so that you would stroll around in the Piazza and lounge around the marketplace with the idlers. . . . Someone asked me, "How is your Antonio doing?" I answered, "He's in Florence studying," and another replied, "He was at the circus, and he can't study very much, because I never see him except in the Piazza or around town."[32]

Antonio's replies to these attacks show his growing independence and self-confidence. Cut off my funds if you wish, he wrote his father, but "I will see that I have what I need, so there is no need for you to scold me. I don't want you to think that I can't live without you."[33] By the

---

[30] Letter of M° Marco to Antonio (27.viii or ix.1458): "lla villa fa grosse bestie e lla città fa valenti uomini." Cf. Paolo da Certaldo, *Libro di buoni costumi*, no. 103. Note that the risks of city life were also felt to be great, particularly in the matter of morals. M° Bartolomeo felt compelled to warn Antonio of the pitfalls of life in Florence: "Toto meo vite tempore ullam civitatem orbis unquam inveni sicut quam noscis tot fraudibus ac vitiis redimitam" (letter of 27.iv.1460).

[31] Letter of M° Marco to Antonio (26.ix.1458): "E ti bisognia inghiottire di choteste pillore se vuoi venire a perfetione di virtù, chè quanto più tosto serai valente in forma ti possi dottorare, potrai stare a medichare a chasa tua e stare negli agi tuoi."

[32] Letter of M° Marco to Antonio (15.xii.1458): "sono avistato che'l minor tenpo che ttu ispenda sie in istudiare e in ischuola e il magiore è in Piaza e in Merchato Vechio. La'ntentione perchè tu sse' chostà mia è perchè tu studi e chon sollecitudine adoperi le tue forze in diventare valente, e non è perchè tu stia in Piaza a piazegiare e in Merchato Vechio dove istanno i ghiottoni." Letter of 22.xii.1458: "Uno mi domandò, Che è d'Antonio vostro, ed io rispuosi, Egli è a fFirenze a studiare, et e' mi fu risposto per un'altro che era al cierchio e deba studiar pocho, perchè io no'l'truovo mai se nonn è in Piaza o per Firenze."

[33] Letter of Antonio to M° Marco (xii.1458): "e tanto farò ch'io arò il bisognio mio,

spring of his second year Antonio had abandoned all plans to visit Pistoia before completing his arts studies and was eager to leave Florence for the farther shores of Bologna and Padua.

The transition to the city and the university was probably difficult at first for most students. But once the jump was made, the attractions of city life were hard to ignore. This applied particularly to doctors and lawyers, for whom the city and the university offered not only intellectual and cultural stimulation but also a forum for their ideas and a market for their services. *Onore* and *utile* lived in the cities.

ESTABLISHING A REPUTATION: TEACHING AND WRITING

Once the physician had received his doctoral insignia from the hands of the bishop or the bishop's representative, he faced the decision of what to do with his newly won credentials. Many young doctors elected to return home, marry, matriculate in the guild, and begin building up a practice. But for those who were willing to sacrifice domestic stability and financial security temporarily in order to make a name for themselves—who in the language of the time coveted *utile* less than *onore*—another course beckoned. The path to a real medical reputation lay not in practice but in teaching and writing, and the place for that was the university.

This attitude underlies a letter from one of the most illustrious medical theorists of the early fifteenth century, Maestro Ugo Benzi da Siena. Maestro Ugo was at the peak of a brilliant medical career. He had already taught arts and medicine at Pavia, Piacenza, Bologna, Siena, and Parma, had disputed at Padua and Perugia, and was currently lecturing at the University of Florence.[34] The government of his native city had made several attempts to force him back to Siena; finally, in January 1423, Maestro Ugo formally asked the Consistory of Siena to allow him to remain at the University of Florence. "I pray you," he wrote,

> to permit me through your grace to continue my teaching career without interruption, as I have done to date, with God's help, for twenty-seven years; and I have never left off—not, I think, to the

---

sichè per questo non bisognia che voi facciate vituperio, e non voglio però che crediate ch'io non possa vivere senza voi."

[34] On the biography of M° Ugo see Lockwood, *Ugo Benzi*, chap. 2 and appendices I and II; supplementary documentation in the less reliable accounts of Garosi, "Alcuni documenti," and Castiglioni, "Ugo Benzi."

shame of our glorious city. Think, therefore, Magnificent Lords, how difficult it would be for me to abandon this noble and famous and liberal occupation and to give myself into the servitude of treating a lord, which, although perhaps profitable, is nonetheless obscure and without glory.[35]

We do not know to which "lord" Maestro Ugo was referring or why the Consistory wished him home. Nonetheless, the tenor of his letter is clear: medical practice, even at the highest level, was inferior to teaching, because it was only in teaching and writing that medicine was elevated from a mechanical to a liberal occupation and from an art to a science.[36] Thus the diminished monetary returns of teaching and writing were more than balanced by the increased nobility and honor.

Benzi may have been unusually successful in the field of academic medicine, but he was expressing an attitude which shaped the early careers of many fourteenth- and fifteenth-century Florentine physicians. It was common for those who could afford the lost income and face the prospect of a temporarily unsettled and hand-to-mouth existence to teach for a while between finishing the M.D. and entering practice. (Such physicians usually began by lecturing on the relatively elementary subject of logic before moving up to philosophy and finally to medicine.)[37] One of the best documented examples of a Florentine doctor who chose to launch his medical career in this ambitious manner is Maestro Lorenzo d'Agnolo Sassoli da Prato, who left a large number of letters from this period in his life.[38]

Maestro Lorenzo finished his studies at the University of Padua and was elected, even before his *conventus*, to read medicine there for the coming academic year (1401/2)—a flattering appointment in view of his youth and Padua's reputation.[39] The next year he was invited to

---

[35] Transcribed in Castiglioni, "Ugo Benzi," doc. VII (99-100), and Garosi, "Alcuni documenti," 92n. On this episode see Garosi, "Alcuni documenti," 102-11. Benzi may also have been swayed by the uncharacteristically large salary of fl. 600 voted him by the University of Florence; see Park, "Readers, 279-80.

[36] This was a commonplace in academic medical writing of this period; see, for example, Siraisi, "Taddeo Alderotti and Bartolomeo da Varignana," 27-39.

[37] A typical Florentine example is Mᵒ Donato d'Agostino Bartolini, who received his M.D. from the *Studio fiorentino* in the fall of 1431 and was successively elected to read logic (1431/32), philosophy (1432/33), and medicine (1438/39). See Alessandro Gherardi, *Statuti*, 414; Park, "Readers," 288, 290, 295. Such postdoctoral teaching differed in degree and kind from the *repetizioni*, or review tutorials offered by students like Antonio di mᵒ Marco da Pistoia (see note 28 above).

[38] For the biography of Mᵒ Lorenzo see Guasti, *Intorno alla vita*, 3-8.

[39] Letter of 1.vi.1401: "considerando che in sì piccola età io sia posto a sì fatta letura

read at both Bologna and Ferrara, choosing the latter after much agonizing.[40] In his letters home to Francesco Datini, a Pratese merchant he had adopted as parent and confidant after his father's death in the plague of 1400, Maestro Lorenzo emphasized that he had elected to teach in the interests of reputation: "The *onore* is great, even if the *utile* is less good, because honor comes before money."[41] He had in fact made a number of sacrifices in order to enhance his professional name. He was forced—without any discernible regret—to put off plans for marrying, and his letters from these years reflect an unstable and peripatetic existence. He moved four times within three years, and each decision caused considerable anxiety.[42] But the main hardship was financial: the stipends of beginning lecturers were always small and often unreliably paid, particularly to foreigners. (Annual salaries of fl. 30 or less were common at the University of Florence, hardly enough to live on.) Maestro Lorenzo complained frequently about his financial situation; he sold off portions of his patrimony and borrowed sums of up to fl. 100 from Datini.[43] Financial worries finally forced him to abandon his ambitious plans for establishing a reputation in the heady field of academic medicine. In August 1403 he informed Datini of his unwilling decision to abandon teaching for medical practice, vehemently cursing his luck: "And I am moved to such wicked words not only because of the material loss but because all my honor and my desires pull me in the other direction. I thought with part of my inheritance and with the small salaries they give young readers like me that I could stay for a while in the universities, in order to acquire a little poor

---

come quella di medicina, et maximamente in tale studio come è questo, il quale al dì d'ogi è'l più famoso studio che noi abiamo in Italia." Note that a large part of the honor lay in in Maestro Lorenzo's appointment to read medicine without passing through the lower ranks of logic and philosophy.

[40] See letters of 8.vi.1402 and 7.x.1402. M° Lorenzo was *conventuatus* in medicine on 14.x.1402 (Gloria, *Monumenti*, 2:395). He apparently turned down the offer from Bologna because of the unstable situation in the university there; see letter of 30.viii.1402: "Io non ò ardire d'andarvi per le diavolerie e sospecti di costà, chè per altro rispetto vi posso andare liberamente, per quello che io sono informato di là; onde io sto confuso e con maninconia e non so che partito pigliarmi, maximamente vegiendo questo studio [Padua] ancora dovere andare male, e di studio non vorrei se io potessi fare altro uscire, perchè mi sta troppo buono usare con gli scolari a rispetto dell'atre [*sic*] usanze del mondo. Spero che idio non mi abandonerà in questo punto."

[41] Letter of 7.x.1402: "L'onore è grande posto che l'utile non sia sì grande, perchè prima ne viene l'onore che l'utile."

[42] See letter of 27.x.1401 and that of 30.viii.1402, quoted in note 40.

[43] See letters of 15.xi.1401, 12.ii.1401/2, 8.vi.1402, 30.viii.1402, 19.x.1402, and 20.vii.1403. M° Lorenzo was also constantly having to defend himself from Datini's charges of extravagance.

honor. .... But I have no alternative, since the heavens turn against me."[44]

Although not all Florentine doctors saw their hopes of academic success dashed as early as Maestro Lorenzo, none from this period achieved either the widespread fame or the distinguished university career of Maestro Ugo Benzi, who abandoned teaching exclusively for private practice only at the ripe age of fifty-six, to become the court physician of Niccolò d'Este, marquis of Ferrara. Nor could any match the oeuvre of commentaries, treatises, and *consilia* which were the product of Maestro Ugo's career.[45] But there were several doctors with strong Florentine ties who achieved a certain eminence in the world of the universities. As we will see in Chapter Six, three—Maestro Iacopo di maestro Bartolo da Prato, Maestro Lodovico di Bartolo da Gubbio, and Maestro Giovanni Baldi, a naturalized Florentine from Faenza—taught primarily at the second-rate *Studio fiorentino* and achieved modest local fame through their lecturing and their writing. But two others—Maestro Tommaso Del Garbo, from Florence, and Maestro Antonio di maestro Guccio, from Scarperia—gained real eminence as academic physicians.

Maestro Tommaso, son of the even more illustrious medical professor, Maestro Dino Del Garbo, lectured at Perugia, Bologna, and Padua for many years before returning to Florence just after 1348 to teach in the newly established university.[46] His younger contemporary Filippo Villani sang his praises:

> He was a very great philosopher and famous in medicine. And because his name was known all over Italy, he acquired such esteem and such a reputation for learning and conscientiousness in practice that the most powerful lords, in which Italy abounds, felt that they would die if Tommaso himself did not treat them. Idol-

[44] Letters of 20.vii.1403 and 15.iii.1403/4: "Or pensate che consolatione io posso avere, che io priego idio che ciò che io vo' vada come andò Sodoma, e così le carni e l'avere di chi n'è cagione, aciò che io esca di tante angoscie. E a sì villano parlare non mi muovo solamente per lo danno, ma perchè io mi vego ongni mio onore e pensieri andare al contrario, inperochè io pensavo con parte della mia entrata e con quegli picoli salari e quali si danno a' miei pari giovani che legono potere stare un tenpo per gli studi aciò che io m'aaquistassi un poco di povero onore. .... Or io non posso altro poichè il cielo per me volge alla contraria."

[45] Lockwood, *Ugo Benzi*, 30. For an exhaustive treatment of the manuscripts and printed editions of Benzi's works see Lockwood's appendices IV, V, VIII-XIII.

[46] Biographical information on M° Tommaso del Garbo is still remarkably scarce, considering his social and intellectual eminence. For a rough outline of his life see Corsini, "Nuovo contributo"; Cappellini, "Date importanti" and "Ancora di Maestro Tommaso."

ized by the Italians almost as another Esculapius, he became extremely rich through large fees and enjoyed a splendid and luxurious life, so that he was sometimes considered negligent.
Nonetheless, he did not leave the academy or his studies. . . . He
composed many works on theoretical and practical medicine, which
because of their utility are constantly referred to in the universities.[47]

Here, as in Benzi's letter to Siena, we see the primacy of academic
medicine. The fame which sparked Maestro Tommaso's successful
practice had its roots in his teaching and writing. Realizing this, he
never entirely abandoned theory for practice; according to Villani, at
his death in 1370 he was still at work on a commentary on Aristotle's
De anima as well as a medical summa, which was to be his crowning
achievement.[48]

It is important to emphasize that academic medicine never developed in a vacuum; throughout their careers Maestro Tommaso Del
Garbo and his colleagues at the *studio* supplemented their teaching
salaries by income from medical practice, particularly in their later years,
when they were sought after by popes and princes impressed by the
reputation they had established in the Italian universities. But the university was not the only place a doctor could acquire credentials as a
theorist and scientist, as opposed to a mere technician. This was also
possible when private practice was combined with writing and public
disputation; thus even non-academic physicians could prove themselves particularly competent in medicial theory and therefore worthy
of special respect and courtly appointments, as another set of doctor's
letters illustrates.

Maestro Naddino di Aldobrandino da Prato had been living and
working in Florence. In the fall of 1386 he traveled to Avignon, seat
of the court of the schismatic pope Clement VII, where there was a
substantial Pratese trading community, with a letter of recommendation to Piero Corsini, cardinal of Florence.[49] By the spring of 1387 he

[47] Filippo Villani, *Vite*, 30-31.

[48] Ibid. For a discussion of M° Tommaso's *Summa* see below, Chapter Six. His *De anima* has been lost, if indeed it ever existed.

[49] On M° Naddino and his correspondence see Brun, "Quelques italiens." He had matriculated in the Florentine Guild of Doctors, Apothecaries, and Grocers in 1373 and had apparently established a residence and a practice in Florence, since he was active in the guild in the late 1370s and appears in the city tax records by 1379. (See AMS-9; Ciasca, *Statuti*, 304; Prestanze-368, fol. 48v.) On the links between Prato and Avignon and the situation in Avignon in this period see Origo, *Merchant of Prato*, chap. 1, esp. 6ff.

had begun to establish himself as a doctor of some repute in ecclesiastical circles. In a letter home from April of that year he referred to the high intellectual standards that his cultivated patients required of their personal doctors. "Every day they question me on medicine or on philosophy. And I know the score, because if I did not study day and night, I—with all my experience—would not be able to fence with them.[50] This theme often reappears in Maestro Naddino's letters. The next month he was lamenting that the chests containing his books had not yet come from Prato, because their arrival was crucial to advancing his reputation: "And if I had had my books I could have performed some pretty scientific turn which would have done me honor." Maestro Naddino did not specify the "turn" he had in mind, but he was probably referring to a public disputation resulting in a written *questio* on a medical subject or to a *consilium*, a short analysis of an interesting case with a diagnosis and prescription for treatment.[51] Either would have enhanced the reputation for theoretical expertise he had acquired during consultations with his illustrious and demanding clients.

We know that the Guild of Doctors, Apothecaries, and Grocers sponsored medical disputations in Florence, and it would certainly have been possible to make a name, at least locally, through public performance. But the surest way to win fame outside the university was by writing. Short *questiones* and *consilia*, especially *consilia* written for highly placed clients, brought a certain amount of honor; the real fame, however, was reserved for those who produced longer works: commentaries, treatises, and summas. The most celebrated Florentine doctor in the fourteenth and fifteenth centuries, for example—with the possible exception of Maestro Tommaso Del Garbo—seems never to have been associated with a university or to have disputed publicly. Maestro Niccolò di Francesco Falcucci da Borgo San Lorenzo was apparently Maestro Tommaso's own doctor.[52] His reputation was based on a single enormous medical treatise, variously called the *Practica* or *Sermones*, a work which acquired considerable renown; it is mentioned by contem-

---

[50] Letter to Monte Angiolini (11.iv.1387): "Tucto giorno pongono questioni o in medicina o in filosofia. E so ben come'l fatto va, chè io ch'ò pur vedute delle cose, se non fosse il grande studio ch'io fo di dì e di notte, non mi potrò scharmire di loro." See also the letter of 7.i.1386/7: "Sono sempre in su' libri e mai non escho."

[51] Letter to Monte (30.v.1387): "E avendo auti libri are' fatto qua alcuno bell'atto scientifico che m'arebbe fatto honore." On the genres of *questio* and *consilium* see Siraisi, *Taddeo Alderotti*, chaps. 8-9.

[52] See the rather peculiar account in BNF: Magl. XV, 71. On Falcucci's life and work see Ristori, "Niccolò Falcucci."

porary chroniclers and figures in virtually every extant inventory of doctors' libraries from this period.

Such doctors represent the highest levels of the medical profession in Renaissance Florence, and indeed in Renaissance Italy. In all cases their reputation—their professional *onore*—arose less from their practice than from their scientific work, that is, their teaching and writing. Some doctors, like Maestro Lorenzo Sassoli, were content with a modicum of fame; having taught for a few years after earning the doctorate in medicine, they entered private practice with enhanced prestige, although they never became involved enough in academic medicine to produce a medical oeuvre. On a somewhat larger scale doctors like Falcucci, Maestro Tommaso Del Garbo, and Maestro Antonio da Scarperia, the most illustrious Florentine physicians of their time, won their names first within the medical academy itself. But in all three cases their fame soon spilled over into the lay community, making them into general culture heroes—a part of the intellectual patrimony of which informed Florentines were so proud, as we can see in Villani's life of Maestro Tommaso, in Sozomeno da Pistoia's chronicle entry on Maestro Niccolò, or in the communal provision celebrating Maestro Antonio's little pills.[53] In this way, by combining writing and teaching with a flourishing private practice, they acquired not only a great reputation but also a large and affluent clientele.

BUILDING A CLIENTELE: CONTACTS AND CONTRACTS

Relatively few physicians sought to put teaching and writing at the center of their professional lives. Once they had left the university, most effectively severed their ties with academic medicine, and with them their aspirations to an international reputation and the higher reaches of medical *onore*. They chose, rather, to enter the world of practice and of *utile*; returning home or to some other promising town, they married, acquired houses, and set about establishing a practice. This last task was not always easy, particularly for a newcomer to the

[53] See note 47 above. Sozomeno da Pistoia, *Chronicon universale*, 3: "Nicolaus medicus Florentie moritur, opus magnum de omni medicina relinquens ex multis veteribus confectum." Alessandro Gherardi, *Statuti*, 471-72: "et messe [Mo Antonio] mesi quarantadua et più di tempo nella compositione et ricecta di tali pillole, le quali durante la sua vita feciono grandissima utilità a' corpi degli huomini che quelle usavano, perchè con diligentia si componevano, et le cose medicinali che in quelle si mettevano si sceglievono et toglievansi in tutta perfectione, donde ne seguiva, oltre alla salute de' corpi, lo honore dello'nventore, il quale è il premio che dagli huomini savi delle loro honeste et laboriose opere et in vita havere et dopo la vita lasciare a' suoi discendenti si disidera. . . ."

community. In a town like Florence, well supplied with doctors, a young physician with no reputation and no experience could find it initially difficult to attract patients. In the corporate world of medical practice, doctors and patients alike set great store by personal contacts. Thus the new doctor's fortunes depended heavily on connections—family, friends, and other members of the profession. Through them he acquired both private patients and the institutional clients which were the bread and butter of many practices. From letters, diaries, and other archival sources we can reconstruct this process of building a clientele in some detail.

Family ties were among the first and most direct connections exploited by doctors in an effort to establish a practice. Obviously much was done through simple recommendations by relatives and family friends to prospective patients. But because there was a great deal of occupational intercourse within medicine and between medicine and related fields like pharmacy, families were often in a good position to help their junior members break into the profession. Many young doctors had fathers, uncles, in-laws, or other older male relatives who were themselves doctors and apothecaries and who could be expected to pass on clients through referrals or even through a joint practice. (It is hard to believe, for example, that a single fifteenth-century household like that of the Toscanelli, which included two sons and a father who were physicians, would have accommodated three entirely separate practices.)

Many older doctors must also have passed on their entire clienteles to their sons or younger relatives on death or retirement—occasions which, given the shorter life spans and the large gap in age between Florentine fathers and their children, would have happened at a much earlier stage in the young doctor's career than would be true today.[54] Certainly families passed on their institutional connections. Beginning in the first years of the fifteenth century, for example, the hospital of Santa Maria Nuova hired Maestro Giovanni di maestro Ciuccio da Civitavecchia as its bone doctor. It is no coincidence that on Maestro Giovanni's death the position passed to his son, Maestro Domenico, who held it for many years.[55] The same is true, as we have seen, of Maestro Iacopo dell'Ossa da Roma, salaried as bone doctor to the

[54] On these demographic patterns see Herlihy and Klapisch-Zuber, Les toscans, 399-400 and chaps. 14-15. Urban males, particularly those from the higher levels of society, tended to marry in their middle or late thirties. Thus in 1427, for example, M° Paolo (30) and M° Piero (31) Toscanelli were just beginning their careers, while their father M° Domenico (67) was close to ending his (Catasto-65, fol. 96v).

[55] M° Giovanni began his tenure in 1402 (SMN-4453, fol. 102r); by 1427 he was dead, and his son M° Domenico had taken over his position (SMN-4477, fol. 39r).

city's poor in the years before 1348. When he died of the plague, the commune hired two of his sons, Maestro Giovanni and Maestro Niccolò; the latter was replaced in 1365 by the third brother, Maestro Stefano.

The number of sons following their fathers into medical careers dropped in the fifteenth century, but the young doctor could still acquire new clients through professional referrals and personal patronage. Although referrals were common, as Zerbi's *On Precautions to Be Taken by Doctors* and certain rubrics in the statutes of the Guild of Doctors, Apothecaries, and Grocers indicate,[56] probably the most important contribution to the young doctor's clientele was made through a wider lay network of personal recommendation. We can see this process at work in letters concerning the early career of Maestro Lorenzo Sassoli da Prato. When Maestro Lorenzo left the university, his friend and protector Francesco Datini mobilized both institutional and personal connections in Florence on his behalf. Datini began by trying to obtain an ecclesiastical contract. He recommended Maestro Lorenzo first to Fra Giovanni Dominici, Francesco's own confessor and prior of the local Dominican convent of Santa Maria Novella, and then to Ser Lapo Mazzei, his closest friend and notary of the hospital of Santa Maria Nuova. "In your letter of yesterday," Ser Lapo replied to Datini.

> where you talked about the partridge, you reminded me of Maestro Lorenzo. If you see him, tell him that I haven't heard a word from him and that—through my own fault—I haven't managed to see him, but that I have well in hand the matter of his commission to become doctor at the convent of Santa Maria Novella. Now I hear that Fra Giovanni has left, who would have been very useful to him. . . . I am certain that he was one of the ones who was favorable to us. As they say, "Strike while the iron is hot." Tell him so. I think he hasn't said anything to me for fear of bothering me, but I am pleased to help him, remembering that I was similarly helped in my youth. May God preserve him. I also want to talk to him concerning our hospital, to open the door for him.[57]

Nor did Datini and Mazzei stop at institutions; they also recommended Maestro Lorenzo to influential or well-to-do acquaintances

---

[56] See statute of 1349, II, 69-70 (Ciasca, *Statuti,* 184-86).

[57] Letter of Ser Lapo Mazzei to Francesco Datini (n.d.), in Mazzei, *Lettere,* 1:240-41.

they knew to be in poor health. Mazzei touched on this process in another letter several years later:

> Yesterday at my house I spoke with Messer Rinaldo [Gianfigli-azzi], . . . and to hear him talk, he has been sick for five months with a terrible illness and is about to succumb to it. I described the goodness and trustworthiness of Maestro Lorenzo to him; he was very glad to hear about it, and thinks he will send for him from Arezzo. And in order not to offend his other regular doctors, he promised to send for him yesterday under the pretext that he had received a letter from you charging him for your own peace of mind to have Maestro Lorenzo see him. He says that he doesn't know him except through his good name and through what he has heard from you and from some woman, and that he intends to hire him. I told Maestro Lorenzo about all this.[58]

We can see a similar network of personal recommendation in the Avignon career of Maestro Naddino di Aldobrandino da Prato, another of Datini's correspondents. Maestro Naddino traveled to France in the company of a Florentine embassy including Datini's friend Messer Filippo Corsini, who seems to have given the doctor a recommendation to his brother, Cardinal Piero Corsini. Once in Avignon, Maestro Naddino found himself in good hands. The cardinal received him well; one contact led to another and he soon acquired a celestial clientele of bishops, archbishops, cardinals, and finally, in 1393, Pope Clement VII himself.[59]

But as Maestro Naddino's letters home make clear, he did not rely on recommendations alone; he also took pains to advertise himself, treating the social scene with the same seriousness he attached to intellectual display. Thus he seems to have transacted a good deal of professional business over meals. Several months after arriving, for example, he reported: "Thursday morning I ate with the cardinal of Amiens along with several other doctors. I pleased him greatly during our discussion, so that he called me aside before I left and asked me to attend him twice a week and be his doctor. He is powerful and wise and rich, and I hope to have much money and honor from him."[60]

---

[58] Ibid. (1.ix.1408); 2:131. Datini also recommended M° Lorenzo to the prior of the Servite convent; see M° Lorenzo's letters of 12.i.1407/8 and 13.iii.1407/8.

[59] See Brun, "Quelques italiens," 220. Also the letters of M° Naddino to Monte (11.iv.1387, 29.i.1388/9, 7.i.1386/7, ?.vii.1387) and to Datini (7.i.1386/7, 21.iii.1388/9, 13.iii.?); extracts in Brun, "Quelques italiens," 222-28.

[60] Letter of M° Naddino to Datini (7.i.1386/7): "Et giovedì mattina mangiai con cardinale d'Amiense con certi altri medici, e fu in sua presenza certa collatione della

A letter dated two weeks later is equally revealing. In it Maestro Nad-dino put in a large order for things to be sent from home: the miniver lining of his cloak, fifty wheels of good cheese ("for gifts"), silverware ("because I must eat with lords often, and I have had to borrow a knife"), and above all news. "Because I associate a great deal with my lord [cardinal of Amiens] and with other lords here," he wrote, "and I see that they greatly enjoy hearing news from [Italy], I would appreciate it if when you write you would sometimes speak of the things happening in our country, particularly in Florence, such as drawings of the priors or election of embassies or clergy from Genova or from Lucca, or people from Rome, or whatever other news there is."[61] To reach the highest levels of the consulting profession, in other words, the physician had to demonstrate not only medical competence but also something of the culture and the polish of his more influential patients. As Zerbi recommended, "he must appear praiseworthy to the public in his manner, behavior, and dress."[62]

Doctors' diaries and account books give an even better sense of the shape of a medical career, since they sequentially record new contracts, clients, and sometimes even yearly income. The *ricordanza* of the physician Maestro Iacopo di Coluccino Bonavia da Lucca is particularly rich in such financial details.[63] Maestro Iacopo received his doctorates in art and medicine from the University of Florence in January 1366. He practiced for a short while in Florence and its subject town of San Gimignano before returning to Lucca, where he set himself up as a physician. The first folio of his diary contains a list of his annual earnings from medical practice between 1366 and 1408; these figures give a good idea of the progress of his career.[64] Maestro Iacopo's income

---

quale assai piacqui al cardinale, in tanto che mmi chiamò da parte anzi io partisse, e pregò mmi io il vicitasse due volte la septimana e fosse suo medico. Egli è potente singnore e savio e riccho, e spero da llui assai utile e honore."

[61] Letter of Mᵒ Naddino to Monte (21.i.1386/7): "e perchè uso assai con monsin-gnore e con altri singnori di qua, e vegio molto si dilectono d'udire novelle di costà, arei charo quando mi scrivi ne scrivessi alcuna volta delle cose che ocorrono in nostro paese, spetialmente a Firenze, come di tracte di priori o electione d'ambasciate o di quelli cherici da Genova o da Luca sieno, o gente da R[oma; could also be gente d'armi], o d'altra novità vi fosse."

[62] Zerbi, *De cautelis*, 71-72.

[63] Although Mᵒ Iacopo practiced for most of his life in the independent Tuscan city of Lucca, his experience was doubtless very similar to that of many Florentine physicians. On his career see Chiappelli, "Maestro Iacopo di Coluccino da Lucca."

[64] *Ricordanza* of Mᵒ Iacopo di Coluccino da Lucca (ASL: Ospedale di S. Luca-180, verso of first, unnumb. fol.). The figures are as follows (note that Mᵒ Iacopo combined his figures for some years):

from medicine varied greatly from year to year, in response to circumstances and above all to the plague. The figures he cites bear out the accusations of contemporaries that doctors profited from the misfortunes of their patients during epidemics. In 1384, for example, he earned fl. 467, nearly double his income of the previous year, and in 1400, which saw the worst wave of plague since 1348, his earnings soared to fl. 498. Nonetheless, these fluctuations appear superimposed on a regular earning curve which began at a relatively low level, climbed through the 1380s and early 1390s (when Maestro Iacopo would have been in his mid-forties to mid-fifties), and declined gradually during the last years of his practice. The early part of the curve corresponded to the period in which he was establishing a reputation and acquiring a clientele; the central portion to the height of his career; and the last part to his later years, when health and declining vigor forced him to curtail his activities.

We can follow the steps by which a physician built up his clientele even more clearly in the *ricordanza* of Maestro Polidoro d'Antonio Bracali, a physician from Pistoia, who returned to his native town in June 1457 after a twenty-six-year absence. Maestro Polidoro's first move, in August of the same year, was to enter into a contract with an apothecary whereby for £70 a year he was to see patients in the shop and to order them medicines to be supplied on the premises.[65] Maestro Polidoro then began to accumulate a number of institutional contracts which, with the apothecary's salary, provided him with a guaranteed income, partly in currency and partly in kind. In January 1458 he was hired by the local hospital of Santa Maria del Ceppo on a nine-year contract. In April of the next year he was awarded the care of the Abbey of San Michele for six bushels (*staia*) of grain a year and, two days later, the care of the Abbey of San Bartolomeo at the same rate. His next new contract came in 1468, when he became doctor to the convent of the "Nuns of the Virgin" for the same amount. In 1469 he was renewed at the Ceppo, and his salary established at forty-eight

1370-1375: fl. 1246	1382: fl. 267	1388: fl. 420	1397: fl. 711
1376: fl. 184	1383: fl. 264	1389: fl. 358	1400: fl. 498
1378: fl. 385	1384: fl. 467	1390: fl. 282	1401: fl. 478
1379: fl. 239	1385: fl. 182	1391: fl. 321	1402: fl. 210
1380: fl. 274	1386: fl. 177	1392: fl. 278	1405: fl. 343
1381: fl. 324	1387: fl. 362	1394: fl. 378	1407: fl. 115.

[65] ASPist: Sala C, 2° piano, scaff. 238-39, Filza 2a, no. 18 (uninventoried), fols. 1r, 3r.

staia of grain and two pairs of capons.[66] Other, similar positions followed; his last was with the priory of Monteoliveto beginning in 1474, four years before his death.[67]

Maestro Polidoro's accounts reveal less concerning his private patients—those he saw neither at the apothecary's shop nor in the convents and hospital. We must assume, however, that things proceeded well on that front, since in 1473 he had acquired a reputation good enough to be called to treat Carlo Forteguerri, cardinal of Pistoia, during an extended illness.[68] This episode probably marked the height of Maestro Polidoro's career as a local practitioner in Pistoia. Doctors in a capital city like Florence, however, or those with a solid academic reputation, reached a stage in the later phases of their professional lives where they could supplement their daily practice not only with long-term institutional contracts but also with occasional consulting, a much more highly paid activity. If the need was great enough and the patient's finances could bear it, an illustrious doctor might be brought to treat a difficult case in person. More often the consultant gave his advice in absentia; someone, usually the principal attending physician, would write with a full description of the patient and his condition, and the consultant would reply with a *consilium*, or written opinion detailing his diagnosis and recommendations for treatment. A few very famous doctors raised this form of practice to a high art. Maestro Ugo Benzi da Siena, for example, left behind a corpus of more than a hundred *consilia* for important patients.[69]

In other cases, as we have seen, the communal government itself hired doctors as consultants, paying them at exorbitant rates. Such opportunities, however, were generally open only to physicians at the top of their profession.[70] Like Maestro Polidoro, the less illustrious contented themselves with the usual contracts and commissions. Even Maestro Polidoro may have flown a bit higher than most physicians, but his career was certainly typical in its outlines. Like Maestro Iacopo da Lucca, Maestro Lorenzo Sassoli, and many other physicians, he spent time abroad practicing, and possibly teaching, before returning to his native city. Once home, he immediately associated himself with

[66] Ibid., fols. 3v, 6r, 11v. A *staio* was about three-quarters of a bushel. Note that M° Polidoro inherited several of his *condotte* from a single doctor, M° Stefano Tavioli.

[67] Ibid., fols. 14v.

[68] Ibid., fol. 14r. See above, Chapter Three, note 93.

[69] See Lockwood, *Ugo Benzi*, 44-78 and appendices IX-X.

[70] This applies to both academic and nonacademic physicians. Note that it was primarily the former who produced *consilia* and primarily the latter (for example, M° Lorenzo Sassoli da Prato and M° Cristofano di Giorgio) who were hired by the commune.

an apothecary and began to collect ecclesiastical contracts and private patients in increasing numbers.

I should emphasize here, as in the previous chapter, that it seems to have been contracts which formed the core of the doctor's practice and which guaranteed his support regardless of the vagaries of his private clientele and the general health of the population. Neither was there any stigma attached to contractual and institutional work; instead it was often considered more desirable than treating any but the most eminent private patients. This applied even (or especially) to what would at first glance seem the least attractive types of institutional positions— doctors hired by hospitals and local governments to treat the city's poor, aged, and homeless. These contracts were among the most highly prized as both lucrative and prestigious. The bishop of Pistoia, recommending a doctor to succeed Maestro Polidoro at the hospital in 1477, wrote that his candidate "would like, both for *onore* and for *utile*, to be hired to practice in the Ceppo."[71] Maestro Stefano di maestro Iacopo dell'Ossa, Florence's public poor-doctor, left a will which showed him to be a rich man.[72] Other doctors saw such practice as a chance genuinely to serve the poor while acquiring a name for charity and probity, two qualities central to a doctor's reputation. Thus the doctors of the Florentine hospitals were often among the most respected members of the profession.[73] After each hospital-related entry in his *ricordanza*, Maestro Polidoro added a pious ejaculation, such as, "May the highest God give me grace by both the salvation of my soul and the health of their bodies."[74] Some doctors even donated their services, while others, like Maestro Cristofano di Giorgio, collected salaries during their lifetimes but made charitable bequests of any outstanding portions at their deaths.[75]

[71] Letter of the bishop of Pistoia to Lorenzo de' Medici (8.xii.1477); MAP-XXXV, 924: "desiderarebbe, e per l'onore e per l'utile, essere condotto al Ceppo a medicare."

[72] See SMN-60, fols. 336r-38v. M° Stefano's wealth is also attested to by his high *prestanze* assessments; for example Prestanze-156, fol. 20r, where his contribution was fixed at fl. 20 s. 13 d. 4.

[73] For example M° Cristofano di Giorgio was associated with the Florentine hospitals of San Gallo, San Giovanni Batista, and San Paolo. He was also consul of the Guild of Doctors, Apothecaries, and Grocers twenty-one times and one of the only two Florentine doctors in the fifteenth century to wield real political power in the communal government. Cf. Zerbi, *De cautelis*, 59: "Invero i poveri e i bisognosi non si devono opprimere nè denunziare per riguardo almeno alla pietà, poichè da qui nasce la lodevole fama del medico."

[74] *Ricordanza* of M° Polidoro Bracali, fol. 14v: "L'altissimo dio sia quello mi conceda gratia sia con salvamento della anima mia et salute delli corpi loro."

[75] M° Bandino di m° Giovanni Banducci, for example, was taken on in 1446 by the hospital of the Innocenti "at any hour and for any need" without salary; I owe this

One of the results of the ready availability of hospital, communal, and other institutional contracts was that most physicians enjoyed a highly diversified practice, which at any one time could have included patients from all segments of society as well as a mixture of private and institutional clients. This is easily documentable for physicians, with whom this chapter is primarily concerned, but it seems also to have been true for surgeons and nonuniversity trained doctors. Such doctors probably built up their clientele much as physicians did, and many of the factors which shaped the career of the physician would also have come into play in the professional life of the surgeon or empiric. This certainly applies to one of the major decisions facing every doctor in this period: where to live and where to practice.

HOW CAN YOU KEEP THEM DOWN ON THE FARM?

We have already seen that members of the medical profession were geographically mobile. Many doctors who matriculated in the Guild of Doctors, Apothecaries, and Grocers stayed in Florence for only a few months or years, moving on before they appeared in the city tax records or in other government documents. Others of provincial or foreign origin chose to immigrate permanently or at least long enough to acquire property, taxpayers' status, and sometimes citizenship. The patterns of mobility and the motivations involved in such decisions illuminate certain aspects of medical practice and the medical profession. But such patterns and motivations were not exclusive to doctors; they also held for many of the middle-class immigrants—notaries and lawyers, affluent tradesmen, skilled craftsmen—who were so important to the growth and life of Florence in the later Middle Ages.[76]

Although the proportion of matriculated doctors from places outside the Florentine territories ("foreigners") increased steadily after 1348, most of the immigrant doctors permanently resident in Florence in

---

piece of information to Philip Gavitt. See also M° Cristofano's will (the last of three), dated 20.vi.1422, Notarile-F.299 (1422-23), fols. 38r-42v, where among a host of other small pious bequests he left fl. 1 and his outstanding salary to the hospitals of San Giovanni Batista ("Ospedale di Messer Bonifazio") and San Paolo.

[76] There is evidence that in the years after 1348 immigrants were drawn increasingly from the ranks of unskilled laborers rather than from the skilled craftsmen and professionals who came to Florence from the countryside in the later thirteenth and early fourteenth centuries; nonetheless the higher class of immigrant was still very much in evidence. On the changing character of immigration in this period see Herlihy and Klapisch-Zuber, *Les toscans*, 318-20; de la Roncière, *Florence*, 2:726; and Cohn, *Laboring Classes*, Chap. 4.

1450 still came from the countryside and district.[77] These local immigrants varied considerably. Some, mostly from wealthy landed families, as we have already seen in the cases of Maestro Antonio di maestro Guccio da Scarperia or Maestro Giovanni di maestro Antonio Chellini da San Miniato, retained close ties to their native towns, deriving much of their income from property there, returning for the summer, and often retiring there at the end of their lives. Such ties tended to weaken over the generations, as descendants sold off the old family property.[78] The situation was different for local immigrants without holdings in their native towns and without the funds to finance frequent trips back. Thus when poorer doctors arrived from the countryside and district they tended to immigrate definitively. In his *catasto* declaration from 1427, for example, Maestro Giorgio di Niccolò da Arencio di Mugello listed no possessions in or ties to the town where he was born.[79] Foreign immigrants were not, of course, required to list foreign property in their tax declarations, but one gets a similar impression concerning their affairs. If only because of the distances involved, once the family had decided to immigrate, Florence became the effective center of its life, whether the head of the household read medicine at the university, like Maestro Lodovico di Bartolo da Gubbio and Maestro Francesco da Conegliano, or was a simple hernia doctor, like Maestro Antonio and Maestro Francesco di Giovanni da Norcia.[80]

Immigrant doctors came to Florence at varying stages in their careers. Some were brought to the city as children by relatives and were effectively first-generation Florentines.[81] Others immigrated relatively late in life, in their forties and fifties, sometimes with their families. As their tax records show, most of these older doctors were notably poorer than the rest and may have been driven to the city by desperation. The

[77] This statement is based on the origins of the doctors in the *catasto* of 1451 (Catasto-687 to 720). See Chapter Two above for the geographical origins of Florentine doctors.

[78] For instance, Ser Matteo di ser Loro da Radda came to Florence sometime near the beginning of the fifteenth century. His son Mº Guasparre matriculated in the Florentine guild in 1421 and seems to have established himself firmly in the city. By 1447 he had sold the family house in Radda; see Catasto-699, fol. 396.

[79] Catasto-78, fol. 337v.

[80] Mº Lodovico di Bartolo retained some connections in his native region, however. In 1382, for example, the Florentine commune sent him on an embassy back to Umbria; see Vitelleschi, *Relazioni*, vol. 2, no. 510.

[81] Mº Nuto di Bandino da Bibbiena and Mº Giovanni Chellini da San Miniato fall into this category; see Miscellanea repubblicana-98, no. 9, fol. [2r], and PR-63, fol. 33v.

only older immigrants who do not seem to have been in this position were those who, like Maestro Niccolò di Bonaventura da Mantova or Maestro Giovanni Baldi da Faenza, initially came to teach at the *studio* and found Florence congenial enough to settle there. But the majority of immigrant doctors, from the territories or abroad, came to the city as young, single men at the beginning of their careers. Some were medical students in their twenties, while others, slightly older, had completed their medical training (academic or empirical) but had not yet established a practice or a family elsewhere. Maestro Lorenzo Sassoli da Prato is typical. He received his doctorate from Padua in 1404, taught for a year at Ferrara, returned home to Prato for a short time, and was securely established in Florence by the age of thirty. He consolidated his position by marrying a Florentine woman several years later and spent most of the rest of his life practicing in the city.[82]

The decision to immigrate was not always taken independently. Some doctors moved to the city alone, but others arrived in groups or came to follow family and friends. Such groups frequently settled in the same part of the city, often in adjoining houses, and created sizable expatriate communities.[83] There was, for example, a Pratese enclave in the quarter of Santa Maria Novella—the part of the city nearest the road to Prato. The first Pratese doctor to arrive had been the surgeon Maestro Giovanni Banducci, who settled permanently in Florence in 1371. He was followed in 1372 by Maestro Lorenzo di Piero da Prato, and in 1373 by his close friend Maestro Naddino di Aldobrandino; both also rented houses in Santa Maria Novella, as did Francesco Datini, who corresponded with all three.[84] Datini in turn advised his protégé Maestro Lorenzo Sassoli to come to Florence and promised to find him a place to live. Maestro Lorenzo replied saying that the size of the house was unimportant, as long as it was nearby;[85] by 1406 he had joined the others in the same section of the city. Even when Maestro Naddino left Florence for Avignon, he did not break all ties with the Pratese medical community. A year after his arrival in France he was visited by Maestro Giovanni Banducci, who would have settled there permanently had the market for surgeons been better.[86] It was

[82] See Guasti, *Intorno alla vita*, 6-7.

[83] It was very common for immigrants from the countryside to settle in the section of the city closest to the gate leading to their place of origin; see Greppi and Massa, "Città e territorio," 32-34.

[84] See their matriculation entries in AMS-9, and Prestanze-368, fols. 48v, 68r. There are letters from all three in Datini's Carteggio privato.

[85] Letters of Mº Lorenzo to Datini (27.viii.1404 and 18.x.1404).

[86] See Mº Naddino's letters to Monte (11.iv.1387 and 29.i.1388/9).

easy for immigrants from nearby towns like Prato to maintain such networks, but we see the same phenomenon, albeit on a smaller scale, even among foreign immigrants. Many of the empirical doctors from Norcia practicing in Florence, for example, had close ties with one another, including three generations of the family of Maestro Niccolò di Bartolo[87] and including also the two brothers Maestro Antonio and Maestro Francesco di Giovanni, both of whom settled in the same *gonfalone* in the quarter of San Giovanni.[88]

Just as important as the ways in which doctors immigrated are the reasons that pushed them to do so. Although these reasons varied from person to person, there were many common concerns. We can see some of them in a letter from Maestro Ugolino di Giovanni da Montecatini. Montecatini was a medium-sized town in the Florentine district. Maestro Ugolino took his medical degree from Bologna in 1367 and soon thereafter moved to Pisa, where he practiced as a public doctor and personal physician to Pietro Gambacorta, lord of the city. In 1381 he was invited to become the public physician in Pescia, near his native town; at about the same time he was also pressed to try his luck in the capital by Ser Coluccio Salutati, chancellor of Florence and a childhood friend.[89] Faced with these alternatives, Maestro Ugolino found himself in an agony of indecision. In June 1381 he wrote for advice to Francesco di Iacopo Del Bene, the Florentine administrator of the region:

> I was talking with Ser Coluccio about being in Florence and about going, on his recommendation, to stay with him for a few days over the holiday of San Giovanni. I think that if I go there I will not find patients right away. I have seen from experience that some doctors have been there for a long time before becoming known, and I think that if Maestro Tommaso [Del Garbo] had not died so young, he would not have become so famous. The expenses would be great. As an unknown, I would have to show myself in disputation and prove my worth from scratch, even if Ser Coluccio smoothed the way for me. May he pardon me, but I think that I know more about medicine than he does. I recognize that coming in his name I would be hated by the doctors

---

[87] The guild's rolls include M° Niccolò (matriculated in 1396), M° Giovanni di m° Niccolò (1437), and M° Antonio di Iacopo di m° Niccolò (1444)—all three recorded as coming from Norcia.

[88] Catasto-Campioni del Monte-San Giovanni/Drago-427, fols. 604r-5v.

[89] Salutati was a native of Stignano, several kilometers from Montecatini. For biographical information on M° Ugolino see Barduzzi, *Ugolino da Montecatini*.

there, although I do not care about that, since the dissensions there do not equal the ones here [in Pisa]. And if by chance I failed in the first cases confided to me—as yet being without a reputation—I would have to leave with little honor. For our art is one which often depends on luck. For these reasons, I have been in agony ever since Pescia began to look for a doctor. I know that here, with an apothecary's shop, I can earn fl. 400 or more a year without running any risk. I realize that this does me no honor, but also little shame. Imagine that I return to my own region [Pescia], putting what face on it I can. In my free time I could study, being young; four years from now I could go to Florence, and I would be more accomplished and older and more able to afford the expenses. I don't say that I have made up my mind; I have brought up these issues in order to help you advise me.[90]

Maestro Ugolino's objections were not trivial. It was not easy for a young doctor to build a reputation and attract a good clientele in the face of established competition. The financial question was also significant; transferring one's household and family to an entirely new city could cost a great deal in both time and money.

Maestro Ugolino, as it turned out, chose to remain a big fish in a small pond, staying in Pisa for the time being; so we do not know

[90] Letter of M° Ugolino to Francesco di Iacopo Del Bene (5.vi.[1381?]); ASF: Carte Del Bene, Busta 49, no. 201: "Ragionamento avea con Ser. Coluccio d'essere a fFirenze et per suo consilglio andare ad starmi con luy per questo San Giovanni alchuni giorni. Io penso che andando non sarò così tosto richiesto, et per experientiam ò veduto che quelli che vi sono, sono stati assai tempo prima che aveano avuto fama, e credo che se Maestro Tomaxo non fosse si tosto morto, ancora la fama gli dormirebbe. Converrebemi essere possente al sostenere le spese a farle grandi. Sarebe mestieri mostrarmi nelle disputationy, nella pratica, e di me nuova experientia fare come incongnito, bene che Ser Coluccio me la mecta più grassa. Ma perdonimy elli: de' nostri facti io credo più di lui vedere, e conosco bene che venendo in nome [suo?] sarei odiato da' medici, benchè io di questo non mi curasse, chè non vanno al pari quelli odi con questi di qui. Et si per ventura ne' primi caxi che alle mani mi venisseno io avessi vergongna, non avendomi ancora adquistato fama, a mme oviene partirmi con pogo onore. E l'arte nostra è di quelle che spesse volte sta nella ventura. Per queste cagioni, essendo cominciato a fabricarsi a Pescia chiamare medico, io sono stato in questo agonia. E veramente qui vego io potere ongni ano con una botega di spezaria guadangnare di fiorini iiii^c o più, e sono fuori di tucti pericoli. È vero che bene conosco non essermi questo facto onore, ma è di meno vergongna. Considerate che ritorno alla patria, e ad questo daremo di quelli colori che si possono. In questo tempo non occupato alla pratica io posso studiare, e assa[i] sono giovane, e di qui a quatro anni io potrei essere a Firenze, e sarei più perfecto e di più matura età, e potrei sostenere alle spese. Io non dico che questo mio scrivere sia mia determinatione, ma per darvi materia di consilgliarmy ò voluto tocchare queste parti. Io non debo fare se non quello che voi mi consilglerete." On this episode in the life of M° Ugolino see Barduzzi, *Ugolino da Montecatini*, chaps. 1-3, esp. 34-36, and Pieri, "Maestro Ugolino."

whether his fears were justified. We do, however, know something of the problems faced by other immigrant doctors. For one thing, the expenses were indeed great. Maestro Naddino estimated that, between new clothes in the local fashion and new furnishings, it cost him at least fl. 200 just to relocate in Avignon.[91] Doctors with a less exalted clientele would not have required such finery, but for many of the Florentine immigrants there were other, hidden costs not faced by Maestro Naddino. One matter of concern to local doctors was double taxation. Until the *catasto*, and in some cases even after, immigrants from outside Florence with property in their towns of origin were subject to both city and provincial taxes. The acts of the Florentine councils are full of petitions from doctors and other immigrants pleading for relief from either the *estimo* of the countryside or the city *prestanze*. (Maestro Ugolino himself, while teaching in the *studio* years later, was caught between both taxes.)[92] This financial penalty only added to the difficulties of administering one's estates from afar.[93] Another problem which Maestro Ugolino did not anticipate in his letter to Del Bene but which caused difficulties for him and for other doctors on the move was the matter of his family. Some practitioners, like Maestro Salvadore da Sicilia, brought their wives and children with them. Others, like Maestro Antonio di Giannetto da Castelfranco or Maestro Naddino di Aldobrandino, left them at home alone—sometimes for years. In Maestro Naddino's case this led to a whole range of difficulties, from loneliness to the constant recriminations of family and friends and even to accusations of adultery.[94]

Despite these problems, city life had its compensations, for large

[91] See M° Naddino's letters to Monte and Datini (26.x.1386, 11.iv.1387, vii.1387, 21.iii.1388/9).

[92] See also PR-102, fols. 74v-75v, and PR-105, fols. 317v-18v (petitions of M° Lorenzo Sassoli da Prato); PR-87, fols. 329v-31r (M° Francesco di Giovanni da Empoli); PR-88, fols. 197v-98v (M° Guerriere di Michelotto da Pescia, in prison for tax evasion); and PR-89, fols. 28v-29v (M° Iacopo di Francesco Chiarenti da S. Gimignano). The last wished to immigrate with his brother, but they were concerned about the problem of double taxation: "Quod maxime dictus M° Iacobus ob prolem suam motus et similiter dictus Johannes desiderant in civitate Florentie se et eorum familias reducere et in ipsa civitate intendunt continue cum eorum familiis habitare. Sed de oneribus presentibus timent etiam habere onera in terra S. Gimignano pro se et suis bonis. . . ."

[93] On this problem see M° Lorenzo Sassoli's letters to Datini (10.ix.1403 and 8.xii.1403); it was this which finally forced M° Lorenzo home to Prato.

[94] See letter of M° Naddino to Monte (3.iv.1388): "Io non credo che fosse mai alcuno sanza la donna sua che vivesse più honestamente di me e più casto così potrebbe essere. Ma più no' nè femmina tenni nè tengo, nè fo cosa d'avere figliuoli, nè ebbi mia nè avrò figliuoli se non della mia donna, se dio ci dia tanta gratia che noi possiamo vivere insieme." See also Catasto-81, fol. 371r (M° Salvatore); PR-85, fols. 122r-24r (M° Antonio).

numbers of doctors flocked to Florence in search of fame and fortune. Perhaps the most common motivation was economic. Maestro Giorgio di Niccolò da Arencio immigrated, as he indicated on his declaration from 1427, because "he was dying of hunger and is anxious to earn the bread he lacks."[95] And Maestro Antonio di Giannetto da Castelfranco explained in a petition to the councils that "he has a large family, and especially seven small children. He is driven by necessity to practice in the city as well as in the countryside, and sometimes outside the countryside of Florence."[96] Clearly a doctor could expand his pool of potential patients by simply moving from place to place. Some practitioners—mostly specialists, for obvious reasons—made this a way of life; they put up for a few days at a local inn, did some rudimentary advertising, and moved on again when business dried up.[97]

There were good reasons, however, for a doctor in search of *utile* to head for the city. In the first place, only the cities had a real money economy; elsewhere business depended heavily on barter and payment in kind, as Maestro Lorenzo Sassoli found out when he returned home to Prato in 1404 to serve as the communal doctor. "I am well and eating a lot of produce," he wrote to Datini, "because my patients pay me with cheese and fresh eggs, or sometimes a basket of cherries. . . . One of my patients sent me a pair of capons while I was writing this, and being completely fed up with such things, I am sending them on to you."[98] In such a situation the opportunities for making a fortune were limited. In the second place, the city represented a much larger market for goods and services of all sorts. An urban center the size of Florence—one of the largest in Europe—could absorb a large number of doctors before competition began to make itself felt, and doctors would have found more work of all kinds there. The private sector was more highly developed, since the economy and culture of the city generated a class of patients who felt the need for private medical services and were able to afford them. The city government itself of-

---

[95] Catasto-49, fol. 1552r: "muorisse di fame ed à brigha di guadagnarsi il pane che manucha."

[96] PR-85, fols. 122r-23r (26.vi.1396): "magnam habet familiam et maxime septem filios parvulos et ex necessitate cogitur suam artem exercere tam in civitate quam in comitatu et aliquando extra comitatum Florentie."

[97] See, for example, the case of the traveling empirics in Lucca, described in Corsini, *Medici ciarlatani*, 56.

[98] Letter of Mᵒ Lorenzo to Francesco Datini (2.vi.1404): "Io sto bene e tocho d'erbolati però che da' miei infermi io sono pagato di cacio e d'uove fresche, o talvolta d'un paniere di ciriege. . . . Mandovi un paio di caponi, e quali mi furono mandati di uno mio infermo in mentre che io scrivea questa. Sichè avendo io giurato la morte adosso a gli erbolati, gli mando a voi."

fered a number of medical positions, and institutional contracts were in general easier to find; the convents, confraternities, and hospitals which employed so many doctors in Florence were an overwhelmingly urban phenomenon.

It was also only in the cities that one could plausibly court *onore*. Medical reputations were won at the university or in the service of the rich and influential, and this made the countryside and the provincial town unattractive to an ambitious doctor. Furthermore, there was something of a cultural stigma attached to provincial or rural life. As Maestro Marco da Pistoia was fond of repeating, "the country breeds strong animals and the city valiant men." Maestro Lorenzo felt this strongly on his return to Prato: "I arrived at my empty and ramshackle house and wandered around a bit," he wrote to Datini, "and I see better each day how true your advice to me has been. . . . It is as if I had come into the land of the Philistines. Here all joy seems extinguished, and I feel as if I had already been here several jubilees—such pleasure have I taken in my homecoming."[99] A month later Prato was less the "land of the Philistines" than a simple wasteland, "where none lived or was remembered by man."[100]

Maestro Lorenzo's situation must have been a common one for the university-educated physician. Many other Florentine physicians of the period came from minor towns—most of them far more provincial than Prato. While at the university they acquired a taste for the excitement and intellectual stimulation of the city. It is easy to understand the disappointment that Maestro Lorenzo confided to Datini:

> The frustration I feel on seeing myself here makes me lose my senses and my reason in my letters to you and in other things. You must imagine what great glory I feel when I see myself fallen from disputing on philosophy and medicine to disputing whether it is better to sow grass or sorbs. And then, passing on to higher questions, we dispute how much better it is to sow flax in the spring. These are matters of lofty speculation. But don't be dismayed, because if I care to stay I will soon be so well informed that I will be able to answer every question you have on the subject. Up to now I have sought instruction with the professors at

[99] Ibid. (16.v.1404): "Io sono giunto alla mia vota e isgangerata casa, e sono ito alquanto a rimeno per la terra, et ben vego più l'un dì che ll'altro le vostre parole essere vere in ongni caso che con voi mi consiglio. Questo vi dicho perchè a me pare esere venuto in terra di filistei. Qui mi pare spenta ongni allegreza, e par' me che chi qui vive, vergongnia abia dello eser vivo. E quanto a me, pare già eserci stato parechi giubilei, tanta è l'alegreza la quale ò presa della mia venuta. . . ."

[100] Ibid. (13.vi.1404): "dove niuno ne fosse, o richordato fosse degli uomini. . . ."

Padua and Bologna. Now my teachers hold their classes at the Porta Corte.[101]

We can see why so many doctors like Maestro Lorenzo were drawn from the subject towns of the Florentine territories to the capital. (The same process certainly held for Venice, Bologna, Perugia, and other capital cities.) It is less easy to account for the growing influx of foreigners into Florence, doctors from Milan or Rome, who could have enjoyed the benefits of city life without the inconvenience of the move. For these, the decision apparently concerned not just money or reputation but also less tangible factors which we might group under the rubric of "lifestyle." Not all cities—even all capital cities—were created equal. In Maestro Lorenzo's eyes, at least, Venice was supreme for beauty and magnificence; he called it "not a city, but an earthly paradise."[102] But fifteenth-century Florence had its own appeal. There is in the Medici archives a letter from Maestro Vittorino, a Mantuan physician who had apparently been in attendance on Lorenzo de' Medici. Called home on a family emergency, he wrote back to Lorenzo to announce his return. A friend had asked him if he intended to stay in Mantua. "I answered no," he recorded, "because I have experienced the sweetness of the good life in Florence, . . . and I want Florence to be my home."[103]

[101] Ibid. (2.vi.1404): "il dispecto il quale io ò nell'animo nel vedermi eser qui mi fa perdere e sentimenti e l'uso della ragione nello scrivervi e nelle altre cose, inperochè voi dovete immaginare che gran gloria io ò nel' animo di vedermi eser venuto dal disputare di philosophia e di medicina a disputare se gli è il meglio di seminare dello scioverzo o di seminare delle sorbe. E se pur a più alte questioni io passo, vengniamo a disputare quanto sia il meglio da seminare lino stio al vernio. Questi son' dubii di grande speculatione. Ma niente di meno non vene sgomentate, perochè se io curo stare, spero . . . eser sì bene introducto in simil materia che quando arete in ciò alcuno dubio, da me ne sarete chiarito a pieno. In fino a qui sono stato a chiarirmi co' doctori bologniesi e padovani d'ongni mio dubio, ma ora e miei doctori tengono le scuole in Porta Corte." Compare this with M° Lorenzo's earlier description of the pleasure he took in the environment of the University of Padua (30.viii.1402): "e di studio non vorrei se io potessi fare altro uscire, perchè mi sta troppo buono usare con gli scolari a rispetto dell'atre [sic] usanze del mondo."

[102] Ibid. (10.ix.1403): "non città ma paradiso in terra si debbe chiamare, considerando le sue mangnificentie."

[103] Letter of M° Vittorino da Mantova to Lorenzo de' Medici (4.xi.1472); MAP-XXVIII, 644: "Io li rispose che no, perchè io havia provato la dolzeza del ben vivere di Fiorenza, . . . chè io vollia Fiorenza essere mia patria."

· V ·

Doctors in Florentine Society

W E MUST now return from the perceptions of doctors and their families to the social order in which they lived. In previous chapters I have described the conditions and aspirations which governed the professional life of the Florentine doctor; in this chapter I will discuss its economic, social, and political rewards. Aspiring doctors were attracted to medicine and provincial practitioners to Florence by promises of *utile* and *onore*. To what extent were these promises fulfilled?

We can begin to answer this question by looking at the economic status of doctors. Doctors varied strikingly in their personal wealth, but as a group they were well-off with respect to the rest of the city's population and becoming better off during the early Renaissance. Their social status is a more complicated issue. The calculus of family antiquity, reputation, marriage alliances, and political representation which contributed to a family's standing in Florentine society was in itself complex, and it was made even more tricky in the case of doctors by their remarkable social and geographical mobility. A lucrative and respected occupation, medicine was a highly effective social elevator—much more so even than law. The flight of established native medical families from the profession in the wake of the plague opened the field not only to immigrants but also to families and individuals lower in Florence's social hierarchy; within one or two generations many of these families were able to establish themselves within the city's social and political elite. Thus a very high proportion of successful doctors belonged to the *gente nuova*, the "new men" of the later fourteenth and fifteenth centuries, who were seen by many patricians as a threat to the traditional order.

To study the place of doctors in Florentine society is also to illuminate the nature of the society itself. The Florentine social order, as Gene Brucker has written, was shaped by its "forms of association"—not only the legal corporations of guild, commune, and religious association which we have already studied but also more informal coalitions of families and individuals bound by kinship, marriage, neighborhood, friendship, and patronage.[1] If the former governed the economic life of the doctor and his conditions of employment, the latter shaped his social prospects. By tracing the social triumphs and failures of the best documented of the city's doctors we can form some idea of the way this collective order operated and the degree to which it was open to geographical outsiders and social newcomers. Such an approach, for all its limitations, sheds more light on the predicament of the *gente nuova* than either defensive contemporary polemics or studies of the very richest and most powerful new families, both of which yield an unrealistically rosy picture of the process of making it in Renaissance Florence.

WEALTH AND INCOME

The most fruitful sources for the relative wealth of doctors in four-teenth- and fifteenth-century Florence are tax records. Two citywide assessments, the *sega* of 1352 and the *catasto* of 1427, have been ana-lyzed statistically and can serve as a point of departure.[2] The 1352 *sega*, or hearth tax, included just under nine thousand households, each listed under the name of its head and registered by street within the four quarters of the city. If we assume, as seems reasonable, that the tax assessed against each household corresponded roughly to its wealth, we can determine the relative economic standing of households headed

TABLE 5-1
Relative Size of Doctors' Assessments (1352)

Tax (£)	Percentage of City Households	Number of Doctors' Households	Percentage of Doctors' Households
0-10	61	14	37
10½-20	21	13	34
20½-50	12.5	10	26
50½-100	3.5	1	3
100½-	2	—	—

SOURCES: Estimo-306; Barbadoro, "Finanza e demografia," 9:629.

[1] Brucker, *Civic World*, 11. On the changes in this collective order during the early Renaissance see ibid., 15-39.

[2] Less useful is de Roover's breakdown of the *catasto* of 1457/8, since this tax included relatively few foreigners in a period when they were becoming very important in the profession; see his *Medici Bank*, 29-31. On Florentine taxes in general, see Appendix I.

by doctors. Thirty-nine doctors appeared in the rolls of the *sega*; their average assessment came to £17, corresponding approximately to the seventy-seventh percentile of households taxed in 1352. A more detailed look at the assessments of individual doctors gives the results in table 5-1.[3]

As the figures in this table show, the pyramid of wealth for doctors in the mid-fourteenth century was considerably more compressed than for the population as a whole. Doctors were relatively underrepresented among the poor and the very rich; the bulk of them might be described as middle or upper middle class. Furthermore, the figures for doctors varied according to type of practice. As one would expect, physicians as a group tended to be wealthier than surgeons and empirics. Of the twenty-seven doctors with assessments of £20 or less, fourteen are identifiable as surgeons or empirics, while only two are known to be physicians. Of the eleven doctors with assessments over £20, on the other hand, seven are identified in other sources as physicians, while only two were definitely surgeons or empirics.[4]

Finally, the figures for doctors also varied according to place of origin. On the whole, immigrant doctors from the Florentine territories seem to have been the most affluent segment of the profession, while foreigners were the least wealthy. Thus of the doctors identifiable as foreign immigrants, five out of seven paid £10 or less, putting them in the lower levels of the Florentine population. Of those identifiable as immigrants from the countryside and district, on the other hand, six out of eight paid between £20.5 and £50, putting them near the top. Doctors identifiable as Florentine natives were spread roughly uniformly across all the economic levels represented. A second comparison shows that, as one would expect, the immigrants from the Florentine territories were largely physicians, while the foreigners were predominantly surgeons and empirics.

Unfortunately, the *sega* of 1352 gives only a rough indication of the nature and extent of doctors' actual wealth; for such information we must look to the *catasto*, the fifteenth-century successor of the hearth

[3] Estimo-306, fols. 7-184, analyzed in Barbadoro, "Finanza e demografia." I have adopted Barbadoro's tax categories and have included dentists, or "tooth doctors." (Barbadoro's numbers for doctors and surgeons are uninformed and should be disregarded.) These figures may not include the poorest households in the city: as Barbadoro points out, the "*sega*" should probably be considered a *prestanza*, or forced loan, and would not therefore have been assessed against the very poor.

[4] Not all doctors in this tax are identifiable by type, either because the roll includes only their first names or because the doctors themselves are not so identified in the matriculation lists and other documents I have examined.

TABLE 5-2
Relative Wealth of Doctors' Households (1427)

Raw Wealth (fl.)	Percentage of City Households	Number of Doctors' Households	Percentage of Doctors' Households
0-210	50	9	29
211-600	20	6	19
601-3200	24	7	23
3201-	6	9	29

SOURCES: Herlihy and Klapisch-Zuber, Les toscans, 254; Catasto-65 to 83 and Catasto-Campioni del Monte-S. Giovanni-1427.

tax and the forced loan. The books of this tax contain itemized declarations of the complete holdings, in property, investments, and cash, of each household in Florence. Herlihy and Klapisch-Zuber have analyzed the official summaries of the first *catasto*, in 1427. Table 5-2 places the figures for the thirty-one households headed by doctors in the context of the total population of city taxpayers from that year.[5] As this table shows, the position of doctors in 1427 had changed relative to 1352. On the one hand, their overall economic standing had improved: where their average assessment in the *sega* placed them between the seventy-fifth and eightieth percentiles, their average raw wealth in the *catasto* (fl. 2,196) corresponded to a position between the eighty-fifth and ninetieth percentiles. With an average net wealth of fl. 1,856, they were richer than any of the occupational groups listed by Herlihy and Klapisch-Zuber except bankers and wool merchants.[6] On the other hand, these figures mask another change from the situation in 1352: the distribution of wealth among doctors had become much more polarized. In 1352 most doctors occupied the middle range in the distribution of wealth for the whole population; by 1427 almost 60 percent of all doctors appeared in either the lowest or the highest category, with relatively few in between.

This trend toward economic polarization within the profession be-

[5] These figures come primarily from the graph in Herlihy and Klapisch-Zuber, *Les toscans*, 255; the wealth figures have been estimated and should be taken only as approximate values. On the general issue of distribution of wealth in the *catasto* of 1427 see ibid., chap. 9. For the fortunes of individual doctors see my Appendix III. A household's "raw" wealth was the sum of its assets (*sostanza*) before declared debts (*incarichi*) and the personal allowance for the household and dependents (*bocche*) had been deducted. A caveat: Herlihy and Klapisch-Zuber shift quickly back and forth from raw to net wealth (*fortune brute* and *fortune nette*) in chaps. 9-10; the reader must be sure to check which is under consideration.

[6] Cf. my table 4-1 and Chapter Four, note 9, above.

comes more comprehensible when we look at the distribution of doctors' wealth with respect to type of medical practice and geographical origin. Identifiable surgeons and empirics still accounted for most (seven out of nine) of the poorest doctors, while virtually all (eight out of nine) of the richest doctors were physicians. At the same time, six out of seven of the poorest doctors were immigrants to Florence, as were six out of nine of the richest. These results help to explain the nature of the polarization in the ranks of the medical profession. By 1427 well over half of the doctors who were heads of city households were immigrants, and immigrants tended to be either quite rich or quite poor. The poor were by and large surgeons and empirics, often from places outside the Florentine territories, who had come to Florence out of economic need. The rich were physicians from the countryside and district, like Maestro Lorenzo Sassoli, who were attracted to the city by a combination of reasons involving *utile, onore,* and cultural stimulation; they came from wealthy families in their towns of origin, and much of their wealth was represented by family property there. It was native Florentine physicians who tended to make up the middle ranks of doctors in the *catasto,* and by 1427 they were, as we have seen, a distinct minority.

This still leaves us with the question of scale. What do the categories in table 5-2 mean in terms of income and lifestyle? Herlihy and Klapisch-Zuber offer rough definitions.[7] The half of the population (and the 29 percent of doctors) with raw wealth of fl. 210 or less was starkly poor. Their only assets were small amounts of cash, household furnishings, or money owed by others. They rented the houses they lived in and were chronically in debt. As de la Roncière's study of wages and prices has indicated, members of such households were probably regularly undernourished, particularly in times of scarcity.[8] Maestro Giorgio di Niccolò da Arencio could well claim to the tax officials that he was "dying of hunger."[9] Herlihy and Klapisch-Zuber denote the next 20 percent of the population (19 percent of doctors) as enjoying a "very modest living." Maestro Taddeo di Cambino is typical. Aged twenty-seven, he stayed with his mother and fourteen-year-old wife in a rented house and recorded a number of debts; but he also owned a

[7] Herlihy and Klapisch-Zuber, *Les toscans,* 258.

[8] De la Roncière, "Pauvres et pauvreté," 2:674-79. For similar estimates see Pinto, "Personale," 145-60. Doctors in this position included Mº Giovanni di Bartolomeo da Montecatini (Catasto-76, fol. 307v), Mº Giorgio di Niccolò da Arencio di Mugello (Catasto-Campioni del Monte-S. Giovanni/Leon d'oro-1427, fol. 573r), and Mº Salvadore di mº Niccolò da Sicilia (Catasto-81, fol. 371r).

[9] Catasto-49, fol. 1552r.

small amount of rent-bearing property, a farm and a house, which provided a cushion against illness or famine.[10] The 23 percent of doctors and 14 percent of the population in the next bracket (raw wealth from fl. 601 to fl. 3,200) represented the city's solid middle classes. They tended to own their own houses and, apart from practice, drew income from rents from several houses and farms, business investments, and modest holdings in the Monte, or public debt.[11] The rich, finally, who represented almost a third (29 percent) of Florence's doctors, indicated in their declarations significant amounts of property of all the types mentioned above as well as thousands of florins in cash and outstanding loans.[12]

The records of the *catasto* are less helpful in giving a sense of the doctor's total income, as opposed to his wealth, because they are mute concerning earnings from investments and practice. The latter, at least, could be considerable. It is striking, for example, that although the surgeon Maestro Giovanni di maestro Piero da Norcia appeared in the *catasto* of 1427 as one of the very poorest doctors in terms of property, he nonetheless recorded no debts; furthermore, his oldest (and illegitimate) son Niccolò eventually went to university and became a physician. Similarly, although the young physician Maestro Bandino di maestro Giovanni Banducci showed a very modest net worth of fl. 441, he was assessed the relatively high tax by "composition" of fl. 1.[13] One would guess that in these cases, and doubtless in the case of most Florentine doctors, medical training acted like hidden capital: neither assessable nor taxable, it nonetheless assured the practitioner a significantly higher income than most others in the same wealth bracket.

It is difficult to estimate a doctor's income from what we know about fees and salaries, because, as we saw in Chapter Three, most doctors patched together a practice from a variety of private and in-

[10] Catasto-75, fol. 421r-v. Mº Francesco di Giovanni da Norcia was in a similar situation; see Catasto-52, fol. 267r.

[11] Examples of doctors in this wealth bracket include Mº Domenico di mº Giovanni (Catasto-81, fols. 251v-52v), Mº Bartolomeo di Cambio (Catasto-78, fol. 262r-v), and Mº Antonio di Giovanni da Norcia (Catasto-Campioni del Monte-S. Giovanni/Drago-1427, fols. 604-5).

[12] See, for example, the *catasto* summaries of Mº Antonio di mº Guccio da Scarperia (Catasto-78, fols. 1r-7r), Mº Domenico di Piero (Catasto-65, fols. 92v-96v), Mº Galileo di Giovanni Galilei (Catasto-69, fols. 114r-15r), and Mº Giovanni di mº Antonio Chellini da S. Miniato (Catasto-79, fols. 47r-49v). For an analysis of the categories of property involved see Goldthwaite, *Private Wealth*, 235-49.

[13] Catasto-67, fol. 310v (Mº Giovanni). Catasto-76, fol. 258 (Mº Bandino). For Mº Niccolò's credentials as a physician see Diplomatico-Monasteri diversi-22.xi.1441. Composition was the process whereby a householder with a negative net worth was assessed.

stitutional clients. We can only guess what this situation might have meant for the average doctor—particularly since, as the *catasto* figures show, the medical profession was extremely stratified. The annual contractual income of a medium-level physician or surgeon might have broken down as follows:

contract with apothecary	fl. 30
contract with two hospitals	fl. 15
contract with two monasteries	fl. 8
total	fl. 53

His earnings from private practice would probably have put him comfortably over fl. 100 for the year.

The most successful and established physicians could make much more. A good example is Maestro Iacopo da Lucca, who recorded his earnings in his personal diary. During the thirty-three years between 1370 and 1403 he averaged an income from practice of about fl. 250 a year. He had also formed a partnership in the apothecary business with Giovanni Sercambi. Maestro Iacopo's share of the profits for the five years the company lasted (1379 to 1384) averaged about fl. 120 a year, in addition to the fl. 300 (his initial investment) he received on the dissolution of the company.[14] Thus for those years his total annual income from medicine and related business approached fl. 400. This impressive sum was not atypical, as we can see from the letter of Maestro Ugolino da Montecatini quoted in the previous chapter, where he claimed that in Pisa he could "earn fl. 400 or more a year with an apothecary's shop."[15] This did not even include the landed and investment income the higher class of physicians collected each year. According to Martines's calculations for the same period, the professional earnings of the most successful doctors were roughly commensurate with, or only slightly lower than, those of the most successful lawyers.[16] A yearly income of fl. 400 plus rents and dividends was certainly not princely—it did not compare with the income of the richest members of the Florentine patriciate—but it was nonetheless consid-

[14] ASL: Ospedale di S. Luca-180, recto of first, unnumb. fol., and fols. 27, 40. M° Iacopo's salary from his apothecary amounted to about fl. 40; see fol. 41r-v. Cf. Chapter Four, note 64, above.

[15] Letter of M° Ugolino to Francesco d'Iacopo Del Bene (5.vi.[1381?]); Carte Del Bene, Busta 49, no. 201. See Chapter Four, note 90.

[16] Martines, *Lawyers*, 103-5. Messer Ricciardo Del Bene, for example, earned an average annual income of fl. 320 from his legal practice during the three years between November 1403 and February 1407; Messer Benedetto Accolti seems to have enjoyed an income of fl. 500-600.

erable. If we recall that an annual income of fl. 50 or 60 was enough to provide an adequate, although not luxurious, living for an average household, we can appreciate the relative affluence of the middle and upper ranks of the medical profession.[17]

SOCIAL ORIGINS AND SOCIAL STANDING

By 1427 almost a third of all doctors active in Florence belonged to the elite 10 percent, the small group of wealthy Florentines from which the men who dominated the city's politics and society were drawn.[18] It is tempting to take the next step: to conclude that doctors at the top of their profession were disproportionately represented among these powerful men. This was not in fact so. As a number of historians have recently shown, the correlation between the wealth of the individual Florentine household and the social standing of its members was at best tenuous: what counted was the wealth of the "family," in its broader sense of lineage, clan, *consorteria*.[19]

The Florentine *consorteria* was a patrilineal descent group, extended in both space and time. At any time it was composed of one or (usually) more households, which could differ greatly in structure, size, and wealth but which were bound to varying degrees by blood, money, law, politics, and tradition. For practical purposes, the Florentine ruling class consisted not of individuals but of *consorterie*—about three hundred by the first half of the fifteenth century.[20] The aggregate social status of a family depended on a number of variables which can be simplified into three categories: wealth, political office, and a miscellany of intangibles including family image, antiquity, and associates.[21] Virtually all families in the Florentine patriciate had a tradition of old and honorably acquired wealth, and they tended to look askance at those whose affluence had been recent or sudden. Similarly, most had a long history of participation in the public life of the Florentine commune; for generations they had supplied men to the city's highest

[17] Pinto, "Personale," 160.

[18] Martines, *Social World*, 108. Martines estimates that the bulk of officeholders came from the 10% of wealthiest households in the city, while the inner core of the ruling group was drawn mainly from the top 3%.

[19] See, for example, Dale Kent, "*Reggimento*," 596-600. On the household/consorteria distinction see F. W. Kent, *Household and Lineage*, 3-17.

[20] Dale Kent, "*Reggimento*," 587-89.

[21] See Martines, *Social World*, chap. 2, and F. W. Kent, *Household and Lineage*, chaps. 3-5.

offices: the priorate, or Signoria.[22] Finally, patrician families acquired through their political and business dealings a reputation or tradition of authority, which resided in the lineage as a whole but which could be both added to and drawn on by individual members. The most concrete repository of this tradition was the family name, its "public and formal badge of membership."[23]

It is striking that of the thirty-seven doctors represented in the official summaries of the *catasto* of 1427 only five, or fewer than 14 percent, registered family names, in comparison with a citywide incidence of almost 37 percent. Of these five only one, Maestro Galileo di Giovanni Galilei, possessed a surname with patrician resonances. This statistic is particularly telling in that family names were heavily concentrated among the wealthier inhabitants of the city, a group to which a disproportionate number of doctors belonged. In Florence—as in Venice—there was an obvious discrepancy between the wealth of a significant portion of Florentine doctors and their social obscurity.[24]

The most obvious explanation for this obscurity lies in the doctors' geographical origins. Many were immigrants, and in the course of leaving their native towns, most immigrants, even those of impeccable local stock, seem to have shucked off both their family tradition and the name which embodied it, or rather could not make an unfamiliar name stick in the tightly ordered social world of the capital city. Maestro Giovanni di maestro Antonio Chellini, a wealthy doctor from San Miniato, is typical. Both Maestro Antonio and his son matriculated in the Guild of Doctors, Apothecaries, and Grocers using their family name. By the fifteenth century this name had virtually disappeared from communal records. When the family appeared in high public office near the end of the century, it was under the toponymic

---

[22] The eight priors, headed by the standard-bearer of justice, were the highest executive officers of the Florentine republic and comprised the Signoria. They were assisted by two small councils—the Twelve Good Men and the Sixteen Standard-Bearers of the Militia. These officers were elected to short terms in office by a complicated process of scrutiny and sortition; for details see Brucker, *Florentine Politics and Society*, 59-69. For lists of Florentine priors from 1282 to 1386 I have used Stefani, *Istoria fiorentina* (in *Delizie*, vols. 7-17); from 1386 to 1411 Ser Naddo, *Memorie storiche* (in *Delizie*, vol. 18); from 1411 to 1437 Giovanni Morelli, *Ricordi* (in *Delizie*, vol. 19); from 1437 to 1500 Giovanni Cambi, *Istorie* (in *Delizie*, vols. 20-21). My lists of consuls of the Guild of Doctors, Apothecaries, and Grocers to 1353 come from Ciasca, *L'arte*, doc. X; after 1353 from AMS-46.

[23] F. W. Kent, *Household and Lineage*, 254. Family names were acquired by an informal process of public recognition. On their changing nature see Cohn, *Laboring Classes*, 45-51.

[24] Herlihy and Klapisch-Zuber, *Les toscans*, 537-43, esp. 539. On Venice see Ruggiero, "Status of Physicians and Surgeons," 183-84.

alone; this was eventually transformed into the entirely new family name of Samminiati.[25]

But even among the doctors of Florentine stock in the *catasto*, family names were rare, and those that made it into the summaries were not by and large out of the top drawer. The simple fact is that by 1427 most wealthy doctors came from immigrant families without a Florentine tradition, while most doctors of Florentine stock—even the rich—came from the socially obscure orders of the petty bourgeoisie, the *mezzana gente*. The situation was of relatively recent origin. A hundred years earlier doctors had been represented in the higher ranks of the Florentine patriciate.[26] This was no longer true after 1350. Martines's threefold categorization of the social origins of Florentine lawyers is useful here, both as a model and for contrast. Martines divides lawyers into scions of the old patriciate, social newcomers, and immigrants; whereas the bulk of his lawyers came from the first group, most prominent doctors in the later fourteenth and the fifteenth centuries were members of the last two.[27]

To begin with the patriciate, there were only three doctors, out of approximately one hundred and fifty active in the period which concerns us, who could be considered of good, old, Florentine families. Furthermore, all three were somewhat anomalous. Maestro Ciango di Dino Compagni was the son of one of the city's leading statesmen in the years around 1300. With his brothers, Ciango had continued his father's silk business after Dino's death in 1324. It was only with the bankruptcy of the concern in 1348, after Ciango had reached a comparatively advanced age, that he seems to have gone into medicine.[28]

---

[25] AMS-7, *ad litteram* A (1386-1408) and *ad litteram* G (1386-1408); *Delizie*, 21:74 (Bartolomeo di Bartolomeo da San Miniato, nephew of M° Giovanni). For the final transformation of the name see Mecatti, *Storia genealogica*, 95, and Maddalena, "Archives Saminiati." Other immigrant doctors who lost their family names included M° Domenico d'Agnolo Accennati da Montegonzio, M° Francesco Mercadelli da Conegliano, M° Michele Onesti da Pescia, and M° Lodovico di Bartolo Accorambuoni da Gubbio; the son of the last appeared in the *catasto* of 1457/8 as Batista di m° Lodovico Bartoli (Catasto-837, fol. 65v).

[26] For example both the Fagni and Salviati families had taken their surnames from doctors of their lineage illustrious in both medicine and the political affairs of the city. M° Fagno di Spigliato (Fagni) was prior many times in the last years of the thirteenth century and first decades of the fourteenth, as was M° Cambio di m° Salvi (Salviati).

[27] Martines, *Lawyers*, 62-78 and appendix.

[28] He matriculated in the guild shortly after 1353, was taxed in the *sega* of 1359, and died soon after. See AMS-7, *ad litteram* C (1353-86); Prestanze-5, fol. 59r. On his earlier career see Del Lungo, *Dino Compagni*, 1/2:977-1012, passim. Del Lungo maintains that Ciango matriculated in the guild only because his default in the silk business deprived him of legal membership in the Arte della Seta. This explains neither why he

The career of Maestro Piero di Barna de' Pulci, who matriculated in 1371, was more typical, but his family was less usual. The Pulci were old feudal nobility and as declared "magnates" were excluded from all but a handful of communal offices and consequently from the mainstream of patrician life.[29] The only doctor to come from a lineage we can identify as belonging to the solid, *popolano* (nonmagnate) patriciate was Maestro Galileo di Giovanni Galilei. But even his family circumstances were unusual. Once part of the old and respectable Bonaiuti clan, which had supplied generations of priors to the city government, Maestro Galileo's branch had apparently broken away and taken its new name sometime in the first half of the fourteenth century. With the break had come comparative political obscurity. It was only in the generation of Maestro Galileo and his brother Michele (a silk retailer) that the Galilei family attained the political prominence which matched its heredity.[30]

The only other doctors of Florentine stock who could claim a "family" in the more distinguished sense were obvious members of the social group identified by contemporaries as "new men." This group was composed of lineages which had acquired both wealth and political standing after the middle of the fourteenth century, when the demographic upheavals of the plague and the political vicissitudes of the years between 1343 and 1382 had acted sporadically to expand the city's ruling group.[31] About fifteen doctors came from families of this

---

chose the Guild of Doctors, Apothecaries, and Grocers nor why he appeared in their lists as well as in the *sega* of 1359 as *Maestro* Ciango. There were a number of doctors in the guild's list who lacked the honorific, but there were no other men in it who enjoyed the title but were not doctors.

[29] See Giovanni Villani, *Cronica*, IV, 13, 1:152. M° Piero was made a *popolano* in 1380 but does not seem even afterward to have been active in politics above the guild level.

[30] See the genealogy in ASF: Archivio Galilei, Inventario. Antonio Favaro rejects the Bonaiuti connection in his "Ascendenti e collaterali," 349-54; his proposed genealogy, however, contradicts the patronymics contained in M° Galileo's name as it appears in Seta-7, fol. 79r. M° Galileo's grandfather, Tommaso di Bonaiuto, seems to have held high office only once, as one of the Twelve Good Men (see note 22 above). His father, Giovanni, who followed Tommaso into the family silk business, does not seem to have been politically active. M° Galileo, on the other hand, was prior in 1430 and 1435, standard-bearer of justice in 1446, and was elected to virtually all the other important bodies within the city (Otto di guardia, Dieci di libertà, Ufficiali della condotta, etc.); see Tratte-80, fols. 14v, 18r, 38r, 41v, 87r. M° Galileo was followed in public affairs by his grandsons and his sons, one of whom married into the Medici family. See Tratte-80, passim, and Litta, *Famiglie*, vol. 2, fasc. 17, tav. VII (marriage of Bernardo di m° Galileo and Lucrezia di Cambio di Vieri di Cambio de' Medici).

[31] These issues have been treated at length by Brucker in *Florentine Politics and Society*. The process was not wholly arrested after 1392; it continued through the fifteenth

kind. A few examples can stand as typical. Probably the most visible of the new families to produce medical men was the Del Garbo. The name appears at least as early as the beginning of the fourteenth century in the guild matriculation entries of Maestro Buono and his son Maestro Dino Del Garbo, both illustrious doctors and professors of medicine at the University of Bologna. Maestro Tommaso di maestro Dino returned permanently to Florence by 1348, when he began to teach at the newly established Florentine *studio*. His great wealth and outstanding professional reputation soon bore political fruit: he served first as consul of the Guild of Doctors, Apothecaries, and Grocers and then repeatedly as prior—the highest and most visible of the commune's elective offices. His success enhanced the social and political fortunes of the entire family; the sons, grandsons, and great-grandsons of Maestro Tommaso and his brother Torello reappear frequently in the lists of priors and other major officeholders throughout the fifteenth century.[32]

Maestro Tommaso was not the only doctor to emerge from a new family and to contribute to its political, social, and economic rise. The Solosmei, for example (first prior 1364), produced two doctors: the physician Maestro Ambruogio di Bartolo and his surgeon son Maestro Giovanni, many-time guild consul and prior in 1377 and 1390. Their descendants continued to appear in important city offices.[33] Maestro

century, but at a slower pace. See Molho, "Politics and the Ruling Class"; and Dale Kent, "*Reggimento*," 593-96, 611-17.

[32] Biographical information in Francesco Guido, "Cenni biografici su Dino e Tommaso Del Garbo"; Cappellini, "Date importanti"; Siraisi, *Taddeo Alderotti*, 55-60; and Filippo Villani, *Vite*, 30-31. Villani claimed that M° Tommaso derived his wealth from practice. For a confirmation of his fortune see Estimo-306 (S. Croce/Bue); Prestanze-5, fol. 41v; Prestanze-94, fol. 29r; Prestanze-130, fol. 29r. M° Tommaso was guild consul in 1343, 1348, 1351, 1355, 1359, and 1364; prior in 1358 and 1363 (the first of his lineage to hold that office); and standard-bearer of justice in 1368. His brother Torello, for example, was elected prior in 1373, three years after M° Tommaso's death, and Torello's daughter Lisa married Simone Capponi, a prominent statesman in the decades before 1400; see Litta, *Famiglie*, vol. 10, fasc. 164, tav. II.

[33] Dale Kent, "*Reggimento*," 631; Brucker, *Civic World*, 256-57; AMS-46 (1359, 1362, 1365, 1369, 1373, 1377, 1385, 1387). Neither M° Giovanni nor his father used the surname Solosmei, unlike other contemporary members of the family, but it was adopted by M° Giovanni's sons; see Tratte-79, fol. 125r. Another, similar case was that of the physician M° Piero di Giovanni, elected to the Signoria in 1386 and many times guild consul. His family origins are obscure; his father was a civil servant in the Florentine bureaucracy (Estimo-306: S. Giovanni/Leon d'oro: "Giovanni di Benino qui moratur ad gabellam"). M° Piero tried to adopt the family name Benini (see, for example, his matriculation entry in AMS-7, *ad litteram* P, 1358-86), but it did not stick; he consistently appears only as M° Piero fiorentino, and even his grandson, Brancazio di Giovanni di m° Piero, appears in the list of priors without a surname (*Delizie*, 21:33).

Fruosino di Cino Della Fioraia came from a similarly new, though wealthier, family. The Della Fioraia produced their first prior in 1371; although Maestro Fruosino never held that office himself, he was prominent in the guild, and his son Filippo, a silk merchant, consolidated the family's position in the social and political elite.[34] But perhaps the most impressive and most interesting of the doctors who can be called new men was Maestro Cristofano di Giorgio. Son of a retail clothes merchant (*rigattiere*) matriculated in the Silk Guild, Maestro Cristofano could lay claim to neither gentility nor wealth. Nonetheless he quickly emerged as a man of great ability and influence, first within the Guild of Doctors, Apothecaries, and Grocers and then within the city government; consul twenty-one times between 1382 and 1425, prior four times, and standard-bearer of justice once, he was one of the small number of men who made up the "inner core" of the Florentine regime in this period.[35] His sons and grandsons continued his political success, although on a somewhat reduced scale.[36]

In some respects these doctors were typical of Florence's new men; in others, however, they were unusual. One of the striking things about them is that, with the exception of the Del Garbo and Maestro Fruosino Della Fioraia, none could claim any significant personal wealth; their success was primarily political, and only secondarily social or economic. In this they differed noticeably from the third and largest group of prominent doctors: the outsiders, themselves immigrants to the city or products of recently immigrated families.

Only among immigrant doctors can we see a social pattern that resembles the one identified for lawyers by Martines. Like lawyers, the successful immigrant doctors after the middle of the fourteenth century tended to come from a distinctly higher class of family than their Florentine counterparts: "professional or landed families, houses of solid merchants or manufacturers or bankers, old county families, and

[34] AMS-46 (1351, 1358, 1360, 1363, 1368, 1371, 1376, 1380); Tratte-45, fol. 24r-v; Tratte-46, fol. 164v; Tratte-79, fols. 17v, 42r, 65v, 71r, 100v; *Delizie*, 19:60, 101. The same was true of Mº Zanobi di mº Lorenzo, whose son Lorenzo first became prior in 1419, and Mº Simone di Cinozzo Cini (or Cinozzi), son of a Florentine apothecary, whose son Piero, a linen merchant, became the first of his family to serve in the Signoria in 1481.

[35] See Brucker, *Civic World*, 269. Mº Cristofano's family name was Brandolini (or Brandaglini), but it was rarely used by him or his children and grandchildren. Mº Cristofano's relatively small *prestanza* assessments were hardly commensurate with his political prominence, and his means, even at the end of his life, were surprisingly modest; see his will (Notarile F.299, 1422-23, fols. 39r-42v). Mº Cristofano married Foresina di messer Rosso Orlandi, from another new, professional family.

[36] See Tratte-79, Tratte-80, passim; *Delizie*, 19:52, 85; 20:276, 332, 373.

not rarely the old nobility—all at least 'respectable' and some very 'grand.' "[37] As one would expect, immigrant doctors from local families—natives of the *contado* and occasionally of the district—were the most successful in assimilating economically, socially, and politically. They had full access to their (often very large) landed holdings, their origins were more easily traceable, and they were more quickly eligible for public office.

A typical example of this kind of immigrant was Maestro Lorenzo d'Agnolo Sassoli da Prato, whose medical career we examined in the previous chapter. Maestro Lorenzo came from a good *contado* family. His great-grandfather Sassolo di Cione had been prior of Prato in 1309. His father, Agnolo di Tura, was a successful spice merchant and apothecary, whose financial worth was assessed in the *estimo* of 1393 at the respectable sum of fl. 2,500. Maestro Lorenzo, as we have seen, experienced some financial difficulties in the first few years after his father's death in 1400 and eventually immigrated to Florence in 1406 under the protection of the very wealthy Pratese merchant Francesco Datini. There, with the help of Datini, his own patrimony, and a successful high-level practice, he quickly accumulated a substantial fortune and married into one of the oldest and most distinguished of Florence's noble families, the Cavalcanti.[38] When he died in 1437 his wealth was divided among his many sons, some of whom found themselves without a trade or prospects and emigrated from the city, while others remained in Florence and prospered. His daughter Caterina was perhaps the family's most striking social success. Her first marriage was to Antonio di Marsilio Vecchietti, an important politician, Medici associate, and scion of an ancient "consular" family; after his death she became the wife of Luca di Bonaccorso Pitti, builder of the Pitti palace and one of the wealthiest and most influential men in mid-fifteenth-century Florence.[39] Maestro Lorenzo, like many successful immi-

[37] Martines, *Lawyers*, 74.

[38] Guasti, *Intorno alla vita*, 3-5. M° Lorenzo showed a raw wealth of over fl. 6,400 in 1427, primarily in the form of cash and land in and around Prato; see Catasto-77, fols. 168r-69v (*campione*), and Catasto-47, fols. 79r-81v (*portata*). His declaration shows that a number of his pieces of property in Prato had been bought recently and were not family property. His wife was Piera di Schiatta di Buglione Cavalcanti; his wife's sister married Francesco d'Averardo de' Medici; Litta, *Famiglie*, vol. 2, fasc. 17, tav. III.

[39] Guasti, *Intorno alla vita*, 15-16, and Catasto-836, fols. 85v, 88r, 89r, 99v, 102v, and 107v (1458). The most famous son was Sassolo, a minor humanist and follower of Vittorino da Feltre; details in Guasti, *Intorno alla vita*, 8-26, and below, Chapter Six. On the Vecchietti see Dale Kent, *Rise of the Medici*, 146, and Rubinstein, *Government of Florence*, 24. On Luca Pitti Dale Kent, *Rise of the Medici*, 59; Rubinstein, *Government of Florence*, 155-66; and Brucker, *Civic World*, 360ff.

grants, could not immediately transform his financial and social triumphs into political capital; he himself was ineligible by birth for city offices. Only in 1453, twenty-six years after his death, did the first male in his line qualify for the Signoria.[40]

Similar forces shaped the career of another doctor from a wealthy *contado* family, Maestro Giovanni di maestro Antonio Chellini da San Miniato al Tedesco. Maestro Giovanni had been brought to Florence by his father toward the end of the fourteenth century. With his two brothers, both notaries, he eventually inherited his father's large fortune.[41] He married Nanna di ser Francesco d'Ugolino Grifoni, whose father had also immigrated from San Miniato to study for the notariate, had been made a Florentine citizen in 1367, and had held a number of important foreign offices. Furthermore, as his account book and *catasto* declarations show, Maestro Giovanni had impressive connections in Florentine society. He regularly lent large sums of money to highly placed Florentines, and he owned a great collection of silver plate which was frequently borrowed by families like the Rucellai, Carnesecchi, Strozzi, and Capponi for banquets to celebrate marriages and political appointments; his most important associates were Giovanni Rucellai and Gino di Neri Capponi, to whose son Neri he stood as godfather in 1452.[42] Maestro Giovanni's only surviving son, Tommaso, himself made an illustrious marriage to the daughter of Andreolo di Niccolò di Franco Sacchetti, and Tommaso's two daughters in turn married into the patriciate. Maestro Giovanni's nephew, Bartolomeo di ser Bartolomeo, heir to his uncle's fortune, made his family's first appearance in the Signoria as prior in 1478.[43]

[40] Dale Kent, "*Reggimento*," 637.

[41] Miscellanea repubblicana-98, no. 9, fol. [2r]. Mº Antonio seems to have supplemented his medical earnings with traffic in banking and loans; he was condemned in 1416 for usury and made to give back fl. 5 in excess interest. His *catasto* declaration of 1427 showed him as having raw wealth of nearly fl. 10,000 in land, cash, and outstanding loans. By 1451 Mº Giovanni had all but abandoned his medical practice, content to live from rents and interest. See Catasto-79, fols. 47r-49v; Catasto-53, fol. 1059; and Catasto-715/I, fol. 293: "Dell'arte mia non fo ghuadangnio nessuno se non la benivolenzia de' cittadini." By 1458 his *catasto* assessment of fl. 33 s. 6 d. 10 put him in the top 1% of Florentine householders; Catasto-837, fol. 76v, and de Roover, *Medici Bank*, 29.

[42] See the numerous entries in his *ricordanza*; Università Bocconi (Milan): Istituto di storia economica, cod. 2 (new numeration), esp. fols. 13r, 98v, 144v, 150v, 170r-171v, 172r (for the baptism of Neri di Gino Capponi), 173v, 174r, 175v, 196v, 198r, 199v; also Lightbown, "Giovanni Chellini," 103. On his father-in-law, Ser Francesco, see Salutati, *Epistolario*, 3:192-94.

[43] *Delizie*, 21:74. See also Battistini, "Giovanni Chellini," 108; Martines, *Social World*, 336; and Brucker, *Civic World*, 279-80. Mº Giovanni's daughter Lisabetta became the

Maestro Lorenzo Sassoli and Maestro Giovanni Chellini were undoubtedly the most socially successful of the immigrant doctors. Nonetheless, there were a number of other doctors from the Florentine countryside and district—including Maestro Niccolò Falcucci, Maestro Antonio di maestro Guccio da Scarperia, and Maestro Michele di maestro Piero da Pescia—who on immigration married into patrician families or the *gente nuova,* or who otherwise found a niche among Florentines of respectable standing.[44] The barriers were more formidable for foreigners—doctors from families outside the Florentine territories—but even those barriers yielded, given the proper combination of wealth, luck, ambition, and birth. The surgeon Maestro Lodovico da Gubbio, for example, whose family, the Accorambuoni, seem to have been Umbrian nobility of wealth and antiquity, quickly found a place in Florentine society; of his sons, Messer Guasparre became an illustrious lawyer, Maestro Bartolomeo a physician, and Piero a silk merchant, while Batista, an apothecary, married into the patrician Machiavelli family.[45] On a more modest scale, Maestro Domenico di maestro Giovanni, son of an immigrant bone doctor from Civitavecchia, became a physician and married the daughter of Ser Niccolò Pierozzi, a successful notary and new man prominent in the city government in the years before 1400.[46]

Reviewing our three categories of socially prominent doctors, then, we can make the following tally. Of roughly one hundred and fifty Florentine doctors settled in the city between the mid-fourteenth and the mid-fifteenth centuries, only three—Maestro Piero Pulci, Maestro

---

wife of Pandolfo di Bernardo di Tommaso Corbinelli, and Nanna married Carlo di Bernardo di Piero Rucellai: Miscellanea repubblicana-98, no. 9.

[44] M° Niccolò Falcucci da Borgo San Lorenzo, who came to Florence in the middle of the fourteenth century, earned a fortune through medical practice and managed to marry at least three of his children into important patrician families, the Corsini, Tolosini, and the Raugi; see Ristori, "Niccolò Falcucci," 262-63. M° Antonio di m° Guccio da Scarperia immigrated with his brothers sometime near the end of the fourteenth century, developed a prestigious practice, and married Angela di Migliore Migliori, from a prominent new Florentine family, while his son married into the Del Pace, who were of comparable standing; see Baccini, "Maestro Antonio di Guccio da Scarperia," esp. 242-44. M° Michele di m° Piero da Pescia married Ginevra di Leonardo di Salvestro Rimani (Catasto-705, fol. 563; Pupilli-7, fol. 46r); his son Niccolò became prior in 1488 (*Delizie*, 21:49).

[45] See Martines, *Lawyers*, 72; I have found no mention of the brother referred to by Martines as M° Iacopo. On Batista's marriage see his *catasto* declaration from 1451: Catasto-715/I, fol. 783.

[46] Catasto-61, fols. 708r-9r. By 1451 his sons had adopted the surname Del Corso, presumably after the street in which they lived, Corso degli Adimari; see Catasto-720, fols. 362, 488r.

Ciango Compagni, and Maestro Galileo Galilei—came from families identifiable with the Florentine patriciate. A second group of about fifteen, both physicians and surgeons, belonged to native families which rose to social and political eminence after the middle of the fourteenth century, especially during the fifty years between 1343 and 1393. (It is worth noting that even these men, like their counterparts in the patriciate, were somewhat anomalous; with the exception of Maestro Tommaso Del Garbo and Maestro Fruosino Della Fioraia, they were relatively poor and lacked the stable family tradition reflected in a surname.)

The third group was the largest; we can count about twenty-five doctors as socially prominent immigrants. These men were economically successful, and they and their children married into the upper classes—both the native new families, as in the case of Maestro Antonio da Scarperia, and the older patriciate, as in the case of Maestro Lorenzo Sassoli or Maestro Giovanni Chellini. A few even reaped political success for themselves and their descendants: the grandson of Maestro Antonio da Scarperia and the sons of Maestro Michele da Pescia, Maestro Antonio Chellini da San Miniato, and Maestro Lorenzo Sassoli da Prato eventually qualified for the Signoria and were elected to the priorate. It is worth noting that almost all these men were physicians and enjoyed the prestige of a university degree. Furthermore, the much smaller number whose families actually attained political power were aided and protected by powerful patricians. In this respect the case of the Chellini is typical: Maestro Giovanni di maestro Antonio established strong ties of business, friendship, and marriage with men who were among the most powerful and influential of their time, and it was largely their patronage which assured the social and political success of his family.[47] In general, the immigrant doctors who enjoyed the greatest social success in Florence tended to come from old and powerful families in their own towns, families of a higher class than those of the native Florentine doctors. In this sense their success amounted less to social climbing than to finding their own social and economic level.

Of the hundred and fifty doctors, therefore, we can identify about forty as being of some social standing. What of the other three-quarters of the profession? The main quality they shared was their origin in families of no political importance, which left no mark on the state or on contemporary Florentine society. A few surgeons and empirics

---

[47] On the importance of patronage in Renaissance Florence see Weissman, *Ritual Brotherhood*, 23-26.

were sons of artisans—a leatherworker, a cobbler, a smith.[48] Many came from families of smaller Florentine merchants active in the trades governed by the greater guilds: cloth and, especially, spices and drugs. But the largest group was composed of the sons and daughters of professionals, above all doctors and notaries. Thus most doctors came from the petty bourgeoisie—lesser members of the greater guilds and small property owners, occupying a secure if not illustrious place in the social hierarchy of the city. Such men may have occasionally held one of the lower guild offices, but they played no real part in the communal government.[49]

This is not to say that these socially obscure doctors were homogeneous in wealth and prospects. A number, particularly among the immigrants and empirics, were poor, while a few were very rich. Maestro Francesco di Ridolfo paid very large *prestanze* in the years around 1400, for example, while Maestro Domenico di Piero had the largest net wealth of any doctor in the *catasto* of 1427. The origins of both are obscure; neither ever held high political office, and it is not even known what their fathers did or how they acquired their wealth.[50] Such doctors and their children married among each others' families or on their own social level—a level at which even foreign immigrants were quickly assimilated into the life of the city.

In conclusion, the social composition of the medical profession changed in two important ways over the century after 1348. In the first place, economic and social stratification increased. The most obvious casualty was the occupation of surgeon. Although surgeons were on the whole less wealthy than physicians throughout the period, nonetheless in the fourteenth century a number of the most successful and influential members of the medical profession were surgeons. Of the seven doctors who qualified in the scrutiny of 1382 as eligible for the priorate, for example, four (Maestro Zanobi di Iacopo Mangani,

---

[48] The father of M° Giovanni di Paolo di Piero is recorded in the *prestanza* of 1379 as a leatherworker, or *galigaio* (Prestanze-368, fol. 77v). The father of M° Benedetto di Francesco di Michele was a shoemaker, and that of M° Arrigo di Ricco a smith (Estimo-307, fol. 134r).

[49] See Brucker, *Civic World*, 260-61.

[50] See Martines, *Social World*, appendix II, tables I-IV (*prestanza* of 1403); Prestanze-1787 to 1790 (1399); Prestanze-2901 to 2904 (1413); and Catasto-65, fols. 92v-96v. M° Francesco was elected guild consul only once, in 1420; from his successive *prestanze* it seems that he acquired his wealth himself rather than inheriting it. M° Domenico di m° Piero is a real puzzle; neither he nor his sons, M° Piero and M° Paolo Toscanelli, appear in the various scrutinies to 1433 as even legally eligible for office. I have found no evidence that M° Domenico's father was a doctor, as claimed by Martines in *Social World*, 333-34.

Maestro Giovanni di maestro Ambruogio Solosmei, Maestro Francesco di ser Niccolò, and Maestro Banco di maestro Latino) were surgeons. (Maestro Zanobi, captain of the Parte Guelfa at his death and politically the most promising of the four, was probably an empiric: the contemporary chronicler Stefani refers to him as a "poultice doctor.")[51] The bone doctor Maestro Stefano dell'Ossa had one of the highest assessments in the profession in the *prestanza* of 1369, and one of the richest doctors in the 1380s and 1390s was the surgeon Maestro Lodovico da Gubbio.[52] The next generation, however, saw a distinct drop in the number of politically and economically successful surgeons. Surgeons supplied no Florentine priors and only one among the consuls of the guild during the entire fifteenth century. In 1427 only one surgeon, Maestro Giovanni di ser Bartolo da Radda, fell into the upper bracket of wealth, and his age of seventy placed him closer to the previous generation than to most of his contemporaries.[53]

In the second place, the balance among the three groups of socially prominent doctors—patricians, new men, and immigrants—changed dramatically. Whereas in the first half of the fourteenth century a significant portion of prominent doctors came from old and respected families, the number had dropped to one (Maestro Galileo Galilei) by the middle of the fifteenth century. The number of new men in the profession peaked in the 1370s and 1380s and declined into the fifteenth century as the number of immigrants continued to rise.

The effect of these changes was a steadily decreasing presence of doctors within the effective ruling class. We have already seen the results within the guild: the number of doctors holding consulships declined dramatically through the fifteenth century.[54] The effect was even more marked within the city government. Whereas doctors accounted for thirty-eight priors during the sixty years after the establishment of the Ordinances of Justice in 1282, doctors were drawn for that office only eight times between 1343 and 1392, and only six times during the entire fifteenth century. (Those six terms were split by two physicians, Maestro Cristofano di Giorgio and Maestro Galileo Galilei, each

---

[51] Stefani, *Istoria fiorentina*, in *Delizie*, 17:7. Mᵒ Zanobi never fulfilled his political promise; he was murdered at an early age in a dispute over the rent owed on a shop owned by the Parte Guelfa. The scrutiny list for 1382 is edited in *Delizie*, 16:125-260; on the scrutiny process see Dale Kent, "Reggimento," 589.

[52] Prestanze-156, fol. 20r (Mᵒ Stefano); Prestanze-1264, fol. 107v; Prestanze-1789, fol. 10r (Mᵒ Lodovico).

[53] Catasto-79, fol. 235v.

[54] See table 1-3.

of whom served three times.)[55] If we look not at the priors themselves but at the men scrutinized as eligible for the Signoria in the years between 1382 and 1450—a more accurate reflection of the actual holders of political power—the picture is the same: fewer and fewer doctors qualified by family and reputation for political office, although the exceptions, notably Maestro Cristofano and Maestro Galileo, were both men of considerable influence.[56]

These changes are certainly due partly to the closing of the ruling classes in Florence, following the era of sporadic democratization which had begun in the early 1340s and lasted fifty years. After 1393 new families, both immigrant and Florentine, found it more difficult to break into the regime of politically active families.[57] But there was another factor in play—one which specifically affected doctors. As we saw in the first two chapters, the period after 1348 was marked by recurring waves of plague, each of which recalled the impotence of the medical profession and the danger of the doctor's work. Doctors from traditional medical families began to send their sons into other occupations. The few men from prominent medical families who did elect medicine as an occupation became physicians rather than surgeons, who were the doctors most in demand during plague epidemics. In fact, the image of the surgeon, who worked with his hands, was becoming a liability in an age when the liberal occupations were increasingly prized precisely because of their nonmechanical and nonmanual character. But the issue of the fates of doctors' sons brings up a different question—that of social mobility.

SOCIAL MOBILITY

Social mobility in late medieval Florentine society was relatively high as compared with other parts of Europe in the same period. Florence was a large city in a highly urbanized region. Endowed with a diversified economy and institutional structure, it enjoyed a high degree of what one historian has called "structural differentiation":[58] with its

[55] Martines observed the same pattern among notaries; see *Lawyers*, 49-50. He neglected immigration as an explanation.

[56] Both spoke frequently in the communal *pratiche*, or select advisory councils convened by the Signoria—one of the principal criteria used by Brucker for determining the composition of the core of the Florentine political elite; see Brucker, *Civic World*, 264-65.

[57] See Brucker, *Civic World*, 255-59, and Najemy, *Corporatism and Consensus*, 280-300.

[58] Hopkins, "Elite Mobility," 16-17.

bureaucracy, its court system, its university, its ecclesiastical foundations, and its wealth of trade, commerce, and industry, it offered the able man a wide variety of occupations, each with different requirements for entry and success, in which to build a fortune or a reputation. Furthermore Florence's inhabitants, like those of all medieval cities, were more exposed to disease than the inhabitants of the more sparsely settled countryside. The city's population maintained its numbers or expanded only through constant immigration from the surrounding province—another pattern historically associated with a relatively high degree of social mobility.[59]

This last tendency was greatly exaggerated by the series of plagues and famines which racked many European cities in the course of the fourteenth century and the resultant demographic collapse; this was especially acute in Florence, where the population had already begun to strain the resources of the region as early as 1300.[60] The enormous losses on all levels of Florentine society created gaps which the enterprising and the lucky, both citizens and immigrants, rushed to fill. The rise to social prominence of new or previously obscure families was further encouraged by the episodes of political openness and democracy which marked the fifty years between 1343 and 1393. The sudden expansion in the class of officeholders allowed large numbers of new men the opportunity to participate in Florentine government and to enjoy the social fruits of political activity.[61] The last decade of the fourteenth century saw the reestablishment of a more strictly oligarchical form of government and the erection of ever higher barriers to citizenship and office for immigrants. By 1400 the period of high social mobility had come to an end; new men and new families did manage to make a place for themselves in Florentine society during the fifteenth century, as we saw in the case of doctors like Maestro Lorenzo Sassoli or Maestro Giovanni Chellini, but such cases were more exceptional than they had been fifty years before.[62]

It should be emphasized, finally, that in Florence, as in other European cities, social mobility was a game of both snakes and ladders. There has been a tendency in recent historical writing to concentrate

[59] Thus Hopkins has argued that an important mechanism for social mobility in the Roman Empire was the assimilation of leading provincials; see ibid., 23-24. For a general discussion of social mobility in late medieval Europe see Nicholas, "Patterns of Social Mobility," 84-96, and Herlihy, "Social Mobility," esp. 645.

[60] See Herlihy and Klapisch-Zuber, Les toscans, 173-77.

[61] Brucker, Florentine Politics and Society, chaps. 3-6 and 8, passim; Najemy, Corporatism and Consensus, 146-52, 166-67, and chaps. 7-8.

[62] See above, note 57; also Martines, Social World, 75.

solely on individuals and families which managed to improve their condition. As Herlihy has recently shown, that tendency is misleading. Because the upper classes reproduced themselves at a higher rate than the population as a whole and because most medieval societies were essentially static in the overall distribution of wealth and power, the dominant direction of social mobility was ultimately downward: "the threat of losing status, which particularly pressed the lower but still propertied classes in the countryside, reached into much higher social levels in the city. The urban patriciate had to find careers for its plentiful children or watch them sink to lower social positions."[63] Thus the movement of individuals from one social level to another should be seen not as an inexorable rise but as a gradual recycling, in which the change was more or less rapid in one direction or the other, depending on the conditions prevailing at the time.

What was the role of medicine in this process? Were the professions in fact social elevators, as various historians have proposed?[64] Martines has challenged this view, at least as regards Florentine lawyers, showing that in the fourteenth and fifteenth centuries law functioned less to improve than to consolidate a family's social status. Thus, among the men of nonpatrician origins who entered the legal profession, most came from families which had made their political and economic fortunes in trade or commerce one or two generations before and which only afterward went on to produce one or more lawyers.[65] Martines's observations do not appear to hold for doctors. The medical profession in early Renaissance Florence conforms much better to the traditional interpretation. Medical education was a way to enhance one's social position. Thus not only did a far higher proportion of doctors than lawyers come from new or previously obscure families, as we have seen above, but virtually all those families acquired their new status during the doctor's lifetime, often as a direct result of his career.

This pattern becomes clearer if we go back and examine our successful doctors' careers in the light of the different components of social standing—wealth, political office, family tradition, and the like. To begin with native Florentine families, again and again a doctor, sometimes the product of several generations of doctors, was the first member of a family to become economically or politically visible. Both Maestro Francesco di Ridolfo and Maestro Domenico di Piero, for

[63] Herlihy, "Social Mobility," 645.

[64] For example, Stone, "Social Mobility in England," 35, on the law.

[65] Martines, Lawyers, 68-71. The main exceptions to this pattern were notarial families, who had a foot in the legal profession already and tended to enter law at an earlier stage in their family histories.

example, were men of obscure origins who amassed large personal fortunes during their lifetimes—whether entirely from medical practice or partly through business investments is unknown.[66] Maestro Tommaso Del Garbo not only made a fortune in medicine, according to Filippo Villani, but in 1358 became the first of his lineage to sit in the Signoria. Maestro Piero di Giovanni and Maestro Cristofano di Giorgio, while far from rich, were both responsible for their families' rise to political prominence. Even in those families such as the Della Fioraia and the Solosmei, in which a doctor was not the first to occupy high communal office, the first prior antedated the doctor by less than a generation.[67]

The pattern is slightly different for those medical families which eventually attained a position of social and political consequence in spite of not being native to Florence. None of the first-generation immigrant doctors ever held high communal office, although a few were active in the politics of their guild. Rather, it was their sons or grandsons who first acceded to the priorate. But in each instance the reputation and earnings of the doctor-ancestor were instrumental, and the political success of his descendants was largely a consolidation of his own achievements. The case of Maestro Antonio di maestro Guccio da Scarperia is typical. Maestro Antonio immigrated toward the end of the fourteenth century and managed to make both his name and his fortune through a combination of teaching and practice. He himself was many times consul of the guild; his sons held various minor communal offices during the early and mid-fifteenth century, but it was not until 1478 that one of his grandsons, Iacopo di Francesco di maestro Antonio, was elected to the priorate.[68]

There was good reason for doctors to occupy a crucial place in their families' histories. A successful medical practice could be highly profitable, far more so than the average cloth enterprise. The wealth accumulated by a doctor like Maestro Domenico di Piero could lay the foundations of a family fortune. But how to account for the political success of doctors who, like Maestro Cristofano di Giorgio, had nei-

---

[66] Both began with modest *prestanza* assessments early in their careers, but by the end were in the highest tax bracket in the city. M⁰ Francesco di Ridolfo, for example, was assessed only s. 15 d. 12 in 1379 (Prestanze-367, fol. 39r); by 1413 he was paying forced loans of fl. 45 (Prestanze-2902, fol. 40r).

[67] See notes 32 to 35 above.

[68] M⁰ Antonio's career in Baccini, "Maestro Antonio di Guccio da Scarperia," 339-41. The same pattern holds for the family of M⁰ Giovanni Chellini da San Miniato. The process was accelerated in the case of M⁰ Michele di m⁰ Piero da Pescia, whose own sons, Niccolò and Francesco, were elected to the priorate near the end of the fifteenth century.

ther personal wealth nor family tradition to boost them into civic visibility? Brucker has provided at least a partial answer in his analysis of the evolution of the Florentine government in the decades around 1400. Noting that a disproportionate number—ten out of seventy-six—of the men he identified as the "inner core" of the Florentine government in the first years of the fifteenth century were professional men, he has hypothesized that although access to office was determined on the whole by one's social background, access to real power increasingly depended on personal qualities—presence, strength of character, expertise in speaking, intellectual skills—that were likely to be developed in the course of professional training and practice. Thus Maestro Cristofano's abilities, which made him a suitable candidate for a physician's career in the first place and which were developed by his own experience, were largely responsible for his rise from political obscurity. He seems in fact to have had all the qualities of a high achiever. As a contemporary commented during Maestro Cristofano's term as prior in 1399, "he is the most, the best, and the greatest in the office, and is almost the whole priorate."[69]

Thus doctors were well placed to advance the social fortunes of their families: members of a traditionally respected profession, they had ample opportunity in the course of their practice to cultivate patrons among the upper classes of the city, the most reliable pool of private patients. Their work was lucrative, and doctors who qualified for government office often found themselves, because of their special skills and abilities, in positions of political prominence. But in order to appreciate the extent to which a doctor was able to advance his family's fortunes, we must consider not just his own successes but also those of his sons and grandsons.

We can begin by looking at the occupations chosen by doctors' sons. As we saw in the first chapter, medical careers often ran in families, especially if we include other fringe medical personnel like barbers. Medical families often also included notaries and apothecaries. In addition, a sizable number of doctors' sons went into the cloth business (wool and silk), both as importers and as retailers, or into banking; a smaller group chose law or the Church.[70] Finally, we find a scattering

---

[69] CS-78, 315, unpag.: "Egli è il più, el meglio e il da più che sia nelo uficio, e quasi il tutto." Quoted in Brucker, *Civic World*, 269n; see in general ibid., 269-72.

[70] The doctors, apothecaries, notaries, cloth merchants, and bankers are too many to enumerate. Lawyers included Messer Monte di m° Bartolomeo di Bernardo, Messer Guasparre di m° Lodovico (da Gubbio), and Messer Niccolò di m° Giovanni Banducci (da Prato); the last two were surgeons' sons. Among those that entered the Church was Messer Baldassare di m° Antonio da Scarperia, canon of San Lorenzo.

of doctors' sons in a miscellany of other occupations—a professional humanist, for example, a goldsmith, a painter, a weaver, a woolcarder, and two shoemakers. (Note that it was not only surgeons and empirics' sons who went into artisanal trades; the fathers of the last four were all physicians.)[71]

When we examine the records, a number of patterns emerge. First, as is to be expected, sons of doctors tended to move either upward or sideways within Florence's occupational hierarchy. Virtually all entered areas governed by the greater guilds. (Those few that did not, but became artisans, tended to maintain their matriculation in the greater guilds, presumably for political purposes; thus the cobblers Giovanni and Piero di maestro Piero di Giovanni, whose tax assessments show them to be well-to-do, joined the Silk Guild.)[72] A number clearly rose in occupational rank by entering high-income or high-status fields—the wool business, banking, or the law—that did not normally supply sons to the medical profession. A special case of this upward movement took place within the profession itself or on its outskirts, as sons of surgeons, empirics, or even barbers, like Maestro Bandino di maestro Giovanni Banducci, Maestro Domenico di maestro Giovanni and Maestro Bonagiunta di Bartolomeo, went to the university and matriculated in the Guild of Doctors, Apothecaries, and Grocers as physicians.[73]

A second striking regularity is the increasing flight of doctors' sons from medical careers. Whereas it was extremely common in the first half of the fourteenth century for sons of doctors to appear in the guild's lists as doctors themselves, this became increasingly rare during the century after 1348. There are variations within this pattern. Sons of empirics or surgeons were more likely to choose medical careers than sons of physicians, as were sons of immigrant doctors, although not *their* sons; immigrants presumably enjoyed a smaller range of connections in the world of Florentine affairs outside the medical field.

[71] Sassolo di m° Lorenzo Sassoli da Prato was a humanist, Carlo di m° Bartolomeo di m° Lodovico a goldsmith, Mercatino di m° Bartolo di Mercatino a painter. Piero di m° Michele (da Colle) a weaver, and Gerardo di m° Niccolò d'Andrea a woolcarder. Piero and Giovanni di m° Piero di Giovanni were shoemakers.

[72] Seta-7, fol. 104v; Catasto-836, fol. 96r. On the Florentine occupational hierarchy in this period see Herlihy and Klapisch-Zuber, *Les toscans*, 574-75.

[73] M° Giovanni Banducci was a surgeon from Prato who immigrated in the 1370s; M° Giovanni di m° Ciuccio was a bone doctor from Civitavecchia who matriculated in the guild in 1385. Other examples of physicians whose fathers were immigrant surgeons include M° Bartolomeo di m° Lodovico (da Gubbio), whose father lectured on surgery in the *studio* for many years, and M° Niccolò di m° Giovanni di m° Piero (da Norcia). M° Bonagiunta di Bartolomeo was the son of a barber.

This hypothesis is confirmed by the fact that whereas the majority of native doctors' sons leaving medicine went into the cloth business or banking, most sons of immigrant doctors chose the spice trade—governed by their father's guild—or the notariate and law, two fields traditionally open to non-Florentines. We have already speculated on the role played by the plague in rendering medicine unattractive and provoking a flight from the profession. But other considerations also pushed ambitious sons of successful fathers toward certain nonmedical occupations. Although doctors on the whole made a good living, wool merchants and bankers, on average, made a better one.[74] Furthermore, as Martines has shown, lawyers and notaries were active on all levels of the Florentine government; it may have been that those two occupations were particularly promising for immigrant families who wished to join the officeholding class.[75]

In any case, the results of such career decisions by doctors' sons and later generations of descendants were predictably mixed, although mixed in an unpredictable manner. The richest descendants of doctors were those who became doctors themselves, followed by those who entered commerce in one of the areas governed by the greater guilds, notably cloth and spices. A typical case is that of the two surviving sons of Maestro Agnolo di Germoglo, a physician from the *contado* town of Bibbiena who matriculated in Florence as a physician around 1385. His son Maestro Lionardo di maestro Agnolo built up an aristocratic medical practice and reaped its financial rewards; he appeared in the *catasto* of 1427 with a raw wealth of nearly fl. 8,000. Maestro Lionardo's brother Giovanni became a successful wool merchant, although his raw wealth of fl. 5,000 in 1427 compared unfavorably with Maestro Lionardo's. A generation later Giovanni's sons, who went into medicine, the wool business, and law, were still prosperous.[76] But it was not only immigrant doctors' families which managed to multiply, or at least conserve, their fathers' talents. The citizens Benedetto and Lorenzo di maestro Bartolomeo di Cambio, for example, who appeared as *lanaiuoli* (wool merchants) in the *catasto* of 1451, and Maestro Piero and Maestro Paolo, the physician sons of Maestro Domenico di Piero, were also in the process of expanding their families' patrimony.[77]

---

[74] See table 4-1.

[75] See Martines, *Lawyers*, esp. 70-72, 106-12, and chap. 9.

[76] On Mº Lionardo's patrician clientele see Ugolino da Montecatini, *De balneis*, passim. His *catasto* summary from 1427 appears in Catasto-67, fols. 106v-8v; for that of his brother see Catasto-67, fol. 122r-v, and for those of Giovanni's sons Catasto-693/II, fols. 308-9, 352-54, 361, 363.

[77] See Catasto-713, fol. 24, and Catasto-688, fols. 641r-44v.

On the whole, however, such cases were in the minority. By and large the economic fates of doctors' descendants confirm Herlihy's estimate that the predominant movement among the sons of the upper classes was downward. A fairly typical case is that of the descendants of Maestro Lorenzo Sassoli, whose raw fortune amounted to an impressive fl. 6,400 in 1427. Maestro Lorenzo died intestate in 1437, leaving three unmarried daughters and ten sons, none of whom, with the exception of Sassolo, a disciple of Vittorino da Feltre, seems to have inherited their father's ability and drive. By the middle of the century many of the surviving sons were doing no more than surviving. The eldest, Ruberto, found himself in Valencia in 1442 "without a job," and back in Florence in 1451 "without possessions." Marsiglio and Antonio were "without houses and furniture" and subsisting on meager salaries. Most of the other sons were either living off the shrunken and divided remains of their father's estate or involved in one or another struggling business enterprise.[78] We can see this same process at work in the careers of the sons and grandsons of several of the most prominent and successful doctors in Florence, including Maestro Francesco di Ridolfo.[79] In all these cases a combination of a large number of male heirs, unfortunate forays into cloth and banking, and a taste for high living off rents acted to dissipate the fortunes built by medical practice.

It is worth noting, however, that the political fortunes of doctors' families appear to have been less volatile than their economic fortunes. Benedetto, an impoverished son of Maestro Galileo Galilei, was more active politically than his more prosperous brothers, serving as prior three times.[80] The same holds for certain descendants of Maestro Tommaso Del Garbo, Maestro Cristofano di Giorgio, and Maestro Antonio di maestro Guccio da Scarperia; although their financial positions were at best modest, they nonetheless were successful as officeholders, consolidating their families' political gains while wasting their patrimony.[81]

[78] Guasti, *Intorno alla vita*, 8-26; Catasto-709, fols. 358, 478-79, 494, 507, 512, 514. Sassolo died in 1449 at the age of thirty-two. By 1458 Antonio had apparently enjoyed some success, to judge by the size of his *catasto* assessment; Catasto-836, fol. 420. See also note 39 above.

[79] See, for example, Catasto-81, fols. 372r-73r (Tommaso di m⁰ Banco, wool merchant); Catasto-697/I, fols. 162, 179, 388 (descendants of M⁰ Tommaso); and Catasto-699, fol. 553 (Francesco di m⁰ Francesco di Ridolfo). The case of the last is particularly striking. Francesco sold his share in a cloth business in 1433. From that year on, he lived off the progressive alienation of property left to him by his father.

[80] Compare their declarations in 1451: Catasto-697/I, fol. 96, and Catasto-697/II, fols. 724, 815.

[81] Tratte-81, passim.

If, in conclusion, we compare the results for doctors with what Martines has observed for lawyers during the same period, we notice a great difference between medicine and the law. Martines found that the legal profession in Florence served not as an agent of social mobility but as its reward. Lawyers came either from old patrician families or from families which had previously established themselves, usually in trade: "the great majority of lawyers listed as new men came from families that had acquired wealth and some political estate one to three generations before there was a lawyer in the household."[82] The medical profession, in contrast, conforms better to our preconceptions regarding the professions and social mobility. After 1350 almost no men of patrician stock chose medicine as a career. Of the doctors that we can identify as new men, both natives and immigrants, the great majority were the first to put their families on the Florentine social and political map. The same holds for those doctors' families too obscure politically and economically to appear on the map at all; it was in the doctor's generation that the family reached its economic peak or turning point. Few doctors of any class or any kind saw their families decline during their own lifetimes.

A second contrast with law involves the sequence of occupations visible from generation to generation within doctors' families. Martines found that lawyers' families tended to have established themselves in trade; once their social position was secure, they then began to produce generations of lawyers. Thus legal dynasties became common only in the later Renaissance, after the middle of the fifteenth century.[83] Again, the reverse holds for doctors. The great age of medical dynasties was the first half of the fourteenth century, extending into the second half of the century for immigrant families. After 1348 it became increasingly rare to find doctors' sons following their fathers into the profession; instead they took their patrimony and invested it in trade, usually in cloth, banking, or spices. If in spite of everything they elected to enter a profession, it was law or the notariate rather than medicine.

How successful were doctors' sons politically, socially, and economically? In general terms, success seems to have depended on the social level of the family. Paradoxically, most doctors' descendants of modest social standing found it easier to consolidate their fathers' gains; notable in this category were the sons of immigrant surgeons like Maestro Giovanni di maestro Ciuccio da Civitavecchia, Maestro Giovanni

82 Martines, *Lawyers*, 68.
83 Ibid., 75.

di Piero da Norcia, Maestro Lodovico di Bartolo da Gubbio, or Maestro Giovanni Banducci da Prato; these men became physicians, with the boost in income associated with that shift, or successful shopkeepers. The Florentine social pyramid seems to have been more slippery the closer one got to the top, however. A study of the economic fortunes of well-to-do doctors' sons tends to look more like an essay on the volatility of wealth in Renaissance Florence, or at least on the unpredictability of banking and the cloth trade. Virtually all the doctors in question were new men, without a stable tradition of family wealth; their fortunes were more easily dissipated than those of patrician families, whose assets were long established and spread out over a large number of households. By and large, however, even the families hardest hit financially managed to maintain or even extend their political influence.[84] It seems to have been far easier to lose one's fortune than one's political eligibility for the Signoria.

DOCTORS AND THE GENTE NUOVA

The old Florentine patriciate did not as a whole welcome the accession of new men and new families to the priorate and other high offices. While some patricians hastened to ally themselves with the new elements, many others deplored the successes of artisans and immigrants who, in their eyes, were usurping the power and prestige due the older aristocratic families. Their complaints became increasingly vocal after 1343, a year marked by the short-lived tyranny of the duke of Athens and subsequent electoral reforms which led to a significant democratization of the city government.[85] Among the most notable critics of the situation were Matteo Villani and his son Filippo. "Every lowly artisan in the city," wrote Matteo in his *Cronica*, "aspires to the rank of the priorate and the highest offices of the commune, . . . as do other citizens of little understanding and recent citizenship."[86] Filippo developed this theme in his continuation of his father's work:

[84] A plausible connection exists between political success and economic failure; the more time one spent on public affairs, presumably, the less one attended to one's own business. This may account, for example, for the disastrous performance of Benedetto di m° Galileo Galilei's silk shop; see Catasto-697/II, fol. 724.

[85] On the reform of 1343 and its political significance see Najemy, *Corporatism and Consensus*, chap. 5. On the reaction of entrenched interests Najemy, *Corporatism and Consensus*, 202-9; Brucker, *Florentine Politics and Society*, 52-53; and Becker, *Florence in Transition*, 1:177-86.

[86] Matteo Villani, *Cronica*, II, 2; 1:120.

in those times the government of the city of Florence had come in no small part to men newly arrived from the countryside and district of Florence, little experienced in public affairs, and to people come from much farther away. Such men had settled in the city and, finding themselves in the course of time rich with money made in trade and commerce and usury, married into any family they pleased. They promoted themselves so well with gifts, banquets, and petitions, both hidden and open, that they were drawn for office and placed in the scrutiny.[87]

It is in passages like these that we find the origins of the category of *gente nuova*, or new men, which has become so important in recent work on Florentine politics in the later fourteenth and the fifteenth centuries. Guided by the initial insights of Gene Brucker and Marvin Becker, a number of historians have attempted to analyze statistically the influx of new families into public office.[88] While this literature illuminates the evolution of Florentine government in the early Renaissance, it sheds less light on the *gente nuova*—their origins, their predicament, and their aspirations. The tendency has been to adopt the blanket characterization found in contemporary observers like the Villani and to write indiscriminately of the " 'new men' who had recently migrated to Florence from the *contado* and beyond" or "risen from the ranks of the urban poor."[89]

We should be wary, however, of confusing political commentary with social description. The portrayal of the *gente nuova* in the works of fourteenth- and fifteenth-century Florentine writers was neither objective nor coherent; like the complaints of many a beleaguered insider, it imposed a false homogeneity on what was clearly a diverse group.[90] Furthermore, the use of the term saw a distinct shift over the period in question. Where early fourteenth-century authors tended to stress the rural origins of the new men (Dante complained of "the stink of the peasant" which the new citizen brought with him from the Flor-

[87] Filippo Villani, *Cronica*, XI, 65, in ibid., 2:452.

[88] Brucker, *Florentine Politics and Society*; Becker, "Essay," "Florentine 'Libertas,' " and *Florence in Transition*, esp. vol. 2, chap. 2. The more statistically oriented studies are Molho, "Politics and the Ruling Class"; Dale Kent, *"Reggimento"*; Witt, "Florentine Politics"; and Najemy, *Corporatism and Consensus*, 195-202.

[89] Brucker, *Civic World*, 33.

[90] See Rubinstein, *Government of Florence*, 65, 192, and Najemy, *Corporatism and Consensus*, 202-7. Najemy has introduced a much greater degree of precision by discussing in concrete social and economic terms the important political divisions within the guild community; see his "Guild Republicanism." He does not, however, deal with the issue of immigration in any detail.

entine countryside), writers from the next century identified them not with immigrants but with the city's native lower orders: in the words of Piero Cavalcanti, "the ignoble who have attained the consulate in the lesser guilds, as well as that part of the lower craftsmen which has been drawn for the priorate."[91] This shift, however, was a gradual one. During most of the period which concerns us, aristocratic writers tended to conflate the two groups—to join in one breath "lowly artisans and foreigners,"[92] or "mechanic citizens" and immigrants from the *contado*.[93]

It was only natural for aristocratic spokesmen to group together those they regarded as politically threatening; but we must ask whether the class backgrounds, aspirations, and achievements of socially successful recent immigrants and of upwardly mobile natives of artisanal families were similar enough to warrant such an identification. Prominent Florentine doctors provide an interesting test case for this question, coming as they did almost wholly from these two groups. At least as far as they are concerned, the answer seems to be negative: although there was of course some small overlap and intermarriage, the two groups differed markedly in almost every respect.

Thus, if we look at the social origins of those doctors—both native and immigrant—classifiable as *gente nuova*, we immediately notice differences between the two. Becker, Plesner, and Martines have emphasized the upper-class origins of many of the successful immigrants to the city; scions of "the wealthiest and most influential classes of the *contado*," they had much in common culturally, socially, and economically with the Florentine patriciate, lacking only antiquity of lineage and political experience in the city.[94] This was certainly true of the immigrant doctors who enjoyed the greatest social and political success during the fourteenth and fifteenth centuries.[95] Almost to a man, they

---

[91] Quoted in Rubinstein, *Government of Florence*, 322. (Cavalcanti was commenting on the scrutiny of 1484.) Cf. Dante, *Paradiso*, XVI, 49-57.

[92] Anon., "Discurso del principio, e di alcuni fatti notabili del priorato (1377)," in *Delizie*, 9:278. See also the quotation from Matteo Villani in note 86 above.

[93] Cavalcanti, *Istorie fiorentine*, III, 2; 1:78. On this speech of 1426, attributed by Cavalcanti to Rinaldo degli Albizzi, see Brucker, *Civic World*, 474n, and Dale Kent, *Rise of the Medici*, 216-20.

[94] Becker, "Essay," 37-45, and *Florence in Transition*, 1:178 (source of quotation), 221. Becker is writing primarily of immigrants in the first half of the fourteenth century, but the generalization applies equally well to politically and socially successful immigrants in the following period, at least as far as doctors are concerned. See also Plesner, *L'émigration*, 129-57, and Martines, *Lawyers*, 74.

[95] The following statements are made on the basis of the careers of the following doctors—all immigrants or sons of immigrants and all men of social or political weight

possessed significant personal wealth on arrival, most often in the form of real estate in their towns of origin, although as they established themselves in Florence they usually diversified their holdings with investments in city property and businesses.[96] The overwhelming majority were university-trained physicians,[97] most of whom came from professional families headed by doctors, or by an occasional notary or lawyer, and had a number of other relatives in the professions. Many, like Maestro Giovanni Chellini da San Miniato or Maestro Lorenzo d'Agnolo Sassoli da Prato, belonged to politically significant families in their own towns. Finally, virtually all were natives of the *contado* or district; there is only one foreign doctor, Maestro Antonio da Bologna, whose descendants ever qualified for the Signoria.[98]

In contrast to this homogeneity, the roughly sixteen native doctors we can identify as new men were extremely diverse. To begin with, they covered the entire economic scale.[99] A few, including Maestro

---

in the city and the guild: M° Lodovico di Bartolo da Gubbio (matriculated 1363); M° Bartolomeo di m° Lodovico di Bartolo (1398); M° Lionardo di m° Agnolo da Bibbiena (ca. 1400); M° Antonio di m° Gherardo da Bologna (ca. 1350); M° Gherardo di m° Antonio di m° Gherardo (by 1363); M° Ugolino di Piero da Pisa (1423); M° Guido di ser Cambio da Pontormo (before 1340); M° Antonio Chellini da S. Miniato (ca. 1405); M° Giovanni Banducci da Prato (1371); M° Bandino di m° Giovanni Banducci (1418); M° Antonio di m° Guccio da Scarperia (ca. 1395); M° Niccolò di Francesco (Falcucci) da Borgo San Lorenzo (ca. 1360); M° Francesco di messer Niccolò (Mercadelli) da Conegliano (1365); M° Guasparre di ser Matteo da Radda (1421); M° Michele di m° Piero (Onesti) da Pescia (1429); M° Iacopo di m° Bartolo da Prato (ca. 1340); M° Lorenzo d'Agnolo Sassoli da Prato (ca. 1405); M° Simone di m° Iacopo da Figline (before 1340); and M° Tommasino di m° Simone di m° Iacopo (1370).

Criteria for inclusion in this list include more than one term as consul of the Guild of Doctors, Apothecaries, and Grocers; a descendant in the Signoria; or particularly successful marriages for themselves or their descendants.

[96] The only exceptions were M° Niccolò Falcucci and M° Bandino Banducci. M° Niccolò soon acquired a large fortune through practice and inheritance. M° Bandino was comfortable throughout his life but never rich.

[97] The only surgeons were M° Lodovico da Gubbio and M° Antonio da Bologna, both of whom matriculated before 1365.

[98] Antonio di m° Gherardo di m° Antonio became prior in 1433.

[99] The following statements are based on the careers of these doctors: M° Giovanni di m° Ambruogio (Solosmei) (matriculated in the 1340s); M° Cristofano di Giorgio (Brandolini) (1371); M° Banco di m° Latino (1340s); M° Benedetto di Ciango (ca. 1340); M° Tommaso di m° Dino Del Garbo (ca. 1348); M° Dino di ser Martino (well before 1340); M° Fruosino di Cino Della Fioraia (ca. 1350); M° Francesco di ser Niccolò (ca. 1350); M° Giovanni di Giusto (1366); M° Lorenzo di Francesco (1432); M° Piero di Giovanni fiorentino (1363); M° Simone di Cinozzo di Giovanni Cini (1429); M° Piero di m° Domenico (Toscanelli) (1425); M° Paolo di m° Domenico (Toscanelli) (1425); M° Zanobi di Iacopo Mangani (1371); and M° Zanobi di m° Lorenzo (1371).

The criteria for inclusion in this list include three or more terms as guild consul,

Tommaso Del Garbo and Maestro Piero and Maestro Paolo di maestro Domenico, were frankly rich; they inherited fortunes from their fathers and multiplied them during their own lifetimes. Several more, for example Maestro Fruosino Della Fioraia, Maestro Dino di ser Martino, Maestro Simone di Cinozzo, and Maestro Lorenzo di Francesco, were at least well-to-do, whether because, like Maestro Fruosino and Maestro Dino, they had inherited wealth or because, like Maestro Lorenzo, they had earned it. The majority, however—including some of the most politically successful, such as Maestro Cristofano di Giorgio, Maestro Piero di Giovanni, and Maestro Francesco di ser Niccolò—possessed no appreciable personal or family wealth, and some, like Maestro Francesco or Maestro Zanobi di Iacopo, were downright poor.

These upwardly mobile citizens varied also in family background. Half had fathers in the professions, although of widely differing prominence. Maestro Tommaso di maestro Dino Del Garbo's father, for example, was an illustrious physician and medical theorist with an international reputation, important enough to merit a glowing chapter in Filippo Villani's book of famous Florentines. Most of the others, however, were sons of surgeons, obscure notaries, or minor merchants. While most came from the lowest ranks of the upper guildsmen, at least one was the son of an unguilded soldier: Maestro Giovanni di Giusto's father is listed in the *prestanza* of 1379 as a crossbowman.[100] Similarly, the successful native Florentine doctors differed as to medical specialty. At least two—Maestro Banco and Maestro Zanobi—were empirics, while another five had matriculated as surgeons.[101] It was only beginning in the last decade of the fourteenth century that virtually all the prominent native doctors—as had been true throughout for immigrants—were physicians.

Thus, at least regarding social origins, there seems to have been very little in common between the two groups of doctors—immigrants and upwardly mobile native Florentines—who qualify for the name *gente nuova*. Furthermore, there seems to have been little social interaction among them in the way of signal friendships or intermarriage, although we can see such ties among members of either group. What, then, can we say about their prospects? Were their social and political expectations similar enough to close the gap in their different origins? Again, this seems not to have been the case. If we begin with social

eligibility for the Signoria through scrutiny, appearance of a son in the Signoria, or particularly advantageous marriages and social connections.

[100] Filippo Villani, *Vite*, 25-26. Prestanze-369, fol. 121r.

[101] I.e., Mº Giovanni di mº Ambruogio, Mº Benedetto di Ciango, Mº Francesco di ser Niccolò, Mº Giovanni di Giusto, and Mº Zanobi di mº Lorenzo.

prospects, we notice immediately that (as seems only natural) the upper ranks of Florentine society opened much more quickly and easily for qualified immigrants than for upwardly mobile Florentine doctors. Immigrant doctors like Maestro Niccolò Falcucci, Maestro Lorenzo Sassoli da Prato, or Maestro Giovanni Chellini da San Miniato, themselves wealthy and of prominent families in their own towns, had no difficulty in marrying into the patriciate, as we have already seen, or in arranging alliances for their children with patrician families and with the cream of the newly arrived Florentine lineages. But even the best-connected of the native nonpatrician doctors, like Maestro Cristofano di Giorgio, found such opportunities closed to them.[102]

The positions were reversed, however, when it came to political success. Here it was much more difficult for immigrants to break in than for native doctors of comparatively obscure origins and modest means, and the difficulty increased steadily after the middle of the fourteenth century. Thus there was only one doctor, Maestro Tommasino di maestro Simone, who was both the son of a recent immigrant (from Figline) and prior of Florence after 1350.[103] It was somewhat easier for a doctor of immigrant stock to be elected consul of the Guild of Doctors, Apothecaries, and Grocers, but comparatively few attained even this position, and almost none managed to transmit its political influence, such as it was, to his descendants. The new men among the native Florentine doctors were considerably more successful in this respect. Thus, of the eleven immigrant doctors to occupy the consulship of the guild between 1350 and 1450, only five held it more than once, as opposed to twelve out of fourteen native "new" doctors. Of the five immigrant consuls, only two qualified for the Signoria in a standard scrutiny, and only three had direct or collateral descendants who so qualified.[104] Among the twelve Florentine consuls, on the other hand, nine were declared eligible for the city's highest offices, and nine

---

[102] Mᵒ Cristofano married Foresina di messer Rosso degli Orlandi; Messer Rosso was himself a new man. Of their daughters, Letta married a notary, Ser Matteo di ser Niccolò Mazzetti, and Lorenza married two apothecaries in succession, Piero di Guglielmo and Doffo di Doffo, neither of whom had family names. Doctors of limited means, like Mᵒ Cristofano, would have found it nearly impossible to provide the dowries necessary to ensure a brilliant match.

[103] Mᵒ Tommasino served as prior in 1386.

[104] The two doctor-consuls were Mᵒ Tommasino and Mᵒ Bandino di mᵒ Giovanni Banducci. The descendants were Agnolo di Panico d'Agnolo, nephew and heir of Mᵒ Paolo d'Agnolo da Castel San Giovanni; Antonio di mᵒ Gherardo di mᵒ Antonio, whose grandfather immigrated from Bologna; and Francesco di mᵒ Antonio da Scarperia and his son Iacopo. See *Delizie*, 16:145; 19:60, 114; 20:428; Tratte-46, fol. 218r. This statement is based on all the extant scrutiny records for this period.

had eligible descendants.[105] Even if we look as late as 1500, only seven of the priors who were descendants of "new" doctors came from immigrant families, as opposed to twenty from Florentine stock (and this in a period when immigrant doctors outnumbered native doctors nearly two to one). The results show clearly that, as various historians have recently argued, the political and social elites were not identical in early Renaissance Florence but appear, rather, as two overlapping groups. While the patriciate as a social class was apparently contracting and becoming more castelike from the later fourteenth century on, access to political power was to some degree broadening for native Florentines, although the reverse was true for immigrants.[106]

These results also shed light on the special position of the recent immigrant, as opposed to the upwardly mobile native. The citizen parvenus were men without families only in the sense that they lacked the family traditions which marked the more patrician lineages. Nonetheless many of them, like Maestro Tommaso Del Garbo, Maestro Fruosino Della Fioraia, or Maestro Giovanni di maestro Ambruogio Solosmei, as their surnames indicate, headed households which were part of a larger clan located in a single neighborhood or a single *gonfalone*. Such families could provide the social and political reinforcement so important in Renaissance Florence.[107] Most first-generation immigrants, on the other hand, had come to the city alone or accompanied by only a few of their closest relatives. They lived in isolated households, and their family—for Florentine purposes—extended no further than the single hearth. This put them in a tenuous position. Economically and politically, such immigrant households either helped themselves or else relied on patrons among the more established Florentine families. Some, like Maestro Giovanni Chellini, managed to

[105] The nine eligible doctor-consuls were M° Tommaso Del Garbo, M° Dino di ser Martino, M° Fruosino Della Fioraia, M° Giovanni di m° Ambruogio, M° Francesco di ser Niccolò, M° Banco di m° Latino, M° Piero di Giovanni, M° Cristofano di Giorgio, and M° Simone di Cinozzo Cini. The nine with eligible descendants were the above, with the exceptions of M° Francesco di ser Niccolò, who apparently died without male issue, and M° Dino di ser Martino, several of whose sons were exiled or declared politically ineligible because of political misdeeds (Stefani, *Cronaca fiorentina*, 305, 310, and Brucker, *Civic World*, 95); to them should be added M° Zanobi di m° Lorenzo and M° Piero di m° Domenico.

[106] See Cohn's formulation in *Laboring Classes*, 45, based on the research of Molho and Dale Kent. Historians previously tended to connect social and political standing more closely; cf. Martines, *Social World*, 48, 51. The case of immigrants was entirely different, as is made clear in Kirshner, "Paolo di Castro"; Kirshner traces the progressive tightening of citizenship requirements for officeholding.

[107] This is a central point of F. W. Kent's *Household and Lineage*, esp. pt. II; see also Dale Kent, "*Reggimento*," 587-92.

convert that patronage into a solid position. Others, however, were reduced to simple dependency. Such was the fate, for example, of the physician Maestro Iacopo di Martino da Spoleto. Forced by illness in his fifties to curtail his practice, he appeared in the *catasto* of 1427 as a mere appendage to the powerful Castellani family. His only declared assets were a wooden desk, his medical library, fl. 100 worth of shares in the Monte commune, and fl. 170 in loans to various members of the family. He lived in the house of Messer Matteo Castellani, and his assessment of his situation was eloquent: "I am fifty-seven, and I have suffered from dropsy for a number of years. I have spent or am spending to cure myself what little is left to me, and if it were not for Messer Matteo I could not live."[108]

More basic even than the economic and political vulnerability of immigrant families was their biological frailty. In this period of frequent epidemics and high mortality it was not uncommon even for a lineage composed of a number of households to extinguish itself. The isolated immigrant household was much more at risk. Examples of this are not hard to find. Take the case of Maestro Iacopo di Filippo da Bisticci, a doctor active in Florence in the mid-fifteenth century. His father, Filippo di Lionardo, a factor in a textile concern, had immigrated from the *contado*, married a Florentine woman, and produced six children—including four sons to ensure the continuity of his line. But one of Maestro Iacopo's brothers died young; two others, Vespasiano and Lionardo, apparently never married and produced no heirs. Maestro Iacopo's only surviving son, Maestro Lorenzo, himself a physician, died without issue the year after his marriage, and a year later, in 1479, Vespasiano, stationer to the humanists and the only surviving member of the family, retired alone to his country estate in Antella, "land of oblivion," as he described it to a correspondent.[109] The family's house in the city was finally sold in 1485. Nor was Maestro Iacopo's case unusual. A number of successful doctors, including Maestro Giovanni Chellini himself, failed to produce adult male heirs to consolidate their successes. Those who, like Chellini or Maestro Antonio da Scarperia, had immigrated in the company of one or more brothers placed their families in a much more secure position.[110]

---

[108] Catasto-28, fol. 575r: "Sono già d'età d'anni 57. Et già sono più anni me cadde la gocciola. Et ò speso et spendo per guarire, sì che pocho m'è rimaso. Et se non fusse Messer Mattheo non potrei vivere."

[109] See Cagni, *Vespasiano da Bisticci*, 12-40; Vespasiano's letter to Ser Leonardo di Giovanni da Colle (vi.1479) is edited in ibid., 161-62.

[110] Mᵒ Giovanni's two sons died without male issue. He left as heir his nephew Bartolomeo di ser Bartolomeo; Battistini, "Giovanni Chellini," 114; Miscellanea repubbli-

When Maestro Ugolino da Montecatini was debating whether to immigrate to Florence (we encountered him in Chapter Four, agonizing over this choice), his worries were mainly short-term ones involving his own earnings and reputation. If the experiences of other prominent and prosperous immigrant doctors are any indication, those fears were unfounded: the upper levels of the Florentine profession lacked for neither *utile* nor *onore*. The real problems were other, more long-term ones—the difficulty of assuring the biological, economic, and political survival of his family. In Maestro Ugolino's case, such long-term fears would have been justified. He did in fact immigrate to Florence near the end of his life, and on his death in 1425 he left two adolescent sons, Piero and Giovanni. Twenty-five years later, in the *catasto* of 1451, both were dead, and Piero's minor heirs had been constrained to sell most of the family property, including the family house in Montecatini.[111]

Certainly doctors represent only a single, and in some respects unusual, occupational group. It would be unwarranted to use them to construct a comprehensive picture of the successes and frustrations of the new men of Florence. Nonetheless, they do show clearly the obstacles faced by socially and geographically mobile families in a corporately organized society, and in particular the sacrifices made even by the wealthiest middle-class immigrants to the city. Their losses, however, were Florence's gain. For as the examples of Maestro Ugolino, Maestro Antonio da Scarperia, Maestro Niccolò Falcucci, and many others show, these men were among the doctors who made significant contributions to Florentine culture.

---

cana-98, no. 9. It was his grandnephew, Bartolomeo di Bartolomeo, who became prior in 1493, crowning his father's and grandfather's social and economic achievements.

[111] Catasto-77, fols. 135v-38r; Catasto-709, fol. 201r.

Doctors in Florentine Culture

O NE OF the reasons why doctors chose to immigrate to Florence was the city's cultural vitality. We have seen in Chapter Four how educated men like Maestro Lorenzo Sassoli, languishing in the small towns of the countryside, were attracted by its university and its schools, its pool of literate and intellectually active inhabitants, its tradition of public and private patronage of learning and the arts. At the same time the city welcomed the cultural contributions of its doctors. The commune celebrated their discoveries in the acts of its councils,[1] called on them as consultants for artistic projects,[2] and included them in frescoes celebrating its leading citizens.[3] The lives and deaths of prominent physicians appear in works like Filippo Villani's *Lives of Famous Florentines* as well as in chronicles and more humble diaries.[4] Thus Florence treated its doctors not only as a reservoir of cultural judgment and taste but also as part of its intellectual patrimony and a source of communal honor.

[1] See the legislation regarding the "pills of Maestro Antonio da Scarperia" in Alessandro Gherardi, *Statuti*, 471-72; quoted above in Chapter Four, note 53.

[2] In 1428, for example, M° Lorenzo Sassoli da Prato was named as arbiter of the value of Donatello's and Michelozzo's pulpit for the Cathedral of Prato; Janson, *Sculpture of Donatello*, 1:109-110. M° Paolo Toscanelli acted as one of the consultants for the dome and interior of the Florentine cathedral; Guasti, *Cupola*, doc. 202.

[3] For example Giorgio Vasari depicted Paolo Toscanelli in his fresco of Cosimo de' Medici surrounded by illustrious Florentines, in the Palazzo della Signoria; Bargellini, *Scoperta*, 128. Maestro Dino Del Garbo, Maestro Tommaso's father, figured among the saved in Orcagna's *Last Judgment*, painted for the church of Santa Croce; Siraisi, *Taddeo Alderotti*, 62.

[4] See Filippo Villani's biographies of Taddeo Alderotti (d. 1295), Dino Del Garbo (d. 1327), Torrigiano Torrigiani (d. ca. 1319), and Tommaso Del Garbo (d. 1370) in his *Vite*, and the biography of Paolo Toscanelli in Vespasiano da Bisticci, *Vite*, 2:72-75. For a general discussion of portraits of Italian doctors in collective biographies of the Renaissance see Siraisi's forthcoming article in Alistair Crombie, ed., *The Rational Arts of Living*. Sozomeno da Pistoia mentions the death of Niccolò Falcucci in his *Chronicon universale*, 3. Luca Landucci speaks with reverence of Toscanelli; see his *Diario*, 3.

We have been concerned thus far with the institutional and social history of the medical profession in fourteenth- and fifteenth-century Florence. This study would be incomplete, however, without some consideration of the place of doctors in the cultural life of the city. Medicine was an intellectual discipline as well as a practical one, and many members of the profession were equipped by training and inclination to play an active part in the literary and artistic culture of Florence. Virtually all the city's physicians were doctors of arts and medicine. This meant that they had ordinarily spent at least seven years at one or more universities and that they were versed in basic Latin grammar and rhetoric as well as in the theoretical and practical branches of medicine.[5] They might also have studied mathematics and astronomy, and all were literate in both Latin and the vernacular. Furthermore, as we have already seen, doctors were linked by social and intellectual ties to the teachers, clerics, notaries, lawyers, and educated patricians who formed the core of the Florentine intelligentsia.

Florentine culture in the later fourteenth and the fifteenth centuries was shaped both by the nature of the intellectual community and by its intellectual traditions. The city's cultural life unfolded within a complex of formal and informal institutions and relationships. Among the former were its guilds, its private schools, its monasteries and convents, and its intermittently successful university. The latter embraced the various intellectual circles of early Renaissance Florence as well as the rich fabric of private and public patronage, friendship, and discipleship which bound students and teachers, fathers and sons, writers or artists and their audiences. Such institutions and relationships channeled a variety of intellectual traditions. These included, for example, the calculatory tradition of commercial arithmetic and practical astronomy embodied in the work and teaching of men like Paolo Dagomari and Luca Pacioli[6] or the scholastic tradition in logic, natural philosophy, medicine, law, and theology that had its stronghold in the *studio* and the schools of some of the religious orders.[7] Such traditions co-

---

[5] On the requirements for a degree in arts and medicine see Alessandro Gherardi, *Statuti*, 77-78 (University of Florence: statute of 1387/8, II, 69); Malagola, *Statuti*, 274-76 (University of Bologna: statute of 1405, 78).

[6] See Goldthwaite, "Schools and Teachers," and von Egmond, "New Light."

[7] This Florentine tradition has never been fully examined in its own right, although some information can be pieced together from studies on the relationship between humanism and scholasticism, on intellectuals like Luigi Marsili, and on the libraries and schools of the convents of San Marco, Santa Croce, and Santa Maria Novella. See in particular Garin, "Cultura fiorentina"; Vasoli, "Polemiche occamiste"; and Davis, "Education," esp. 420-35, as well as other literature cited in the second and third sections of this chapter.

existed with—and were at times challenged by—the new movement of humanism which was beginning to consolidate itself in the decades around 1400; this had its roots in the private circles of friends and admirers forming around men like Marsili, Chrysoloras, Salutati, and Traversari, in the convents and libraries of Santo Spirito, Santa Maria degli Angeli, and Santa Croce, and in the chancery of the Florentine commune and the intermittently resident papal court.[8]

In examining some of these institutions and traditions, however, we should be aware of the limited scope of our study. During the early Renaissance, university-educated physicians and surgeons comprised less than half of the profession, and there is no evidence that other doctors, many of whom may have been only marginally literate, played any part in Florence's high culture. Even among the university-educated doctors, only a few (and those overwhelmingly physicians) participated actively in the city's intellectual and artistic life. Thus in this chapter I have tried less to construct an exhaustive collective portrait than to interpret the motives and the contributions of the relatively few Florentine doctors who appear as culturally active in the extant records.

This approach requires some revaluation of Florentine intellectual life in the later fourteenth and the fifteenth centuries. Most historians of Florentine culture in this period have concentrated on the movements associated with humanism and the new art, to the virtual exclusion of the other intellectual traditions mentioned above. Their account does particular injustice to scholastic learning, which was after all the dominant form of high intellectual culture: they tend either to ignore it entirely or to reduce it to the uninspiring backdrop against which the originality of the early humanists stands in high relief. The example of medicine, however, shows that the scholastic tradition was still vital. Writers like Tommaso Del Garbo or Ugolino da Montecatini (in deference to their celebrity we can refer to them without their honorific titles) saw themselves as part of a continuing enterprise of medical discovery. Their works testify to the interest and sophistication of the scholastic tradition as well as to its ability to generate new problems and new forms.

At the same time physicians also participated in the literary and artistic culture of the Renaissance, although in a more marginal way,

[8] The literature on early Florentine humanism is vast. For a lucid introduction focusing on the social and institutional context see George Holmes, *Florentine Enlightenment*, and also the studies of Paul Oskar Kirsteller and Eugenio Garin cited in the Bibliography.

as patrons, book collectors, and aspiring classical philologists. Their example argues against the common assumption that humanist and scholastic scholars were hostile and unreceptive to each others' forms of learning, an assumption based largely on the literal reading of a few polemical texts by Petrarch and Salutati. But polemics are notoriously unreliable as historical sources. If we move from these texts to the social and institutional world from which they sprang, the continuities reassert themselves and the ruptures seem less abrupt. Despite their differences, many physicans and humanists shared not only a broad common culture but also common interests, experiences, and ambitions—as immigrants, as *gente nuova*, and as intellectuals with a professional education—and these are as important for our understanding of Florentine culture as polemics and treatises. In this chapter, then, we will begin by looking at the intellectual culture of the Florentine medical profession as revealed in the books they owned and read. We will then examine the culture of both academic medicine and medical practice through the works of the more important and prolific Florentine medical writers. Finally, we will study the place of doctors in the cultural movements of the early Florentine Renaissance.

DOCTORS' LIBRARIES

A man's library is no sure index to his culture. Doctors doubtless owned books they never read, although this was probably far less common before the invention of printing in the mid-fifteenth century, when manuscripts were relatively rare and expensive. They certainly read books they never owned: as their account books show, borrowing and lending manuscripts was a matter of course. Nonetheless, the inventories of doctors' libraries, supplemented by their accounts, are the best available source of information concerning the intellectual life and interests of the profession as a whole.[9]

Even in a cultural center like Florence, manuscripts were difficult to come by and large private libraries unusual. Only the rich could afford to hire scribes to produce books for them; others either assumed the laborious task of copying texts themselves or bought them secondhand from stationers, friends, teachers, and the various religious foundations

[9] Samuel Hough at Brown University is in the process of studying this subject in more detail.

which received libraries as bequests.[10] There are still no statistical studies of book ownership in Florence; nonetheless it seems likely, by analogy with other parts of Europe, that the groups most likely to possess manuscripts included the clergy, university teachers and students, lawyers, notaries, and doctors, together with a smaller proportion of merchants and tradesmen, whose holdings have recently been studied by Christian Bec.[11]

As their *catasto* declarations show, doctors in fact had a high rate of book ownership relative to the rest of the city's population. Of the thirty-six doctors resident in Florence in 1427, nineteen lived in households which declared books as part of their assets.[12] Of these, eighteen were physicians—a fact which confirms the impression that surgery was for the most part a craft learned by apprenticeship. The only surgeon to own any books at all was Maestro Piero di Feo da Arencio, doctor to the communal prison. Evidently he seldom referred to them, for all four were on deposit at a local bank, presumably as security for a loan; assessed at fl. 10, they were the smallest medical collection in the *catasto*. Conversely, the only physician without a library was Maestro Giovanni di Bartolomeo da Montecatini, a marginal figure who had the distinction of being the poorest doctor in the city and being burned for heresy.[13] While three physicians' libraries in the *catasto* were valued at fl. 100 or more, most of the rest fell between fl. 20 and fl. 50; these were considerable sums at the time, but they reflected not so much extensive libraries as the high cost of manuscripts, which could run to fl. 5 or 6, although the average was more typically fl. 1 or 2. In a period when the salary of a junior lecturer in arts or medicine amounted to only fl. 20 or 30, such prices demanded considerable sacrifices by younger and less prosperous physicians. The libraries declared by some of the poorer doctors in 1427 represented 15 or 20 percent of their net wealth.

To judge by the contents of three libraries inventoried for the *catasto* in 1427, the smaller collections owned by doctors were similar in extent and range. They consisted typically of seven or eight books, vir-

[10] On the Florentine book market in this period see De la Mare, "Shop of a Florentine 'Cartolaio' " and "Messer Piero Strozzi," and Carabellese, "La compagnia di Orsanmichele."

[11] Bec, *Les marchands écrivains*, 407-15; also Febvre and Martin, *Coming of the Book*, 263.

[12] See Appendix III for details.

[13] Catasto-88, fol. 178r (Mᵒ Piero); Catasto-76, fol. 307v (Mᵒ Giovanni). On the latter's trial and execution see Uzielli, *Toscanelli*, 212-14.

tually all of them medical texts, and a few notebooks on logic, grammar, and philosophy copied by the owner and declared without value.[14] The notebooks and many of the books were probably acquired while the owner was a student; the titles of the latter include the standard texts on which the medical curriculum was based: Avicenna's *Canon*; the *Articella* (a collection of Greek and Arabic treatises on medicine), with associated commentaries; and medical works by the Arabic authors Rhazes, Mesue, and Isaac Israeli.[15] In addition Maestro Lionardo di maestro Agnolo da Bibbiena owned the *Surgery* of Guglielmo da Saliceto, a thirteenth-century Italian author, while Maestro Giovanni Chellini da San Miniato declared a volume of Aristotle's logical works and another of the "philosophy of Aristotle, with the *Physics* and other books pertaining to that philosophy." Only Maestro Domenico di maestro Giovanni explicitly mentioned expanding his library after he had left the university; his list included a copy of the *Conciliator* of Pietro d'Abano purchased three years earlier. Maestro Giovanni Chellini was alone in declaring any books on nonprofessional subjects: he owned several volumes without value, "for pleasure."

Thus doctors' libraries had a strong professional cast. While merchants, if they collected manuscripts at all, tended to own devotional

---

[14] The three inventories in question are those of M° Lionardo di m° Agnolo da Bibbiena, M° Domenico di m° Giovanni, and M° Giovanni di m° Antonio Chellini da San Miniato (Catasto-25, fols. 95r-96v; 61, fols. 708v-9r; 63, fol. 646r). M° Giovanni's collection, for example, included the following works:

Avicenna, *Canon*, I and II (in one volume)	fl. 2
Avicenna, *Canon*, III and V (in one volume)	fl. 5
Avicenna, *Canon*, IV, with other short works	fl. 2
Articella, including Hippocrates' *Aphorisms*, Galen's *Art of Medicine*, and other short works	fl. 3
Mesue (probably *Antidotarium*)	fl. 2
Rhazes, *Ad Almansorem*	fl. 2
"Several notebooks written by his own hand, useful to him, but of no value"	—
"Certain notebooks and short works of logic which he has written himself, of no value, since they cannot be bought or sold"	—
"Some books for pleasure"	—
Aristotle, *Physics*, and other works of philosophy	fl. 3
Aristotle, *Logic*, and other works of logic	fl. 1
	fl.20

For a similar collection from the 1480s see Verde, *Studio fiorentino*, 2:255-56.

[15] On the *Articella* and the medical curriculum of the late medieval Italian university see Kristeller, "Bartholomaeus, Musandinus, and Maurus of Salerno," Siraisi, *Taddeo Alderotti*, 98-107.

works, elementary grammar texts, and occasional works of classical and contemporary literature—most or all in Italian[16]—the books owned by physicians were almost exclusively Latin medical texts. This does not imply that doctors never read outside the field of medicine, but it suggests that the price of manuscripts was high enough to prevent many of them from acquiring books on other subjects except on loan.

The practice of borrowing books was in fact widespread among doctors, as we can see from the account books of Don Giovanni di Baldassare, a Vallombrosan monk, and Maestro Giovanni Chellini da San Miniato, both of whom were active lenders of medical and philosophical manuscripts.[17] Don Giovanni's *ricordanza* runs from 1396 to 1400. Many of the men who borrowed books from him during that time were students in arts and medicine at the University of Florence; they consulted a wide variety of works on medical theory, logic, and natural philosophy, with an emphasis on recent Latin authors: Heytesbury, Swineshead, Blasius of Parma, Marsilius of Inghen, Albert of Saxony, and others. Most of those who borrowed from Maestro Giovanni, on the other hand (he had added significantly to his *catasto* collection by the 1450s, when he began to lend manuscripts in large numbers) were practicing Florentine physicians. Their interests, unlike the more theoretical concerns of the students, were limited almost entirely to practical medicine. There are references, for example, to both Bernard Gordon's *Lily of Medicine*, a widely used compendium, and Serapion's *Practica*; the work in by far the most demand, however, was the *Medical Sermons* or *Practica* of the Florentine doctor Niccolò Falcucci (d. 1412), a massive and systematic catalogue of particular diseases and their causes, symptoms, and cures. Chellini owned two copies of this work, which he repeatedly lent by section to local physicians wishing to consult it on specific topics and to copy relevant passages. "He said he wanted to read about the diseases of the gall bladder," runs a typical entry in the account book, or "to read about the diseases of the womb," "to read about hysteria," "on fevers."[18]

Practicing physicians may well have found compendia like Falcucci's *Sermons* more useful than the more theoretical treatises and commentaries they had used at the university. According to a contemporary admirer of Falcucci, "while at the *studio*, every doctor studies Avi-

[16] Bec, *Les marchands écrivains*, 407-12. These smaller merchants' libraries typically consisted of between one and ten books.

[17] Brentano-Keller, "Il libretto"; *Ricordanza* of Mᵒ Giovanni Chellini, Università Bocconi (Milan): Istituto di storia economica, cod. 2 (new numeration), fols. 1r-201r.

[18] Chellini, *Ricordanza*, fols. 174r-v, 175v, 196v, 200r. For an introduction to this literature see Demaitre, "Scholasticism."

cenna, Galen, Hippocrates, and many worthy medical authors. But then they abandon all such writers, pawn their books, and take with them only the *Practica* of Maestro Niccolò, which explains all remedies to perfection."[19] Thus when Maestro Galileo di Giovanni Galilei, a prominent and wealthy Florentine physician, filed his *catasto* declaration in 1427, he felt compelled to explain to the city officials why he owned only fl. 30 worth of books. "For twelve years," he wrote, "I have had in my possession a work by Maestro Niccolò, in which, with great clarity and understanding, he has collected and summarized the opinions and teachings of almost all the authorities, as well as many beautiful speculations and experiences and useful things from his own mind. The book itself is made up of twelve hundred great folios and is the most useful work on medicine to have been written in the last five hundred years."[20]

Surgeons also borrowed books, although such references are much rarer and the works in question are almost always in the vernacular. In the years around 1400, for example, Ser Piero Mini, head of the hospital of Santa Maria Nuova, lent two manuscripts to Maestro Giovanni di ser Bartolo da Radda, a "book of medicine in Italian" and a homilary, and Maestro Giovanni Banducci da Prato borrowed three from Don Giovanni di Baldassare: "the fourth book of the Holy Fathers," "a book of school stories on the Old Testament," and "the Boethius" (probably an Italian translation of *The Consolation of Philosophy*).[21] In their nonmedical reading surgeons seem to have resembled physicians. Thus, if we supplement our small sample of Florentine

---

[19] BNF: Magl. XV, 71: "et fe' maraviglosi libri, i quali son' magnifichi. Chiamasi la *Praticha* del Maestro Niccholò di Firenze, in tal modo che in ongni studio ongni dottore studia in Avicena o in Galieno o in Iprograso et molti valenti autori di medicina, et nella fine istanno allo studio più anni, e di poi lasciano tutti i libri e tali autori, solo s'appicano e portano cho' loro libri della *Praticha* del Maestro Niccholò, e che quelli sono aluminati della medicina mostrando profettamente tutti rimedi." Most of the doctors who owned Falcucci's work had only the last six parts; the first, on medical theory, was much less popular, implying that the book was prized precisely for its practical utility.

[20] Catasto-29, fols. 235r-36r: "Da dodici anni in qua io ò tenuto uno libro il quale fece il Mº Niccholò, nel quale con grande ordine e grande intelletto racholse ed abrieviò le sententie e i detti quasi di tutti gli autori e appresso di suo intelletto molte belle spechulationi e isperimenti e utili chose. Ed è il detto libro di volume di mille dugiento fogli reali, ed è il più utile libro a medichare che ssi facesse da cinqueciento anni in qua." Mº Galileo had also excerpted various medical writings himself.

[21] SMN-31, fols. 5, 9 (entries from xii.1399 and ii.1400/1); Brentano-Keller, "Il libretto," 143, 150, 155. The vernacular Boethius appeared commonly in merchants' libraries; see, for example, the inventory of Ugo Vecchietti's fourteen manuscripts in Bec, *Les marchands écrivains*, 412.

booklists with inventories of physicians' libraries from other northern cities, we can find a sprinkling of nonmedical manuscripts:[22] the *Golden Legend* of Iacopo da Voragine (a popular collection of saints' lives); portions of the Bible (usually the Gospels or the Psalms, sometimes with commentary) or compilations of biblical stories; and an occasional copy of the *Divine Comedy*—the same mix of works of devotional and vernacular literature which were also owned and read by Florentine merchants.[23] In this respect the Florentine doctor was also part of the general lay culture of his time.

As Maestro Giovanni Chellini's account book shows, however, a few Florentine physicians were bibliophiles and serious collectors of manuscripts. (Recall Maestro Ugo Benzi da Siena's comment on his own books: "I prize them like half of my soul.")[24] Like Benzi, some of these men were associated with the university; Maestro Ugolino da Montecatini and Maestro Agostino di Stefano Santucci da Urbino, for example, both taught medicine at the Florentine *studio*.[25] Others, like Maestro Lorenzo Sassoli da Prato and Maestro Mariotto di Niccolò da Castiglione Aretino, were practicing doctors, while Maestro Paolo Toscanelli and Chellini, both of whom possessed sizable collections, had abandoned regular practice for other pursuits.[26] These larger libraries typically contained from fifty to a hundred titles and were assessed at between fl. 100 and fl. 175. Their contents varied according to the special interests and background of the owner; a physician with

[22] Here and in the rest of this section I am drawing for comparative material on the inventories contained in the following: Ceccarelli and Manara, "Livello di cultura"; Leporace, "Biblioteche mediche"; Cipolla, "Valore," 8-11; Lazzarino, "I libri," 26-32; Gloria, *Monumenti*, 1:112-13 and 2:385; Billanovich, "Giacomo Zanetini," 29-40; Corradi, "Biblioteca"; Biadego, "Medici veronesi," 578-84; Lazzareschi, "Ricchezze," 117-26, 137-39; Mazzi, "Studio," 35-48; Garosi, "Codici di medicina," 227; Dorez, "Recherches"; and Sambin, "Cristoforo Barzizza."

[23] See Bec, *Les marchands écrivains*, 407-13.

[24] Quoted in Garosi, *Inter artium*, 10.

[25] Inventories and biographical sketches in Bombe, "Hausinventar," 228-38; Battistini, "Contributo"; and Ristori, "Libreria," 35-37.

[26] The inventory of M° Lorenzo's library is not extant, but it was clearly a very large collection; in the *catasto* of 1427 he declared fl. 150 of "libri di mio uso di medicina e d'altre scienze"; Catasto-47, fols. 79r-81v. M° Mariotto di Niccolò was the doctor first of Piero de' Medici and then of the hospital of Santa Maria Nuova; see the list of medical books he donated to the library in SMN-75, fol. 353v. The contents of Toscanelli's library are presently unknown, although Uzielli claimed to have found a list of his Greek manuscripts; see his *Toscanelli*, 656. In 1427 Toscanelli's father, M° Domenico di Piero, declared medical books worth fl. 160, most of which probably belonged to his two sons, who had recently returned from their studies at Padua; Catasto-65, fols. 92v-96v. Information about Chellini's collection can be gleaned from the entries in his account book; see note 17 above.

a degree from the University of Bologna tended to own more works of Bolognese authors, for example, while others might have a particularly strong collection in astronomy, alchemy, or mathematics. But even these libraries were very strongly oriented toward medicine and its ancillary disciplines, although they embraced a much wider range of texts than those of the average physician. Of the hundred and fifteen manuscripts belonging to Maestro Ugolino da Montecatini at his death in 1425, for example, all but fourteen were works of medicine or natural philosophy. The rest were theological and devotional—parts of the Bible; commentaries on the *Sentences* of Peter Lombard by Aquinas, Durandus de Saint-Pourçain, and others; a treatise by Hugh of St. Victor; "a pamphlet on the body of Christ"—with the exception of a single, secular volume: the travels of Marco Polo.[27]

Maestro Ugolino was unusual in the strength of his religious interests. By the mid-fifteenth century the nontechnical portion of most large medical libraries was devoted to classical and contemporary literature. Thus the seventy volumes of Maestro Agostino di Stefano Santucci, inventoried in 1468, included besides the usual array of scholastic texts two elementary books of grammar and rhetoric (doubtless relics of his school days); a work on the art of memory; the *Aeneid*; the *Facta* of Valerius Maximus, with commentary; Petrarch's Latin treatise *On the Remedies of Both Kinds of Fortune*; and Dante's *Comedy*.[28] Maestro Giovanni Chellini owned several other classical works, notably Bruni's Latin translation of Aristotle's *Ethics*, a book by Pompeius Festus, presumably *On the Signification of Words*, and Diogenes Laertius' *On the Lives of the Philosophers*.[29] With the exception of Maestro Paolo Toscanelli, the contents of whose library are unknown, and of Maestro Antonio Benivieni, who was active toward the end of the fifteenth century, we can hardly call these Florentine doctors and book collectors humanists:[30] for every volume of Vergil or Petrarch they owned five of Avicenna, and on the whole their tastes did not go beyond the most conventional of classical authors.[31] Nonetheless, they had not only a reading knowledge of Latin but also a passing interest

[27] Battistini, "Contributo," 145-47.

[28] Ristori, "Libreria," 35-37.

[29] Chellini, *Ricordanza*, fols. 152v, 161r, 172r.

[30] Benivieni's library is catalogued in Bindo de Vecchi, "Libri," 297-301; see also Dorez, "Recherches," on the library of Mᵒ Pierleone Leoni da Spoleto. Other fourteenth- and fifteenth-century doctors whose book collections testify to humanist interests include Mᵒ Giovanni Dondi da Padova and Mᵒ Giovanni Marco da Rimini; see Lazzarino, "I libri," and Baader, "Bibliothek."

[31] See Bec, *Les marchands écrivains*, 411; the classical authors most commonly read in translation were Boethius, Cicero, Ovid, Sallust, Valerius Maximus, Livy, and Vergil.

in classical culture, and at least Chellini showed an awareness of the new philology flourishing in the city.

The libraries of most Florentine physicians, however, were confined to works of theory which they had studied at the university and compendia of use in medical practice, and the mere lists of titles give little sense of the richness and variety of academic medicine in this period. If we turn to the medical works written by Florentine doctors, we find a much more dynamic intellectual tradition than inventories can reveal.

The Culture of Academic Medicine

The writing of Florentine doctors, like their reading, centered on the discipline of medicine and, to a much lesser extent, the related fields of natural philosophy, astronomy, and mathematics. Yet the intellectual world of medical culture was a wide one; it embraced medical students and their professors as well as practicing doctors and their clients, and the texts it produced reflected the varied institutional and social world of medicine itself. Thus doctors wrote for three main groups of readers: an academic audience of students and teachers; a broader professional audience of practicing physicians and surgeons (that portion of them who read); and a lay audience of clients, patrons, and interested citizens. In this section we will look at the works produced by Florentine doctors for the first group, concentrating on the oeuvre of Tommaso Del Garbo, the most illustrious medical writer at the University of Florence in the early Renaissance.

Academic medicine was in many ways the backbone of the intellectual discipline of medicine. Virtually all Italian medical writing of the fourteenth and fifteenth centuries was based on a unified tradition of theory and practice which had its seat in the late medieval universities.[32] By about 1300 medicine had emerged as an autonomous discipline with a recognizable curriculum based on the study of Hippocrates, Aristotle, and Galen, among classical authors, and Avicenna, Rhazes, Averroës, and Haly Abbas, among their Islamic followers; and it flowered in both Italy and the North, although with local differences.[33] In Italy the study of medicine was characteristically secular in

---

[32] On popular alternatives to the tradition see above, Chapter Three.

[33] These developments were prepared at Salerno, the main center of medical study in Italy through the middle of the thirteenth century, but they did not reach maturity until a generation or so later, when Salerno was already in decline; see Kristeller, "School of Salerno." The main source for the formation of Italian medical studies and medical curriculum in this period is Siraisi, *Taddeo Alderotti*, chap. 4; for a general bibliograhical

orientation. Surgery, which in northern Europe was treated mostly as a manual craft, was integrated into the Italian universities, where it was studied by physicians as well as by surgeons in training, and where it developed its own textual and intellectual tradition.[34] And whereas in northern universities medicine usually constituted a separate college, in Italy it was taught in the same faculty, and often by the same professors, as the disciplines known as the arts: logic, astronomy or astrology, philosophy, and (at least in Florence) grammar, rhetoric, Greek, and the works of Dante. This situation gave Italian medicine a certain speculative and philosophical cast.[35]

The two great centers of academic medicine in early Renaissance Italy were Padua and Bologna. Florence had strong political and cultural ties with the latter, its neighbor to the north, and the University of Bologna attracted many Florentine students and scholars. The central figure of the early fourteenth-century Bolognese school of medicine, Taddeo Alderotti, was himself a Florentine, as were two of his most influential pupils, Dino Del Garbo and Torrigiano Torrigiani.[36] Thus it was only natural that when a university was founded in Florence during the last months of the plague of 1348, Dino's son Tommaso was invited from Bologna to occupy the first chair in *physica*. Having voted to establish a university, however, the communal government was unwilling to guarantee it stable and substantial funding during the century after 1348. For this reason the Florentine *studio*, like that of Siena or Perugia, remained a second-class institution in both size and reputation, although it enjoyed episodes of prosperity and vitality.[37] The important medical writers who taught there were almost all foreigners who remained in Florence at most two or three years, unless, like Tommaso Del Garbo, they were bound to the city by other ties.

If Florence produced considerably less significant work in academic medicine than Bologna or Padua, there were nonetheless several medical authors associated with its university in the early Renaissance: Lodovico di Bartolo da Gubbio and Iacopo di maestro Bartolo da Prato

---

survey see Siraisi, "Some Recent Work." For the books prescribed in medicine at Bologna in 1405 see Appendix II.

[34] Siraisi, *Taddeo Alderotti*, 108-10; see also her *Arts and Sciences at Padua*, 166-71.

[35] See Kristeller, "Philosophy and Medicine," 33-35.

[36] See Siraisi, *Taddeo Alderotti*, on the Bolognese school.

[37] On the foundation of the *studio* and its history in the early Renaissance see Brucker, "Florence and Its University." Its best years were the 1360s, 1390s, and the decade or so after 1413; see Park, "Readers," esp. 250-51, 269-71. On the University of Florence in the later Renaissance see Verde, *Studio fiorentino*.

produced commentaries on the surgical sections of Avicenna's *Canon* in the 1360s and 1370s,[38] and Antonio di maestro Guccio da Scarperia taught and wrote on *physica* in Florence in the decades around 1400.[39] These lesser lights were far outshone, however, by Tommaso Del Garbo (d. 1370), who alone of these authors produced a corpus of medical works which was still being reprinted in the mid-sixteenth century.[40]

Despite its small size and precarious funding, the University of Florence played an important part in the intellectual life of the city. Be-

---

[38] Lodovico di Bartolo da Gubbio, Commentary on Avicenna, *Canon*, IV, 3 (BVA: Pal. lat. 1131, fols. 1r-168v). Iacopo di maestro Bartolo da Prato, *De operatione manuali* (BNF: Pal. 811, fols. 1r-25v); this work, which is incomplete and possibly unfinished, is presented as an autonomous treatise for medical students, although it closely follows the organization and subject matter of *Canon*, IV. The same manuscript contains two other short items by the same author: *Responsio ad quandam lecteram quam misit michi Magister Nerius de Senis, in qua reprendebat Dinum et Gentilem super expositione testus 4i Canonis capitulo de medicinis consolidativis* (fol. 26r-v), and *Quae complexio humana sit longioris vite* (fol. 27r-v), based on a question disputed by Iacopo at Perugia. Further copies of *De operatione manuali*, in Wellcome MS 375, fols. 1-73; Wellcome MS 540, fols. 151-76.

[39] Antonio's works include *De signis febrium* (BVA: Pal. lat. 1265, fols. 13r-21v; BR: Ricc. 2153, fols. 61r-101r; Bodleian: Canon. misc. MSS 455, fols. 260v-70r), composed while teaching at Florence in 1392, according to the incipit in Ricc. 2153; all copies more or less incomplete. His *Summa de causis et curis febrium* (BVA: Vat. lat. 4440, fols. 90r-107v) was probably written at about the same time, to judge by the overlap in subject and the author's reference on fol. 98r to practice in the hospital of Santa Maria Nuova. A number of other works by Mº Antonio survive, copied by students while he was lecturing on *physica* at the University of Perugia in 1386-87: *Questio de contraoperantiis* (Vat. lat. 4445, fols. 66r-90r; Vat. lat. 4447, fols. 2r-24v); *Questio utrum digestio et evacuatio que fiunt in morbo . . .* (Vat. lat. 4447, fols. 25r-32v); thirty-three questions on natural philosophy and medicine (Vat. lat. 4447, fols. 257r-94r); Commentary on Hippocrates' *Prognostics* (Vat. lat. 4447, fols. 33r-98v); Commentary on Hippocrates' *De regimine acutorum* (Vat. lat. 4447, fols. 99r-157v); and Commentary on Galen's *Tegni* (Vat. lat. 4448). The first four works are attributed to Mº Antonio in the manuscripts themselves. The main evidence for his authorship of the others comes from the explicit of the commentary on the *Prognostics* (Vat. lat. 4447, fol. 157v: "A.D. in quo legi librum Tegni Galieni et librum Pronosticorum Ypocratis et librum eiusdem de regimine acutorum morborum . . . "); the dates in 1386-87 scattered throughout the last three commentaries; and the incipit of the *Questio de contraoperantiis* (Vat. lat. 4445, fol. 66r): "Incipit questio medicinalis difficilis et profunda de contraoperantiis determinata per egregium artium et medicine doctorem Magistrum Antonium de Scarperia salariatum et electum ad legendum in studio perusino medicinam videlicet ordinarie et de mane . . . sub anno domini 1386."

[40] See below, note 46. The other important medical author associated with the University of Florence in the later fourteenth and early fifteenth centuries was Ugolino da Montecatini, but his works were written for a broader audience and will be discussed in the next section.

cause most cultural historians of this period have concentrated on its art and literature to the virtual exclusion of more traditional areas of study, they have tended to minimize the significance of the scholastic disciplines and the *studio* in the early Florentine Renaissance. Recently, however, Garin and others have emphasized the vitality of the scholastic tradition and its importance for understanding the Florentine cultural achievement of the fourteenth and fifteenth centuries.[41] In academic medicine this vitality is manifest not only in the list of illustrious Italian medical writers who came to Florence to teach—Giovanni Dondi da Padova, Iacopo da Forlì, Marsiglio da Santa Sofia, and Ugo Benzi all stayed for varying lengths of time—but also in documents like Don Giovanni's account book, mentioned in the previous section, which shows, as we have already seen, that Florentine medical students were immersed in the work of many of the most important northern European philosophers and logicians, including Albert of Saxony, Marsilius of Inghen, William of Ockham, Richard Swineshead, and Jean Buridan.[42]

The medical texts produced at the University of Florence show a living, changing intellectual world, in contrast to the conservatism and dogmatism often associated with late scholastic thought. Even the limited repertory of scholastic literary forms embraced a wide variety of methods and approaches, as is clear if we compare the two surgical commentaries by Lodovico da Gubbio and Iacopo da Prato mentioned above. Both works follow the text of the *Canon of Medicine*, IV, 3, by Avicenna, the eleventh-century Arabic writer whose work played an important part in the medical curriculum of the later Middle Ages and Renaissance. Yet Iacopo's treatise is extremely concrete and practical, while Lodovico's is entirely theoretical. Where Lodovico referred his readers constantly to the works of previous surgical authorities (not only Avicenna and Galen but recent writers like Dino Del Garbo), Iacopo informed his students that such authors, being "tedious," "prolix," and difficult to understand, would make no further appearance in his work.[43] Where Lodovico emphasized the philosophical problems

---

[41] For example Garin, "Cultura fiorentina" and "Gli umanisti e la scienza."

[42] Dondi taught at Florence from 1367 to 1368, Iacopo da Forlì between 1357 and 1363, Marsiglio da Santa Sofia in the 1380s, and Benzi from 1421 to 1423; Park, "Readers," 268, 307; Abbondanza, "Atti degli ufficiali," 99-100. On Don Giovanni's account book see Brentano-Keller, "Il libretto."

[43] Iacopo da Prato, *De operatione manuali*, fol. 1r; partially edited in Sudhoff, *Geschichte der Chirurgie*, 2:425: "Est tamen difficile studenti cum reperiatur interpretata de greco uel arabico in latinum in sermone difficili et quia rep[eri]tur transposita in verbis et discontinuatata [sic] in sententijs, obscura brevitate, quandoque tediosa prolixitate

posed by his subject—distinctions between primary and antecedent causes of disease, between the genera and species of various sorts of boil, between the virtual and actual qualities of a medicine—Iacopo dealt only with the immediate diagnosis and treatment of disease. He filled his work with concrete recommendations for the future surgeon: make sure you have an adequate supply of instruments and medicines before you begin practice; do not attempt an operation unless you have already seen it performed; if you are asked to treat a patient with no chance of recovery, say that you will be leaving town shortly and cannot take the case. His concern was not with the nature and causes of disease but with the details of treatment: the color and size of the sore, for example, the proper length and position of the incision required, the correct way to hold one's hands, and mistakes commonly made in particular operations. He referred frequently to his own experience, recalling unusual cases he had treated successfully and the reasons for his success.[44] It is not that Iacopo was unversed in the intricacies of surgical theory—witness his doctorate in medicine and the content of his other works in the same manuscript—but that he chose this approach as most useful to prepare medical students for surgical practice.[45]

The same variety of approaches and modes of inquiry marked academic writing on *physica*, as appears in the writings of Tommaso Del Garbo. Tommaso's principal works were *On the Generation of the Embryo*, a commentary on part of the third book of Avicenna's *Canon; On the Differences of Fevers*, a commentary on Galen's treatise by the same name; and a *Medical Summa*, which he began shortly after his return to Florence in 1348 and left unfinished at his death.[46]

---

sermonis, ex quibus omnibus studens antiquorum uolumina fit dubitans et tediosus in continuando studiique in eis."

[44] Iacopo da Prato, *De operatione manuali*, for example fols. 7v (his experiences in the plague of 1348), 10v (a sore on the knee of one of his patients), and 16r (the case of a seventy-year-old man with an intractable case of *nodae*). Many of Iacopo's specific recommendations concerning conduct were also part of the tradition of deontological writing, on which see Wellborn, "Long Tradition."

[45] On Iacopo's other works see note 38 above. It is interesting that despite his rejection of the scholastic and theoretical mode, Iacopo was trained as a physician and had doctorates in arts and medicine, while Lodovico, whose commentary is so resolutely "academic," apparently acquired his degree only late in his career.

[46] The first two works were composed at Bologna; according to the explicits, *De generatione embryonis* was completed in 1343 and *De differentiis febrium* in 1345. His shorter works from these years include *De restauratione humidi radicalis* and four medical questions: *An per solam digestionem materie putride sit possibile cessare febrem putridam* (Vat. lat. 3144, fols. 15r-16v); *Utrum solutio continuitatis sit per se et immediate causa doloris* (Vat. lat. 4446, fols. 147r-49v; fragments in Vat. lat. 3144, fol. 11r and Vat. lat.

As these works show, Tommaso was strongly influenced by the medical tradition at the University of Bologna, where he had both studied and taught.[47] He referred often to the opinions of Bolognese medical writers, including Taddeo Alderotti, Torrigiano Torrigiani, Bartolomeo da Varignana, Guglielmo da Brescia, Antonio da Parma, and his own father, Dino, although his relationship to the last was marked by equal amounts of pride and intellectual rivalry.[48] Unlike Dino, however, whose interests tended more toward practice, Tommaso wrote almost exclusively on theory. Like the more philosophically oriented of the Bolognese authors, he was concerned to apply the tools of contemporary logical analysis to problems in medicine. But whereas Taddeo and his pupils tended to work within the logical and philosophical framework of the older thirteenth-century tradition, Tommaso added to these the new fourteenth-century methods of Ockham and his followers, arguing throughout in the language of consequence and connotation as well as that of first and last instants or latitude and degree.[49] Many of the *questiones* which make up the in-

---

4445, fol. 242r); *Utrum sanitas membri consimilis que est sibi propria sit idem quam sua bona complexio* (Vat. lat. 2484, fols. 195r-96r); and *An fetus in octavo mense sit vitalis* (Vat. lat. 2484, fols. 211r-12r). From his years at Florence there exist, besides the *Summa*, an oration, *Verbum cecidit inter querentes* . . . , given at the first convocation of the *studio* in 1348 (Vat. lat. 2484, fols. 212r-14r); two short treatises on pharmacological theory (*De reductione medicinarum ad actum* and *De gradibus medicinarum*, composed in the early 1350s); and a short plague treatise in Italian, probably from 1362. The *Summa medicinalis*, *De reductione*, *De gradibus*, and *De restauratione* were published together at Venice in 1506 and 1531 and at Lyon in 1529. The commentary on *De febrium differentiis* went through three editions (Lyon, 1514; Pavia, 1519; and Venice, 1521), and that on *De generatione embryonis* was printed in Iacopo da Forlì et al., *Expositio de generatione foetus*, Venice, 1502, fols. 33r-45r. *De reductione* and *De gradibus* were further published together in *De dosibus*, Pavia, 1579, and in *Opusculum illustrium medicorum de dosibus*, Heidelberg, 1584. Tommaso's plague treatise was reprinted in numerous collections; for a modern edition see his *Consiglio contro a pistolenza*. I have found no record of the commentary on *De anima* referred to by Filippo Villani (*Vite*, 30-31); Villani may have been thinking of the psychological portions of the *Summa*.

[47] Tommaso's other principal teacher was Gentile da Foligno, with whom he studied at Perugia, possibly also a student of Dino's and certainly part of the same tradition; see Siraisi, *Taddeo Alderotti*, xxi n.

[48] On these authors see ibid., chap. 2 and passim. Tommaso referred frequently to his father's status and reputation and always identified himself as "Thomas de Garbo, filius Dyni de Florentia sui temporis principis medicorum," or the like.

[49] On these late scholastic "languages" and on the logical and philosophical context in which Tommaso was working see Murdoch, "Social into Intellectual Factors," esp. 280-312; Wilson, *William Heytesbury*; Clagett, "Some Novel Trends"; and Sylla, "Medical Concepts." Tommaso was aware of the strongly philosophical nature of his work and made frequent reference to it. See for example *Summa*, I, Q. 1, fol. 4r, on the elements: "Et hec sufficient de hac materia ad presens, in qua multa essent discutienda,

complete *Medical Summa* in fact treat issues which belong properly to Aristotelian natural philosophy: the elements, sensation, the nature of the soul. A question concerning the pulsation of the arteries reduces to a discussion of the existence of a vacuum; a question concerning the role of the attractive power in digestion, to a discussion of natural and projectile motion in a void.[50] "And these things are very clear," Tommaso wrote, "to a good logician and philosopher."[51]

Tommaso's frequent references to the Bolognese tradition do not indicate, however, that medicine was for him a static intellectual system; on the contrary, he presented the study of medical theory as an ongoing venture in which many issues remained to be explored, reinterpreted, or reformulated. This is particularly apparent in the *Summa*, written for advanced students who needed no introduction to the basic concepts and phenomenology of physiology and medicine; the format allowed him, as he noted, to concentrate on controversial topics, "leaving out those things about which authorities do not disagree."[52] Thus the *Summa* consists of more than ninety problems, presented in *questio* form, representing issues which, according to Tommaso, had not been raised before or which had not been clearly decided.

Furthermore, Tommaso took these controversial issues and argued them in ways which show him remarkably open to new resolutions. Although he occasionally branded as frivolous writers who rejected accepted opinions without adequate reason,[53] he did not accept tradition and authority as decisive, frequently criticizing the opinions of even those writers on whom he most commonly drew, his teacher Gentile da Foligno and his father, Dino. At times he proposed ideas which seem radical in their rejection of tradition, expressing real skep-

---

quia tamen hunc librum in medicina componimus; non intendimus in physicis puris ex toto omnia pertractare."

[50] Tommaso, *Summa*, I, QQ. 41 and 60 (fols. 39v-40v and 50r-51r). These were hotly debated issues in mid-fourteenth-century physics; see, for example, Grant, *Physical Science*, chaps. 4-5, and Murdoch and Sylla, "The Science of Motion." Tommaso also used the characteristic modes of argumentation of contemporary physics, including thought experiments (e.g., I, Q. 3; fol. 7v), speculation "secundum imaginationem" (e.g., I, Q. 68; fol. 58v), and appeals to the absolute power of God (e.g., I, Q. 13; fol. 14r); see Murdoch, "Social into Intellectual Factors."

[51] Tommaso, *Summa*, I, Q. 41 (fol. 40v): "Et sunt hec multum clara bono logyco et bono philosopho."

[52] Ibid., prologue to II (fol. 87r): "ea que dubia sunt apud doctores inquirendo, ut in primo fecimus libro, pretermittendo ea in quibus discrepationes non cadunt apud doctores, ut clare ab eis determinata sunt, et hoc gratia brevitatis." For an example of a *questio* identified by Tommaso as new see I, Q. 21 (fol. 20r): "Utrum post etatem iuventutis calor diminuatur solum diminutione quantitative, an gradualiter remittatur."

[53] For example ibid., I, Q. 23 (fol. 21r), where he criticizied Torrigiani's position on the number of humors.

ticism, for example, concerning Aristotle's relation between the elements and qualities, one of the cornerstones of contemporary natural philosophy and medical theory: "many writers on philosophy," he noted, "rigidly maintain [the traditional position] using arguments drawn from consensus rather than founded on valid reasons."[54] On this issue, as on many others, he reached only a tentative conclusion.

In fact, the entire tone of Tommaso's *Summa* is anything but dogmatic; it reflects rather the characteristically speculative and questioning nature of mid-fourteenth-century scholastic thought. Tommaso treated the teaching and study of medicine as a process of gradually working out true positions on problematic issues. For example, in the *questio* "Whether all the operations of a temperate complexion are more perfect than those of a distemperate one," he suggested that although some physiological functions, like smell, appeared to work better in a state of distemper, the entire subject needed more investigation. "If the authorities say that perfect operations take place in a temperate body," he concluded, "you may understand this as you wish. Let my remarks serve as an exercise for others . . . ; they will allow those who follow to investigate with greater subtlety."[55] Tommaso's lack of dogmatism is particularly striking when we recall that these *questiones* were close transcriptions of classroom lectures and that he was speaking directly to his students, as the conversational tone makes clear.[56] After stating his own positions, he often encouraged disagreement: "Either position may be defended," he noted, "hold whichever you like," or "If you wish you may maintain another opinion."[57] Intriguing unsolved problems, like the cause of the eunuch's high voice, might be left as an exercise for the student. "You reflect on this," he often concluded, "thanks be to God."[58]

[54] Tommaso, *Summa*, I, Q. 2 (fol. 4v): "a quampluribus philosophantibus ad unguem tenetur cum multis sermonibus ex quadam communitate concessis, potius quam super validas rationes fundatis." In this *questio* Tommaso places in doubt the theory whereby the four elements (fire, air, water, earth) were marked by different pairs of the prime qualities (hot, cold, wet, dry). On this and other issues of contemporary medical theory see Siraisi, *Taddeo Alderotti*, 156-59, and in general chaps. 6-7.

[55] Tommaso, *Summa*, I, Q. 9 (fol. 11v): "Et si auctores dicunt quod in temperato est operationum perfectio, potest intelligi quocumque istorum modorum vis. Et ista dicta sint ad exercitium aliorum, cum in hoc quesito illud breve recitatum communiter inveniatur ab omnibus. Ista autem sequentibus viam dabunt investigandi subtiliora."

[56] See, for example, the end of I, Q. 45 (fol. 35r): "Sum enim hodie fessus, propter quod gratia brevitatis et laboris hic amplius nihil dico. Deo gratias."

[57] These formulas appear many times in the course of the *Summa*. For a flavor see fols. 4r, 10r, 11r, 22r, 37r.

[58] Ibid., I, Q. 37 (fol. 36v): "Secundum autem eam quam Conciliatoris acuitas et gravitas ex alia causa assignatur, et aliter aliqualiter assumuntur, et tu considera. Deo gratias."

The sense of intellectual community and intellectual exchange in these remarks is characteristic of all Tommaso's work and of late medieval medical theory in general. Tommaso conceived of medicine as a collective enterprise and his collaborators as a community extended in time and space. For him, this community included not only the great medical writers of the distant past—classical and Arabic authorities like Galen, Hippocrates, Avicenna, and Averroës—but also contemporary and near-contemporary scholars, like his father and the other Bolognese authors mentioned above, or Giovanni da Penna and Francesco Zanelli, who were alive as Tommaso was writing. The members of this collective enterprise communicated in many ways: orally, in the classroom and private discussion, and in writing, through their works, letters, and marginalia. Tommaso and his colleagues lent each other their manuscripts and commented upon each others' work. ("Dino proposed other interpretations," he wrote in a *questio* on sleep. "I have them in his hand in the margins of my book, which he annotated, and which I then gave to Gentile.")[59] Tommaso collated and compared their opinions, accepting some, rejecting others, keeping intact a web of continuous debate. At the same time he projected this debate into the future; as he introduced his students to the ideas of his predecessors, he informed them of issues left to be explored and invited them to continue the inquiry.

What, then, was Tommaso teaching his students at the University of Florence? On one level, of course, he was conveying medical and physiological information, as he answered such questions as "What is the cause of the pulse?" or "Is it best to exercise before or after eating?" or "Is hair alive?"[60] (Because he was lecturing on theory, not practice, he was not directly concerned with issues of therapeutics and medical treatment.) On another level, however, he was teaching methods of inquiry and, above all, intellectual standards—the standards accepted by the community of medical scholars and by which he expected his students to judge his work and their own. He was concerned, for example, to establish guidelines for the correct use of sources, emphasizing the importance of quoting in context and identifying one's sources.[61] Thus in one of the questions near the end of the first book of his *Summa*, he castigated Francesco Zanelli da Bologna, identified as a correspondent and friend, for his lack of care in this respect: "I

[59] Ibid., II, Q. 10 (fol. 96r): "Alie sunt expositiones quas dedit Dynus, et sunt de sua manu in marginibus nostri libri, quod ipse notavit, quod etiam a nobis habuit Gentilis." (The book in question is probably Avicenna's *Canon*.)

[60] Ibid., I, Q. 40; II, Q. 7; I, Q. 34.

[61] For example ibid., II, Q. 7 (fol. 92v); II, Q. 10 (fol. 96r).

hear from his students," he wrote, "that he repeats faithfully the ideas of others. He should be reproved for recording their opinions without mentioning them and for presenting those opinions as his own."[62] Tommaso also referred frequently to standards for argumentation and proof, counseling his students to avoid prolixity (a quality he attributed above all to his teacher Gentile) and *peditatio*, by which he seems to have meant quibbles over trivial distinctions.[63] Above all, he tried to educate them in the distinction between arguments based on deductive logic and "merely probable" ones based on "opinion" derived from tradition, experience, or incomplete proof; this distinction was crucial for understanding which questions were still open and which had already been determined.

One of the most striking aspects of Tommaso's work is the sense of progress and discovery which informs it. Tommaso did not hesitate either to congratulate himself on solving a particularly difficult problem or to acknowledge a previous error. At the end of his short treatise *On the Restoration of the Radical Moisture*, for example, he wrote, "This is how the truth appears to me now, although I was confused about it for a long time."[64] Indeed, if one of the indices of the vitality of an intellectual tradition is its ability to absorb and generate new ideas, then the medical tradition represented by Tommaso Del Garbo at the University of Florence was in full vigor. A case in point is the group of questions on perception and cognition near the end of the first book of the *Summa*, where Tommaso adopted a set of controversial positions on the soul associated with what came to be known as the "modern way," or *via moderna*. This school of Aristotelian thought had emerged at the universities at Oxford and Paris during the third and fourth decades of the fourteenth century. Relying heavily on the writings of William of Ockham, its adherents used new methods of logical analysis to develop a theology and natural philosophy which frequently incorporated the nominalist rejection of unnecessary distinctions.[65] Tommaso seems to have come into contact with these ideas at

[62] Ibid., I, Q. 80 (fol. 83v): "Et comuniter sic de ipso audio a scolaribus quod ipse est fidelis recitator dictorum aliorum. Reprehendendus ergo est scribens aliorum opinionem nullam de illis faciens mentionem, sed predictam opinionem ponens ac si esset de novo formator illius. . . ."

[63] For example ibid., I, Q. 1 (fol. 3r), on the nature of mixture; I, Q. 40 (fol. 38v), on Gentile's "tedious" discussion of the cause of the pulse.

[64] Tommaso, *Tractatus de restauratione humidi radicalis*, in *Summa*, fol. 99r: "Et hoc est quod de hoc quesito mihi de veritate apparet, in quo longo tempore steti caliginosus in mente." On the problem of radical moisture see McVaugh, "Humidum Radicale."

[65] For an introduction to this tradition see Moody, *Logic of William of Ockham*, and Shapiro, *Motion, Time and Place*.

Bologna, probably through the works of Ockham himself.[66] On several occasions in the *Summa* he defended positions identifiable with the more extreme wing of the *via moderna*. In I, 50, and I, 74, for example, he appealed to the principle of parsimony (Ockham's razor) to deny that the various faculties of the soul were really distinct.[67] In I, 63, he used the same kind of reductive argument to deny that the act of vision required a real image (*species*) to travel between the object and the eye.[68] In I, 73, he maintained that the entities referred to by Aristotle as objects of common sense (shape, number, motion, and the like) could not be sensed per se, since "they do not signify anything outside the soul and are not anything outside the soul other than substance and quality; let this be held as true, as all modern philosophers agree."[69] Furthermore, he used the whole battery of modernist analytical tools—terminist logic, supposition theory, and the language of signification and connotation—to argue these positions.[70]

These issues are complicated and technical, and we cannot explore them here. What is important for our purposes is that Tommaso's work included controversial conclusions and novel forms of argument, which Tommaso himself recognized as such. In the question concerning the objects of common sense, for example, he noted that if his conclusions in the *Summa* contradicted the ideas he had advanced in

[66] See his remarks in *Summa*, I, Q. 63 (fol. 53v), rejecting the reality of *species* in vision: "est opinio quorumdam modernorum, et nos iam Bononie sub quodam magistro in sacra pagina de ordine minorum hanc sustinuimus et defendimus, ubi fuit magna doctorum congeries et multitudo maxima scholarum congregata." Note that Ockham argued this position at length in his work on the *Sentences*; this was probably why Tommaso defended it under a "master of theology." A number of Tuscan Franciscans traveled to Paris to study theology, coming into contact there with Ockhamist ideas. See Moody, "Ockham," 133 and 149 (on Bernardo da Arezzo), and Mattesini, "Biblioteca," 263n, 296 (on Francesco Nerli, who taught theology at the University of Florence).

[67] Tommaso, *Summa*, fols. 45v, 70v-71v; in the latter Tommaso argued that "cognition" and "knowledge" (*scientia*) were connotative terms signifying the soul itself. Tommaso's position on this issue is closer to Ockham's than to the more moderate opinion of Buridan; see Park, "Albert's Influence on Late Medieval Psychology."

[68] Tommaso, *Summa*, fols. 53r-54r. On this issue see Maier, "Problem der *Species*."

[69] Tommaso, *Summa*, I, Q. 73 (fol. 70r): "figura, numerus etc. nullam rem extra animam significant, nec alique res sunt extra animam preter substantiam et qualitatem. Illa superponatur pro vera, sicut in hoc concordant omnes moderni philosophi." On this issue see Shapiro, *Motion, Time and Place*, esp. 20-22.

[70] See, for example, *Summa*, I, Q. 73 (fol. 70r): "Sec illa logicis dimittimus, quorum est hec doctrina terminorum. Et nulli mirum si in medicina illas posuimus conclusiones et per istum modum, quia in quibuscumque scientiis sunt aliquando materie quarum veritas diludicari non potest nisi talia exprimendo; et aliter oportet divisiones multimodas et frivolas formare, intellectum obfuscantes."

a *questio* on pain at Bologna, it was because he had changed his mind, rejecting the older forms of analysis for the more powerful new ones.[71] These issues continued to generate controversy after Tommaso's death in 1370; his opinion concerning the nonexistence of *species* in perception was soon criticized in detail by Marsiglio da Santa Sofia at the University of Padua.[72]

Tommaso Del Garbo was no intellectual revolutionary. Like the other travelers of the *via moderna*, he aimed not to overthrow the system of Aristotelian logic and philosophy and Galenic medicine which dominated medieval and Renaissance universities but to explore that system by pushing it to its limits. In the process, the ideas of even Aristotle, Galen, and their most respected commentators could be criticized and overhauled. In this sense the tradition of scholastic medical theory at the University of Florence was dynamic, open not only to ideas from other Italian medical faculties (Perugia, Padua, above all Bologna) but also to new methods in logic, philosophy, and theology from elsewhere in Europe (most notably Oxford and Paris). This extended geographical frame of reference was reflected in the contents of the larger libraries owned by Florentine teachers of medicine like Ugolino da Montecatini and Agostino di Stefano Santucci. Nonetheless, as the data on libraries recall—and as Maestro Lorenzo Sassoli's laments (quoted in Chapter Four) about his "exile" from Padua to Prato confirm—the faculties of arts and medicine constituted a small, heady world in which very few doctors participated once they had completed their medical studies. The academic writings of Tommaso Del Garbo and Lodovico da Gubbio were of interest mainly to other scholars and medical students. The great majority of physicians, insofar as they referred to works of medicine at all, tended to use works of medical practice.

The Culture of Medical Practice

In addition to the literature of academic medicine Florentine physicians also produced a literature of medical practice intended for a non-academic audience of patients and doctors. This included treatises on various aspects of therapeutics, complimentary works on medical topics offered to aristocratic patrons, and the regimens, *consilia* (medical

---

[71] Ibid.: "quia cum predictam materiam in hoc libro tractabimus, in aliquibus aliter sentiemus quam ibi scripsimus, que credimus veriora." The Bolognese *questio* to which Tommaso refers is *Utrum solutio continuitatis* . . . (see note 46 above).

[72] See Smith, "Disagreement," chaps. 2-4.

opinions), and recipes used in the course of private practice. Such works had close ties with academic writing on the theory and practice of medicine: they were often written by the same men, and they shared the same theoretical base. But they also reflected the broader medical marketplace, which was shaped more by custom and economic interest than by a disinterested concern for the advancement of learning. (It is notable, for example, that Tommaso Del Garbo's collaborative and nonproprietary attitude toward his learning faltered where practice was concerned: he physically assaulted one of his favorite students, Maestro Piantavigna da Ravenna, who had happened to open Tommaso's notebook of medical recipes.)[73] Furthermore, the diversity of medical practice ensured that this therapeutic literature was more varied in form and subject matter than the literature of academic medicine. It reflected nonetheless a restricted intellectual and social milieu; in Florence, at least, all these works were composed by and for physicians, and most of them grew out of the elite private practice to which only very successful doctors could aspire.

As shown by the account books and library inventories discussed above, the most widely disseminated works of this sort were medical *practicae*, compendia of diseases, symptoms, and treatments written for the practicing physician.[74] The success of these compendia in the later fourteenth and the fifteenth centuries resulted from the complexity and sophistication of late medieval medical learning: physicians needed works of high quality which digested the material relevant to practice, selected the most important points, and presented them in accessible form. Rather than leafing through all their commentaries on Avicenna in order to find the specific references to help them in a puzzling case, many preferred to consult the practical encyclopedias which summarized existing medical knowledge on particular illnesses.

The most widely owned Italian work of this kind was the *Medical Sermons* of Niccolò Falcucci da Borgo San Lorenzo, who lived and practiced in Florence in the late fourteenth and early fifteenth centuries. Falcucci and Tommaso Del Garbo were the Castor and Pollux of

[73] Account in Sabbadini, *Giovanni da Ravenna*, 214: "Fuit huic [Tommaso] discipulus ac percarus quidem Plantavigna. . . . Hunc, dum Florentie libellum semel aperuisset, in quo medicus ille ad apothecam remedia conscribebat, indignatus sue singularitatis prodi thesauros, acerbe increpitum alapa percussit."

[74] After the *Sermones* of Niccolò Falcucci, discussed below, the medical works most popular among Italian doctors were the compendia by Bernard Gordon, Serapion, John of Gaddesden, Guglielmo da Varignana, and Gilbert the Englishman. See Demaitre, "Scholasticism" and "Theory and Practice," 113-14.

the Florentine medical firmament in the early Renaissance.[75] Both had their intellectual roots in the Bolognese tradition and shared an interest in Aristotelian logic and natural philosophy. But whereas Tommaso wrote on the principles of medicine and physiology for students and scholars, Falcucci devoted the bulk of his enormous work—it runs to roughly four million words—to a discussion of the causes, symptoms, and cure of all known illnesses, ordered from general to particular and according to the organ affected. The *Sermons* were an immediate success. First consulted widely in manuscript, as Giovanni Chellini's account book shows,[76] they were printed by 1480 and went through several editions in the next fifty years.

Falcucci acknowledged no gulf between theory and practice. He considered medical theory the backbone of therapeutics; it gave a rationale to each medicinal, dietary, and surgical procedure, and this offered specific guidance to the doctor faced with an ambiguous case or a choice of treatments.[77] Medical treatment was always to be guided by an understanding of causal principles; this set the formally trained doctor above the empiric, whose cures he described as due to luck rather than knowledge.[78] Thus Falcucci used the first sermon, on medicine and the human body in general, to introduce his reader to the same concepts and debates—the action of elements in a mixture, for example, or the nature of complexion and its properties—which Tommaso Del Garbo raised in his *Summa*,[79] and he maintained this theoretical frame of reference in later parts on particular diseases. In the section on headache, for example, he noted that to understand headache one had to understand pain, and to understand pain one had to understand sensation. Furthermore, in order to understand how to cure the headache associated with a hangover, for example, one had

[75] For what is known of the life of Falcucci (d. 1412) see Ristori, "Niccolò Falcucci." He probably studied at the University of Bologna and/or the University of Florence under Tommaso himself; he cites Tommaso often and with great respect.

[76] See above, note 18.

[77] Students of medieval pharmacology have tended to emphasize the discrepancies between theory and practice; see Riddle, "Theory and Practice," and McVaugh, "Quantified Medical Theory." But pharmacology represents a special case; for the opposite position see Demaitre, "Theory and Practice," and Siraisi, *Taddeo Alderotti*, 267-68.

[78] Falcucci, *Sermones medicinales*, I, 1, chaps. 5-6 (vol. 1, fols. 3r-4r), on the relationship between theory and practice, and VII, 3, chap. 1 (vol. 4, fol. 43v). Note that all seven sermons are separately foliated. For a more general discussion see Agrimi and Crisciani, "Medici e 'vetulae.'"

[79] See, for example, ibid., I, 1, chap. 27 (vol. 1, fol. 18r); the three questions addressed in this chapter on complexion correspond to Tommaso Del Garbo, *Summa*, I, Q. 9; I, Q. 13; and I, Q. 19.

to learn the physiology of inebriation, the different effects of different alcoholic drinks, and their peculiar interactions with different parts of the body. It was only by knowing that drinking leads to an "obstruction in the cerebral ventricles caused by vapors rising to the head from the inebriating agent" that one could understand why rubbing the feet (which draws the vapors downward) was prescribed.[80]

In his concern for theory, then, Falcucci resembled Tommaso Del Garbo, whom he so admired. Where he differed from Tommaso was in tone. Falcucci's exposition conveys no sense of inquiry and avoids the *questio* form, which emphasized debate and speculation. Debate and speculation were all very well in the classroom, but they had no place in the sickroom. A doctor faced by a patient with a migraine did not want to be told that the pain was more likely to be caused by complexional imbalance than by local motion producing a "dissolution of continuity" within the brain but that, as Tommaso was so fond of saying, "the opposite is also possible, and you may hold whichever opinion you wish." Falcucci's information was complex but rarely equivocal, and he avoided indefinite answers. His concern was not to develop new theories but to summarize the practical knowledge contained in the texts of authoritative writers, particularly the Greeks and the Arabs.[81] This strategy is particularly striking in the section on plague, about which fourteenth-century writers were far better informed than their predecessors. Yet Falcucci's discussion of its causes, symptoms, and treatment came almost exclusively from Galen, Avicenna, Avenzoar, and the like. It was only in the chapter on prevention that he abandoned his authorities in order to suggest measures of which he had direct experience: prayers to Saint Sebastian, avoidance of the sick, flight from the cities. And it was only there that his tone became tentative. Experience confirms, he noted, that it is dangerous to move from an infected to a healthy place; nonetheless "others advise one to leave corrupted air and travel to uncorrupted air, . . . and perhaps," he concluded in a fleeting echo of Tommaso's scholarly ambivalence, "their counsel is better than the other."[82] In general, however, Falcucci was

---

[80] Falcucci, *Sermones medicinales*, III, 2, 3, chap. 9 (vol. 2, fol. 42r).

[81] See ibid., proemium (vol. 1, fol. 1v): "Volo autem aggregationem istam vocari librum sermonum scientie medicine in quo afferam verba auctorum in propria forma secundum quod iacent in textu; valde autem raro afferam dicta eorum nisi secundum quod mea parva facultas poterit enodare." Falcucci cited contemporary authors relatively seldom and only on disputed topics.

[82] Ibid., II, 2, 4, 6, chap. 5 (vol. 1, fol. 133r): "Alii autem consulunt ab [a]ere infecto etiam in processu se absentare et transire non infectum, ne ex longa actione infecti aeris pereant, et fortasse consilium istorum est melius quam primorum."

content to reproduce carefully and clearly the complexities of medical knowledge as it had been handed down from the classical and Arabic texts and elaborated by the writers of the late medieval Italian medical faculties. The fact that the *Sermons* were still being reprinted in the 1520s, more than a century after their composition, indicates the stability of the intellectual tradition they represented.

Not all the works of medical practice, however, stayed so close to academic writing. Writers for a nonacademic audience were not as strongly tied to the conventions which bound their colleagues in the universities, and they could more easily incorporate new content and approaches. For this reason their works often allow us glimpses into the psychological and intellectual world of the practicing physician which are not possible in the more formal commentaries, *questiones*, and treatises. A case in point is Ugolino da Montecatini's *On Baths*, written in 1417, six years after Falcucci's death. Like many natives of the Florentine territories, Ugolino had received his doctorate in medicine from the University of Bologna. Except for two short stints teaching at the universities of Florence (in the mid-1390s) and Perugia (1419-20), he spent his career in various forms of practice: as communal doctor in Pescia, Lucca, and Città di Castello; as court doctor to Pietro Gambacorta, Paolo Guinigi, and Malatesta Malatesta, lords of Pisa, Lucca, and Pesaro; and as a private physician in Montecatini, Bologna, and Florence, where he died in 1425. His other works included *consilia*, a commentary on Avicenna's *Canon*, III, 16, and a treatise on plague.[83]

On Baths was the only work by Maestro Ugolino to circulate widely; although it never had the currency of Falcucci's *Sermons*, it was edited and printed in the sixteenth century. As its title implies, it treats hydrotherapy, a subject which had generated considerable interest among Italian medical writers in the fourteenth century and which had become a patrician fad by the middle of the fifteenth.[84] Ugolino divided

---

[83] Biographical information in Barduzzi, *Ugolino da Montecatini*, chaps. 1-5; Battistini, "Contributo"; and Pieri, "Maestro Ugolino." Titles of his other works are from his library inventory (see Battistini, "Contributo") and from references in *On Baths*; I know of no surviving manuscripts. One *consilium* exists in a modern edition: see F. Baldasseroni and G. Degli Azzi, "Consiglio medico" (original in MAP-LXXXVII, fols. 44-46).

[84] The correspondence of fourteenth- and fifteenth-century Florentines is full of references to trips to baths in the city's territories; these functioned as centers not only for medical treatment but also for socializing and entertainment. See Barduzzi, *Ugolino da Montecatini*, 71; Raspadori, "Legislazioni"; Maguire, *Women of the Medici*, passim, esp. 83-87 and 101-9; Pieraccini, *Stirpe de' Medici*, 1:57-59, 63-68, 86-92, 128-33; Ross, *Lives of the Early Medici*, passim, esp. 112-16, 179-86; and Guerra-Coppioli, *Bagno a Morba*. On the printing history of *On Baths* see Barduzzi, *Ugolino da Montecatini*, 72-

his work into two parts, on "natural baths," or therapeutic springs, and "artificial baths," made by infusing herbs or dissolving minerals; the first part is longer and more interesting, and consists of detailed descriptions of the most important springs in central and northern Italy.

Ugolino's treatise resembles Falcucci's in that it was composed for practicing physicians and was organized systematically for easy reference. There, however, the similarity ends, for *On Baths* is short and strongly empirical. It contains a few brief references to problems of medical theory—what makes thermal springs hot? why do artificial baths help in some kinds of fever and not others?[85]—but these are wholly overshadowed by a practical preoccupation with the springs and their effects. The discussion of the baths at Montecatini is typical. Ugolino was interested above all in the history and archaeology of the earliest thermal establishments found there, the conditions for which they were prescribed (dermatitis, arthritis, digestive problems, kidney stones, and worms), and the ways in which they could be used for treatment.[86]

Ugolino also differed from Falcucci in his lack of concern for medical authorities and the textual tradition. His only contemporary medical source was Gentile da Foligno's own treatise on baths, which he mined for information on several springs he had not been able to visit.[87] Otherwise, his principal source was personal experience: as he noted frequently, "I can testify to what I have seen."[88] For the most part he wrote of springs which he had studied by observing their effects on his own patients and by performing, or causing to be performed, distillation experiments on their waters. When this was impossible, he relied on the knowledge of colleagues and local doctors. "And because I was in Viterbo," he wrote, "I spent the day there with doctors and other people learning about its many springs and their

---

74, and Michele Giuseppe Nardi, introduction to Ugolino da Montecatini, *De balneis*, 18-19.

[85] Ugolino da Montecatini, *De balneis*, 87-89, 131-32.

[86] Ibid., 95-96.

[87] For references to manuscripts of Gentile's *De balneis* see Thorndike and Kibre, *Catalogue*, cols. 789, 1564. Of Ugolino's five or six references to classical and medieval authors, three—to Albertus Magnus, *De mineralibus*, and to the pseudo-Aristotelian *Problemata* and *De proprietatibus elementorum*—did not belong properly to the medical tradition.

[88] Ugolino da Montecatini, *De balneis*, 98: "Ego possum dare testimonium de his que vidi. . . ."

great mineral diversity and the good they have done for various diseases."[89]

As these passages indicate, the tone of *On Baths* is autobiographical, even confessional. Ugolino's choice of subject had clear biographical roots; his native town of Montecatini possessed perhaps the most famous mineral springs in Tuscany, and his descriptions of the area testify to time spent exploring the ruins of the classical baths as well as the springs frequented by local peasants and more recently by the fashionable Florentine establishment. We learn of his wife's infertility, his friends (Coluccio Salutati, Maestro Cristofano di Giorgio, Pier Giovanni, a Florentine apothecary), his clients (not only long-term patrons like Gambacorta or Malatesta but also humbler citizens like Piero del Voglia and Bernaba degli Agli of Florence), and his colleagues, of whom more below.

But perhaps the clearest indication that Ugolino was moving outside the accepted medical tradition—which equated the corpus of valid medical knowledge with what was taught at the university and practiced by duly certified members of the profession—was his interest in the use local inhabitants made of the various baths. Regarding one of the springs at Montecatini, for example, he noted that "most of those that frequent this spring are peasants affected by pains in their joints. . . . They use it without following any rules [i.e., without medical advice and supervision], and they often receive great relief from this practice. They pull up the plants [which grow there] and make a pit, which they enter, mixing the water and mud together, for they say that the water is more effective when mixed with mud."[90] Ugolino considered certain of these empirical practices, such as being buried in mud, inappropriate for his gentle clientele;[91] but where Falcucci scorned them as unworthy of discussion, Ugolino treated them as an important source of information concerning the properties and uses of the baths in question. In this respect his attitude in practical therapeutics resembled that of Tommaso Del Garbo in medical theory: he referred often to thermal medicine as a new and open field.

In addition to illustrating the new approaches which could be gen-

[89] Ibid., 123. See also his remarks concerning the baths of Siena., ibid., 109. Accounts of distillation experiments in ibid., 89-91.

[90] Ibid., 95. Compare Falcucci's attitude in note 78 above.

[91] Ibid., 135 (concerning artificial baths): "Vidi etiam multos rusticos qui propter has et simil[es] passiones se in fimo fatiunt sepellire sicut et equi sepelliuntur cum doloribus intestinales [*sic*] incurrunt. Et hoc est dictis rusticis bestialibus medicamentum sicut meretur, et illis sit medicamentum conveniens bestiale."

erated in the world of nonacademic medicine, the literature of medical practice also illuminates the social and professional relationships informing that world. Ugolino wrote at length about his relations with his colleagues in *On Baths*, and these passages testify to the competitive nature of high-level private practice. At times he collaborated happily with fellow doctors, as when he consulted with Maestro Giovanni da Pisa and Maestro Niccolò da Mantova about the properties of Bagno ad Aqua near Pisa or recommended Maestro Lionardo da Bibbiena to his patient Bernaba degli Agli.[92] But his relations with other physicians ranged from rivalry to frank hostility; he was particularly bitter about Maestro Giovanni Baldi da Faenza's unabashed and luckily unsuccessful efforts to destroy the trust of two of his most illustrious patients, Niccolò di Vieri de' Medici and Malatesta Malatesta da Pesaro, by impugning Ugolino's professional judgment.[93] The same competitiveness also appeared in Ugolino's tendency to drop names and in his preening references to huge fees and remarkable cures.

These propagandistic elements are also pronounced in the writings on practical medicine of Ugolino's rival, Giovanni Baldi himself. (Baldi had come to Florence in the 1380s to teach at the university; he lectured and practiced there until his death in 1424.)[94] But where Ugolino chose to write for his fellow physicians, Baldi went after the source of patronage itself. The main collection of his works appears in a decorated codex—clearly a presentation copy—in the Laurentian Library, transcribed in 1415 and probably presented to the young Cosimo de' Medici, to whom one of the works is addressed. Of the manuscript's five short Latin treatises, the first two, *Whether Natural Philosophy Is Contrary to the Christian Faith* and *On the Extirpation of Wrath*, are dedicated to Malatesta Malatesta and Niccolò di Vieri de' Medici, the two patients for whom Baldi jockeyed so strenuously with Ugolino. The third is a consolatory treatise to the Count of Montegarneli on the death of his son, while the fourth and fifth, *On the Times of Birth* and *On Choosing a Doctor*, treat more strictly medical topics; they are addressed to the Florentine lawyer Messer Alessandro di Salvi di Fillippo and the "noble Florentine youth," Cosimo himself.[95]

The five works share a tone of flattery, exaggerated humility, and

[92] Ibid., 104.

[93] Ibid., 105-6. Ugolino wrote of Baldi, "Semper mecum discordiam habuit."

[94] Capasso, "Baldi, Giovanni dei Tambeni"; Alessandro Gherardi, *Statuti*, 377; Park, "Readers," 305.

[95] BLF: Laur. 19, 30. Extracts from the first in Guasti, *Commissioni*, 3:601-19. One other work of Baldi's is known: his *Disputatio an medicina sit legibus politicis praeferenda* (BLF: Gadd. 74, fols. 102-5).

self-promotion. Baldi referred to his lectureships at Florence and Bologna, his conversance with philosophy and literature, and his friendships with Rinaldo degli Albizzi and other Florentine patricians. His subject matter was conventional and his style clumsy, despite studied humanist echoes in the second and third treatises. In his two specifically medical works, *On the Times of Birth* and *On Choosing a Doctor*, Baldi was concerned to present a readable account of medical problems of clear interest to an educated lay reader. Thus he avoided the complex issues and the empirical argument which marked the works of Tommaso Del Garbo, Falcucci, and Ugolino da Montecatini, couching his account in concrete and dogmatic terms. He used few recent authorities, and he emphasized only those points of interest to a layman: his brief account of the physiology of conception was overshadowed by the far longer sections on fetal presentations, on predicting the character of the child from the length of the pregnancy, and on the times of quickening and birth.[96] In this as in his other works Baldi aimed to provide his reader with a simplified version of the medical learning taught at the universities, to impress and compliment his patrons, and to secure their business and their esteem. Ugolino's references to Baldi's esteemed clientele in *On Baths*, Baldi's steadily growing tax assessments, and his invitation to the papal court in 1419 all testify to his success.

Many of the same social and intellectual issues are reflected in a final body of medical writing by Florentine doctors: short texts generated in the course of medical practice. These include *receptae* and *experimenta* (recipes for compound medicines and proven remedies), *consilia* (medical opinions on particular cases, often delivered in absentia at the request of a patient or his attending doctors), and *regimina* (directions for the regulation of "diet," usually for a particular patient or class of patients, including advice on food, drink, sleep, exercise, and the like).[97] These texts are among the most elusive and problematic medical works produced in the fourteenth and fifteenth centuries; they are often highly technical, and it is unclear how and by whom they were meant to be used. It is enough here to note that Florence produced its share of this literature, in both Latin and Italian, and that most of the surviving examples were the work of physicians also known for their academic

[96] Baldi, *De temporibus partus*, Laur. 19, 30, fols. 40r-44r.

[97] These genres overlapped and were closely related in purpose and origin; longer surveys in Demaitre, "Theory and Practice," 113-14, and Siraisi, *Taddeo Alderotti*, 270-75. On *receptae* and *experimenta* in particular see McVaugh, "*Experimenta*"; on *consilia* and *regimina*, Siraisi, *Taddeo Alderotti*, chap. 9, and Lockwood, *Ugo Benzi*, 44-78 and chap. 6.

and practical treatises.[98] These texts show in particular how the competitive interaction of doctors and patients affected actual medical practice.

Ugolino da Montecatini's *consilium* for Averardo de' Medici, who suffered from catarrh, illustrates the triangular relationship between the consulting physician, the patient, and the doctors who supervised treatment. Ugolino was painfully aware of his double audience. On the one hand, he wrote in Italian so that Averardo might understand his recommendations. He explained technical terms and tried to ensure the patient's cooperation by keeping his advice realistic: "I don't say," he wrote, "that you can do everything [I recommend], but do as much as you can."[99] On the other hand, he also spoke to Averardo's attending physicians, tempering his relaxed tone with references to professional standards and parading his learning on the kinds and causes of catarrh. Thus on several occasions he was constrained to apologize both to Averardo, for including more detail than he needed or wanted, and to his doctors, for writing in the unprofessional and imprecise vernacular: "because *consilia* given by doctors are sometimes seen by other worthy men, I must follow the conventions of our authors and be prolix. And indeed it is difficult to write in Italian; I have done so in order that you may understand everything."[100]

Rivalry, display, and endless prolixity were certainly part of the actual private practice of an ambitious physician like Ugolino. In fact,

[98] The problems of survival for these shorter works are much greater than for the longer ones. The only independent Florentine examples of Latin recipes which I have found from this period are those of Tommaso Del Garbo: Vat. pal. lat. 1284, fol. 121v; 1295, fols. 118r, 156r; and Wellcome MS 724, fol. 79v. See also the recipes attributed to Tommaso and others in the late fifteenth-century collection prepared by the College of Physicians for Florence's apothecaries: *Nuovo receptario*. *Consilia* by Tommaso Del Garbo appear in Vat. pal. lat. 1260, fols. 35r-36r (for a "woman of high status"); 77r-79r (two for Giangaleazzo Visconti, for a foot problem and for a cough); 88r-89v (for Messer Amerigo Cavalcanti's catarrh); and 89v (for a "great merchant"). Ugolino da Montecatini composed an Italian *consilium* for Averardo de' Medici; see note 83 above. I have not seen Falcucci's *consilium* in the Biblioteca comunale e dell'Accademia etrusca di Cortona 110, fols. 183r. For the three plague *consilia* by Del Garbo, Falcucci, and Francesco da Conegliano see notes 101 and 102 below. Examples of vernacular recipes and regimen (by Lorenzo Sassoli for Francesco Datini) in ASP: Archivio Datini-Carteggio privato-1102 (busta).

[99] Baldasseroni and Degli Azzi, "Consiglio," 142. See, for example, his restrictions on the drinking of wine (ibid., 145).

[100] Ibid., 143: "et perchè i consilli si danno per li medici s'ànno ad vedere alcuna volta per altri valenti huomini, mi conviene pur procedere secondo volliono i nostri autori et essere prolisso. Et quello è più faticoso è consilliare per volgare, che tucto ò facto perchè melglio possi et sappi ongni cosa intendere." See also Lockwood, *Ugo Benzi*, 124-25.

the only Florentine physician from this period who seemed at ease writing in Italian for a lay audience was Tommaso Del Garbo, who composed a *Consilium against Plague*, probably in 1362, "for the good health of the inhabitants of the city of Florence."[101] The plague *consilium* had become a standard genre after 1348; we have two other Florentine examples, one by Falcucci and another by Francesco da Conegliano, who taught at the *studio* in the years after 1360, both of them complicated and technical Latin texts filled with physiological and astrological speculation.[102] Tommaso's, in contrast, had a popular orientation. Unlike Falcucci and Francesco da Conegliano, Tommaso barely concerned himself with the disease and its causes, offering instead concrete and practical advise to his lay readers regarding prevention and treatment. He did not assume that they had access to the flower of the medical profession, or even that they were under a doctor's care. He told them what to eat, what to drink, what to wear, when to open their windows, and when to keep them closed. The medicines he recommended were either easily available (for example, "laudanum apple according to the common recipe") or easily made from common ingredients. (In this respect his work resembles the vernacular medical collection of Ruberto di Guido Bernardi discussed in Chapter Two). None of Tommaso's counsels was unusual or surprising; his *consilium* represented a vulgarization of the same practices advised by Falcucci and others. What is remarkable is the complete absence of the claims to status and professional dignity so prominent in the writings of Ugolino da Montecatini and Giovanni Baldi.

It is not hard to understand this difference. Tommaso was a native Florentine from a wealthy and respected family. His father and grandfather had been famous doctors; he himself was rich, celebrated, and politically influential. But Ugolino, Baldi, and Francesco da Conegliano were immigrants. Their names and their livelihoods depended on their professional success; they were not insulated from the vagaries of the medical marketplace by birth, position, or personal wealth, and their competitive inclinations reflected their situation.

Thus the medical works written by Florentine doctors mirrored the social and intellectual world in which they lived and worked. This world was complex and varied, and the literature they produced shared

---

[101] Del Garbo, *Consiglio*, 13: "Ordine e reggimento che si debbe osservare nel tempo di pistolenze . . . massimamente per bene e salute degli uomini, che abitano nella città di Firenze."

[102] Both date from 1382. They are edited in Karl Sudhoff, "Pestschriften," 354-84. I have found no trace of the plague treatise composed by Ugolino da Montecatini, according to his library inventory.

in that variety. The academic discipline of *physica* remained the core of medical learning, at least for those doctors who participated in its written culture. Whether addressing common citizens, patrician clients, or their colleagues, Florentine physicians retained the theoretical framework and practical genres developed in the late medieval university. Yet that system, if stable, was far from static; throughout the early Renaissance it continued to evolve new forms and new approaches in response to changes both within the university and outside it.

DOCTORS AND THE FLORENTINE RENAISSANCE

The intellectual interests of early Renaissance physicians, as expressed in their reading and their writing, were largely shaped by their training in the theory and practice of medicine. Yet the doctors who lived and worked in fourteenth- and fifteenth-century Florence were also surrounded by a vital literary and artistic culture which flourished outside the university and the disciplines taught within its walls. In 1373, three years after the death of Tommaso Del Garbo, Boccaccio was giving public lectures on Dante. In the late 1390s, while Falcucci compiled his *Medical Sermons*, Chrysoloras was teaching Greek to a circle of students which included Niccolò Niccoli and Leonardo Bruni. In 1417, as Ugolino da Montecatini composed his *Treatise on Baths*, Ghiberti was finishing the statute of Saint George for Or San Michele, and Brunelleschi was starting on the Foundling Hospital. It was in these years, in other words, that Florence emerged as the leading center of the artistic and intellectual movements identified with the Italian Renaissance. Many Florentine physicians found themselves caught up in the new Renaissance culture.

The nature and extent of doctors' participation in these movements changed as the movements themselves evolved. In the decades before the middle of the fifteenth century Florentine humanism was largely literary. Poggio, Niccoli, and their colleagues shared a general enthusiasm for the culture of classical antiquity, and they sought out ancient literary and scientific texts with indiscriminate zeal; nonetheless their own intellectual interests, limited to a large extent by the relatively rudimentary state of their Greek, tended to center on the disciplines we identify with the *studia humanitatis*—poetry, drama, history, politics, ethics—and on their Latin sources. These disciplines were largely irrelevant to the professional interests of doctors, and they added little to contemporary understanding of the Galenic and Hippocratic texts which formed the core of scholastic medical learning. It was only after

1450 that the interests of doctors and humanists began to converge, as classical scholars like Poliziano started seriously to study the more technical and philologically demanding Greek texts which constituted the classical tradition in metaphysics, natural philosophy, and medicine. In the same way, it was only toward the end of the century that doctors and artists, led by men like Leonardo da Vinci, began to see how the new knowledge of perspective and drawing could be applied to the medical fields of anatomy and botany.

In the late fourteenth and early fifteenth centuries, however, the period with which this study is concerned, these developments were still in their infancy. Those Florentine physicians who took part in the cultural movements of the Renaissance did so primarily as patrons and interested onlookers rather than as active participants. They dabbled in ethics and classical literature, sent their sons to the fashionable new schools, and commissioned tombs and memorials from leading Florentine sculptors, but their interests in the new art and learning seems as much social, or sociable, as intellectual. There is no sign that they guessed at the ways in which their own disciplines would be transformed by the new texts and methods. The principal exception was Paolo Toscanelli, who abandoned medicine early in his career for mathematics and classical studies. Toscanelli was not typical of Florentine physicians. Nonetheless, his life and work illustrate the potential for future collaboration between humanists, artists, and medical or scientific scholars as well as the intrinsic limits on such collaboration in the early Renaissance.

It is wrong to assume that the compartmentalization of humanist and medical studies in this early period argues a deep hostility between humanists and physicians. It is commonly argued that the representatives of humanist and scholastic learning were implacable adversaries in this period, since the former looked to the cultural ideal of antiquity while the latter put their faith in the authority of medieval Latin and Arabic writers.[103] According to this interpretation, Florence became the main center of early Quattrocento humanism precisely because of the weakness of its university: "it was therefore easier in Florence than elsewhere," according to George Holmes, "to point out the absence of the emperor's clothes and treat the whole subject of scholasticism with derision."[104] Two texts often adduced in favor of this position are Petrarch's *Invectives against a Doctor*, written in the early 1350s,

[103] See, for example, Baron, *Humanistic and Political Literature*, 27-34, and *Crisis*, epilogue.
[104] George Holmes, *Florentine Enlightenment*, 30.

and Salutati's *On the Nobility of Laws and Medicine*, completed in 1399; both are usually interpreted as evidence that the early humanists despised the scholastic discipline of medicine, or at least considered it greatly inferior to the more "humanistic" discipline of law.[105]

A closer examination of these texts, however, suggests that the issues are not so simple. In a letter of 1370 to his friend Giovanni Dondi, who taught *physica* at the University of Padua, Petrarch claimed that he had not attacked medical learning but only the medical profession: "no one can say that I have said a word against medicine," he wrote, "although I have often written and spoken against those who call themselves doctors."[106] Stripped of humanist rhetoric, in fact, much of Petrarch's polemic, and after it Salutati's, echoes criticisms of the medical profession which had become commonplace after 1348: doctors promote themselves shamelessly, making exorbitant claims about their competence; yet when faced by an emergency like plague they can only inveigle the trustful out of their money and watch them die.[107] Furthermore, they destroy religion and the state during epidemics by counseling people to elude Providence by fleeing the cities.[108] Both Petrarch and Salutati gave piquancy to their accusations by appealing to squeamishness and social snobbery. "You frequent gloomy, fetid, dark, and lightless places," Petrarch castigated his opponent in the *Invectives*, "you look into soiled basins, you examine the urine of the sick, and you think about gold. Why is it surprising that you, who have so much to do with things that are gloomy, dark, and yellow, should yourself be gloomy, dark, and yellow?"[109]

---

[105] Petrarca, *Inventive*; see also in that edition Martinelli, "Petrarca," and see Garin, "Petrarca." Salutati, *De nobilitate*, and Garin, *La disputà delle arti*; see also Garin's introductions to both volumes. Also Thorndike, *Science and Thought*, chap. 2; Klein, "Les humanistes"; and Vasoli, "Polemiche occamiste."

[106] Petrarca, *Sen.* XII, 2, in Petrarca, *Lettere senili*, 2:238.

[107] Ibid., *Fam.* V, 19; VIII, 7; XV, 5, in Petrarca, *Le familiari*, 2:43-44, 174-179; 3:144-45. See also *Invective*, 28-29, 32, 80. Cf. Salutati, *Epistolario*, 2:92, and *De nobilitate*, 123-59. The Petrarchan resonances in all Salutati's writing on doctors and plague are extremely strong.

[108] Petrarca, *Fam.* XXII, 12; IX, 1; XIV, 3, in *Le familiari*, 4:135-36; 2:211-12; 3:108-10. Cf. Salutati, *Epistolario*, 1:167-70; 2:80-98, 104-9, 112-30, 221-41; 3:396-99. Salutati was impassioned on this topic, giving the original Petrarchan argument a new political twist. His long letters attacking colleagues for their flight during epidemics of plague engendered equally passionate responses from those who found his arguments against the medical analysis of contagion preposterous; see, for example, Vergerio, *Epistolario*, 399-422.

[109] Petrarca, *Invective*, 57; cf. Salutati, *De nobilitate*, 86. Their castigations of medicine as a mechanical art and Salutati's preoccupation with the social inferiority of medicine to law should be seen in this context.

It would be an exaggeration to deny all intellectual substance to these criticisms of medicine. Petrarch on several occasions expressed his distrust of the Arabic authorities ("I hate their race") and the modern logic used by writers like Tommaso Del Garbo, and Salutati devoted several chapters of *On the Nobility of Laws and Medicine* to arguing that law was superior to medicine insofar as it related to the active rather than the contemplative life.[110] But it is also true that law itself was a scholastic discipline and that other humanists, like Poggio, tended to opt for medicine over law.[111] For our purposes, then, this literature is something of a red herring. Self-consciously polemical, it illuminates the political and religious views of Salutati and Petrarch, and it illustrates the depth of popular sentiment against the medical profession after the Black Death; but it sheds little light on the actual intellectual relations between doctors and humanists in early Renaissance Florence. Far more revealing of these relations are the simple facts that Salutati wrote *On the Nobility of Laws and Medicine* in response to a *questio* on the subject by Bernardino di ser Pistoia and that he was answered in turn by an admiring Giovanni Baldi da Faenza; both of these men were prominent physicians and professors of medicine at the University of Florence.[112] As this exchange indicates and as Garin has more recently argued, it is shortsighted to assume that a wall of hostility and incomprehension separated early Florentine humanism and the older scholastic disciplines; in fact the decades around 1400 saw a lively dialogue between students and teachers at the *studio* and professional and amateur humanists outside.[113]

The evidence for this dialogue is strong in Florence, as elsewhere in northern Italy. Both Petrarch and Salutati, for example, despite their crusades against the medical profession, counted doctors among their colleagues and friends. In 1366 Petrarch corresponded with Tommaso Del Garbo concerning the relative power of opinion and fortune;[114] he had met Tommaso in Milan at the court of Galeazzo Visconti and certainly had him in mind when he wrote, near the end of his life, "I

---

[110] Petrarch, *Sen.* XII, 2, in *Lettere senili*, 2:260-62; *Invective*, 52-53. Salutati, *De nobilitate*, chaps. 22-23; see also chap. 15.

[111] For example Poggio Bracciolini, *Conviviales disceptationes*, 2, in Garin, *La disputà della arti*, 15-33; full text in Bracciolini, *Opera omnia*, 1:37-51.

[112] Pagallo, "Nuovi testi," 469-70; Giovanni Baldi, *Disputatio an medicina sit legibus politicis praeferenda*, BLF: Gadd. 74, fols. 102r-5v.

[113] Garin, "Cultura fiorentina." The groundwork for this reassessment was laid in Kristeller, "Humanism and Scholasticism."

[114] Petrarca, *Sen.* VIII, 3; *Letter senili*, 1:463-74. On the circumstances of their friendship see Levati, *Viaggi*, 5:255-59, and Petrarca, *Lettere senili*, 1:475. I have not seen Tommaso's letter to Petrarch in BVA: Chigiano L.VII.262, no. 23.

have had many doctors as friends, of whom four survive: one in Venice, one in Milan, and two at Padua—all learned and pleasant men, remarkable in conversation, quick in disputation, vigorous in argument. . . . They speak continually of Aristotle, of Cicero, of Seneca, and—amazing to say—of Vergil."[115] (One of Petrarch's main criticisms of doctors was in fact that they paid too much rather than too little attention to poetry, rhetoric, and other humanist studies, neglecting their medical responsibilities.)[116]

A generation later Salutati wrote to Antonio da Scarperia, then lecturing on medicine at the Florentine *studio*, to explicate a passage from Seneca's epistle to Lucilius; he closed by reminding Antonio that he was expecting several books from him, including one by Euclid and two by the fourteenth-century medical writers Torrigiano Torrigiani and Pietro d'Abano.[117] The explicit of this letter reminds us that Salutati himself owned a large number of manuscripts of classical and medieval texts in medicine and science, from Ptolemy's *Almagest* to Egidio Romano's *On the Formation of the Fetus* and Pliny's *Natural History*, copiously annotated, and that he cited many more, including a dozen books by Galen and works of Gentile da Foligno, Pietro d'Abano, and Tommaso Del Garbo.[118]

Thus not only were physicians interested in the new classical literary studies of their humanist colleagues; humanists themselves also had scientific and medical concerns. This is well illustrated in the *Paradiso degli Alberti*, an Italian dialogue by Giovanni Gherardi da Prato, who for many years lectured on Dante at the University of Florence. Set in 1389, the work describes a series of discussions held at a villa belonging to the Alberti family and presided over by Luigi Marsili, the Augustinian friar who linked Petrarch to the Florentine humanists of the

---

[115] Petrarca, *Sen.* V, 3; *Lettere senili*, 1:292-93. The doctor in Venice may have been Guido di Bagnolo da Reggio. One of the two Paduans was certainly Giovanni Dondi, who owned a number of manuscripts which reflect humanist interests, including several works by Petrarch; see Lazzarino, "I libri," 26-32, and Petrarch's letters to Dondi in *Sen.* XII, 1-2.

[116] For example Petrarca, *Fam.* V, 19; *Le familiari*, 2:44: "Iam enim professionis sue immemores et dumetis propriis exire ausi, poetarum nemus et rethorum campum petunt, et quasi non curaturi sed persuasuri, circa miserorum grabatulos magno boatu disputant; atque illis morientibus ypocraticos nodos tulliano stamine permiscentes, sinistro quamvis eventu superbiunt. . . ."

[117] Salutati, *Epistolario*, 3:239-58. See Panizza, "Textual Interpretation," esp. 43-46. Salutati was composing *On the Nobility of Laws and Medicine* in this period and may have wished to consult the two medical works for this purpose.

[118] Ullman, *Humanism of Salutati*, chaps. 9-10, passim.

early fifteenth century.[119] The *Paradiso*'s principal interlocutors were Marsili, Salutati, the musician and poet Francesco Landini, the theologian and mathematician Grazia Castellani, and two professors at the Florentine *studio*, Marsiglio da Santa Sofia and Biagio Pelacani da Parma, who were lecturing respectively on *physica* and natural philosophy. Its minor participants included "numerous doctors, students and teachers in arts, and other noble citizens."[120]

Gherardi depicted as close and cordial the intellectual relations between Marsiglio and Biagio, two of the leading scholastic scientific writers of the day, and the early humanists Marsili and Salutati. Their conversation moved from natural philosophy to theology to ethics to political history to courtly love, with no sense of intellectual antagonism or even of serious disciplinary competition. Rather, the speakers showed themselves fully sympathetic to and conversant in each others' fields. After Salutati, the moral philosopher, had held forth on the formation of the fetus, for example, the physician Marsiglio took up the ethical topic of earthly felicity, claiming the right to cite Ovid because Salutati had already shown his familiarity with medical theory: "considering the extent to which he has referred to our physicians, I will refer to his poets."[121]

The *Paradiso*, in other words, like the letters of Petrarch and Salutati, belies the idea that the late fourteenth and early fifteenth centuries saw a pitched battle between humanists and scholastics or physicians. The impression left by these texts accords with the dictates of common sense: in a city as small as Florence the network of friendships and intellectual ties among prominent and intellectually active inhabitants was not constrained by artificial distinctions of discipline or approach. Doctors and literary scholars, university teachers and men of state, friars and businessmen with a love of letters might differ in their primary interests; nonetheless they shared a broad common philosophical and literary culture which embraced both the traditional fields of scholastic learning and new work in the *studia humanitatis*.

The activities of the next generation of Florentine humanists, the

---

[119] Gherardi da Prato, *Paradiso*. On Gherardi and the dating of the *Paradiso*, which Baron attributes to the early 1420s, see Baron, *Humanistic and Political Literature*, 13-37; Wesselofsky's introduction to Gherardi da Prato, *Paradiso*, vols. 1/1 and 1/2; and della Torre, *Storia dell'accademia*, 171-84. On Marsili's importance see Mariani, *Petrarca*, 66-96. Baron's criticism of the *Paradiso* as unrealistic is based mainly on his conviction that any text portraying humanists and scholastics on terms of amity must be unreliable.

[120] Gherardi da Prato, *Paradiso*, 3:4-5: "più e più medici e artisti e altri nobili cittadini."

[121] Ibid., 3:88.

students of Salutati and Chrysoloras who dominated the movement during the first half of the fifteenth century, show that this intellectual ideal did not die. Guided by Niccolò Niccoli and Ambrogio Traversari, they aimed to revive the culture of classical antiquity in its entirety by systematically seeking out and recovering the textual legacy of Greece and Rome, including its science.[122] Although they had a special interest in the Greek mathematical disciplines of geometry, astronomy, geography, optics, and mechanics,[123] they also looked to classical natural philosophy and medicine. Niccoli had a Greek manuscript of Aristotle's *Physics* as early as 1408, and Traversari wrote to him in 1432 from Rome describing his efforts to acquire a Greek manuscript containing the *Meteorology* and the *Metaphysics*.[124] Two years before, in 1430, Traversari had also undertaken to copy Theophrastus' *On Plants* for Niccoli, but owing to lack of time he was forced to farm the task out to a young friend and Florentine physician, Paolo Toscanelli.[125]

Traversari and his circle also collected classical medical texts. During a trip to Milan in 1431 Niccoli found a copy of the *Fragments* of Cornelius Celsus, whose works were unknown in the Middle Ages.[126] Traversari later wrote to him for a copy of Galen's *On Simple Medicines*,[127] and in 1432 and 1433 he sent Niccoli a series of enthusiastic letters from Venice concerning a local doctor named Pietro Tommasi, who collected Greek coins and owned several Greek medical works by Galen and Paul of Aegina as well as (pseudo-)Plutarch's and Ptolemy's treatises on music, with a commentary by Porphyry. "I spoke to him of Paolo [Toscanelli]," Traversari wrote, "and of his remarkable skill and diligence; he was most grateful and said that he would write him to cultivate his friendship."[128]

Paolo Toscanelli, whose name appears so often in Traversari's correspondence, was an anomalous but crucial figure in the cultural his-

[122] This process is vividly documented in Traversari's letters and those addressed to Niccoli by Poggio Bracciolini; Traversari, *Epistolae*, esp. book VIII, and Gordan, *Two Renaissance Book Hunters*. See in general, Sabbadini, *Scoperte*.

[123] See Rose, "Humanist Culture" and *Italian Renaissance*, esp. chaps. 1, 2 (a revision of his "Humanist Culture"), and 4. Marshall Clagett has examined in detail the *fortuna* of Archimedes in this period; see his *Archimèdes*, vol. 3/3, esp. chaps. 1-2.

[124] Sabbadini, *Scoperte*, 1:54; Traversari, *Epistolae*, VIII, 44; vol. 2, col. 410. In 1438 Traversari wrote Ser Filippo Pieruzzi about a complete Greek Aristotle with commentaries on the major works possibly by Simplicius, which he had been shown by the Greek emperor: Mercati, *Ultimi contributi*, 24-25.

[125] Traversari, *Epistolae*, VIII, 35-37; vol. 2, cols. 394-395, 399.

[126] Sabbadini, *Scoperte*, 1:91.

[127] Mercati, *Ultimi contributi*, 46.

[128] Traversari, *Epistolae*, VIII, 45; vol. 2, col. 412. See also VIII, 46-47; vol. 2, cols. 413-15.

tory of the early Florentine Renaissance. Its most important scientific thinker, he was also the only doctor in Florence to participate actively in the humanist movement of the first half of the fifteenth century.[129] Like his friend Niccoli, he left no real body of letters or written work; his importance lies rather in the way he testifies, through the variety of his interests and intellectual friendships, to the connections in this period between literary humanists and those working on classical science, or between proponents of the new Renaissance learning and adherents to the medieval scholastic tradition.

Toscanelli had returned to Florence in 1424, after finishing his medical studies at the University of Padua. According to Vespasiano da Bisticci's biography, he was already a bibliophile and "had collected a very great number of books in all seven of the liberal arts, both Latin and Greek"—the core of what was to be an important collection at his death.[130] Soon after his return he began to take part in the informal humanist academy presided over by Traversari at his convent of Santa Maria degli Angeli, the heir of Marsili's discussion groups in the later fourteenth century. According to Vespasiano, "the days were few that Maestro Paolo did not meet with Cosimo [de' Medici], Ser Filippo [Pieruzzi], and all those other learned men . . . ; most days Niccolò [Niccoli], Cosimo, Lorenzo [Cosimo's brother], Maestro Paolo, Ser Filippo, and Maestro Carlo [Marsuppini] da Arezzo met at the Angeli, where they spoke of notable things."[131] Toscanelli was particularly close to Traversari, Niccoli, and Pieruzzi, whose religious and mathematical interests he shared, but he was also on good terms with more secular humanists like Bruni and Poggio, and later in the century Landino and Poliziano.[132] In addition he was friendly with several men more marginally tied to early Florentine humanism. The architect Brunelle-

129 The physician Niccolò Leonardi was also of Florentine stock, a friend of Vergerio, and a member of the circle of Francesco Barbaro, but he lived and worked in Venice; see Traversari, *Epistolae*, VI, 20; vol. 2, cols. 299-300. General discussions of Toscanelli in Garin, "Paolo Toscanelli" (original Italian in his *Cultura filosofica*, 313-34); de Santillana, "Paolo Toscanelli"; and the massive study of Uzielli, *Toscanelli*.

130 Vespasiano da Bisticci, *Vite*, 2:75. The contents of Toscanelli's library are presently unknown, although Uzielli mentioned his own intention to publish the list of Greek manuscripts owned by Toscanelli at the time of his death; see *Toscanelli*, 656. His collection was renowned; Ercole d'Este attempted to copy and acquire some of the books (*Toscanelli*, 306-7).

131 Vespasiano da Bisticci, *Vite*, 2:75. On these meetings see Stinger, *Humanism*, 30.

132 Traversari asked Pieruzzi and Toscanelli to edit his correspondence; see Stinger, *Humanism*, xiii and 44-51, and Mercati, *Ultimi contributi*, 34-36. Niccoli appointed Toscanelli as one of the executors of his will; see Vespasiano da Bisticci, *Vite*, 2:75, and Ullman and Stadter, *Public Library*, 7-8. For evidence of Pieruzzi's mathematical interests see Björnbo, "San Marco Handschriften." On Toscanelli's ties to the others Landino, *Scritti*, 1:134-37, and Uzielli, *Toscanelli*, 233-34;

schi consulted him on mathematics and optics as well as on structural problems associated with the cathedral dome and the church of Santo Spirito.[133] Alberti discussed geometry, perspective, and geography with him and collaborated with him on astronomical observations.[134] Toscanelli also corresponded on mathematics with Nicholas of Cusa, whom he must have met as a student at Padua, and attended him at his deathbed in 1464.[135]

Toscanelli was eulogized by his contemporaries as one of the flowers of fifteenth-century Florentine culture. Landino called him "the venerable image of Antiquity" and grouped him with Alberti and Niccolò Falcucci as one of the learned Florentines who had illuminated the city with his erudition, while Ugolino Verino composed a verse epigram praising his knowledge of geometry, optics, and medicine as well as geography and astronomy: "He knew both heaven and earth / And recast the great work of Ptolemy."[136] In fact, medicine seems to have been the least of Toscanelli's interests. These focused instead on mathematics, both the traditional quadrivial disciplines of astronomy (or astrology) and geometry, which he had studied at Padua as part of his work in medicine,[137] and the newer field of geography, which had been revitalized in the late fourteenth century by the recovery of Ptolemy's *Cosmography*.[138]

[133] Contemporary accounts of this friendship by Antonio Billi, cited in Battisti, *Filippo Brunelleschi*, 321; see also Manetti, *Brunelleschi*, 55-56, and in general Uzielli, *Toscanelli*, 40-52. Toscanelli's role in Brunelleschi's development of a system of linear perspective is still unclear; see Klein, "Studies on Perspective," and Edgerton, *Renaissance Rediscovery*, 61-62, 77-78.

[134] Uzielli, *Toscanelli*, 200-207; Gadol, *Alberti*, 70-75, 164-78, 195-97.

[135] Vansteenberghe, *Nicolas de Cues*, 11-12; Meuthen, *Die letzten Jahre*, 99, 101, 246; Uzielli, *Toscanelli*, 240-68; Rose, *Italian Renaissance*, 30-31.

[136] Landino, proemium to his commentary on Dante, in his *Scritti*, 1:117-18. Verino, in BLF: Laur. 39, 40, fols. 50v-51v: "Hic rerum causas et coeli sydera norat; / Phylosophum talem saecula rara ferunt. / Pythagorae ex solido statuam conflaverat auro / Grecia et e Pario marmore pyramidem, / Qui rudibus populis geometrica signa parumper / Ostendit. Quanto doctior iste fuit. / . . . / At Paulus Thuscus terram cognovit et astra, / Et Ptholomeneum grande retexit opus, / Qui prospective formam depinxit et artem, / Quo libro cunctis equiparandus erit. . . ."

[137] Padua was particularly noted for its astronomy and mathematics, in contrast to the University of Bologna: Siraisi, *Taddeo Alderotti*, 139-45, 178. On the Paduan tradition see Siraisi, *Arts and Sciences at Padua*, chap. 3; Favaro, "Lettori"; Marangon, "Miscellanea astrologica," 94-95; and Billanovich, "Giacomo Zanetini," 4-5. Toscanelli's teacher was Prosdocimo de' Beldomandi, on whom see Favaro, "Prosdocimo de' Beldomandi."

[138] Chrysoloras brought a Greek copy of this work to Florence in 1397; the translation was finished by Iacopo di Angelo da Scarperia. See Weiss, "Jacopo Angeli da Scarperia."

Despite the enormous respect in which Toscanelli was held by both humanists and professional mathematicians,[139] his work remains elusive, largely because we have fewer than two dozen folios from his pen. They include, in mathematics, a short letter to Nicholas of Cusa from 1453 or 1454 criticizing one of his attempts to square the circle;[140] in astronomy and astrology, a notebook of loose sheets containing cometary observations made between 1433 and 1472, a reflection on the astrological significance of comets, some exercises in Ptolemaic spherical trigonometry, and some planetary and lunar tables for astrological use;[141] in geography and cartography, a set of tables of the latitudes and longitudes of various cities and a grid for a map (both in the same notebook) as well as a letter from 1474 to the Portuguese canon Fernao Martins describing a western route to the Indies and copied onto the flyleaf of Christopher Columbus's manuscript of Pius II's *Cosmography*.[142] There is in addition a vernacular treatise on optics which has been attributed to Toscanelli on the basis of meager circumstantial evidence.[143]

Taken as a whole, Toscanelli's work shows him as a man with an ambiguous relationship to the movement which aimed to develop a new Renaissance science based on the return to classical texts unmediated by Arabic and medieval Latin versions. On the one hand, Traversari's letters show that Toscanelli participated in the effort to collect new Greek scientific works, and we know that he owned important manuscripts of Archimedes, Galen, and other Greek writers.[144] Re-

---

[139] For an example of the latter see Regiomontanus's comments in the appendix to *De triangulis*, 29 and 56, and in Zinner, *Regiomontanus*, table 26.

[140] Printed in Regiomontanus, *De triangulis*, appendix, 13-14; translated and annotated in Cusanus, *Die mathematischen Schriften*, 128-31. See also Joseph Hofmann's introduction to this edition of Cusanus, xxxii-xxxiii; Jervis, "Mathematics"; Rose, "Humanist Culture," 59-63; and Clagett, *Archimedes*, 3/3: 318-19.

[141] BNF: Banco rari 30 (formerly Magl. XI, 121, fols. 237-58); large portions transcribed or reproduced in Uzielli, *Toscanelli*, 326-28, 356, and tables III and VII-IX. See also Jervis, "Toscanelli's Cometary Observations," and Giovanni Celloria's discussion in Uzielli, *Toscanelli*, chap. 6.

[142] Reproduced in Uzielli, *Toscanelli*, table IV; transcribed and translated in Vignaud, *Toscanelli and Columbus*, 275-303; the map referred to in the letter has not survived. Although Vignaud rejected the letter as spurious, new evidence has confirmed its authenticity, although not that of the forged correspondence between Toscanelli and Columbus. Toscanelli's geographical fragments have generated a vast body of scholarship of uneven quality: reliable introductions in Durand, 258-59, and Wagner, "Rekonstruktion."

[143] Edited in Parronchi, *Studi*, 599-645, from BRF: Ricc. 2110. both Parronchi's arguments and my own examination of the text are inconclusive.

[144] See Uzielli, *Toscanelli*, 656, Rose, "Humanist Culture," 63; and Clagett, *Archimedes*,

giomontanus testified to his concern for their correct translation: "after thorough medical studies you learned Greek," he wrote to the Florentine, "and if you came upon something translated poorly from Greek into Latin, you refined it and thereby educated others."[145] On the other hand, there is little evidence that Toscanelli actually integrated these new classical texts into his own work. The mathematical fragment is too short to allow us to determine whether, like Regiomontanus, he was drawing on Archimedean ideas and methods unavailable through the medieval tradition.[146] But the sources for his astronomical and geographical writing were conventional: Ptolemy's *Centiloquium* and *Almagest*, Marco Polo's narrative, Albertus Magnus's *Mirror of Astronomy*, Alzarkali's *Canons on the Astronomical Tables*, and other medieval sources of Arabic origin and inspiration.[147]

The only element of Toscanelli's work which suggests a creative assimilation of new classical sources is his use of a rectilinear grid to record celestial and terrestrial latitudes and longitudes—a device adopted from Ptolemy's *Cosmography*, which was unknown in medieval Europe before the end of the fourteenth century.[148] Toscanelli seems to have been one of the first Europeans to refine the medieval star catalogue on the basis of new observations and to chart these findings on a large-scale flat star-map using a rectilinear coordinate system. His comet observations may thus represent the earliest astronomical use of charts in the service of precise measurement, as opposed to pictorial representation.[149] The interest and significance of this innovation lies less in its influence—Toscanelli's notebook remained unknown until the

---

3/3: 334, 357n. The Greek manuscripts acquired by Poliziano from Toscanelli's heirs included Galen's *De compositione medicamentorum* and medical excerpts from Aetius, Dioscorides, and Diocles, among others; Perosa, "Codici," 75-79.

[145] Regiomontanus, *De triangulis*, appendix, 56: "post medicinam summopere percognitam, literas graecas didicisses, quo ingenii tui vim abundiorem ostenderes, et si quid somnolento interprete latinitati ineptius forsitan redditum e greco offenderes, ipse limare ac demum caeteros docere posses." Regiomontanus may have been thinking of the much-criticized humanist translations of Ptolemy's *Cosmography* by Iacopo di Angelo da Scarperia and of Archimedes and Ptolemy's *Almagest* by George of Trebizond; see Rose, *Italian Renaissance*, 41-42, 95, 99-102, and Zinner, *Regiomontanus*, table 26.

[146] See Clagett, *Archimedes*, 3/3: 342-83, esp. 381. Clagett contrasts Regiomontanus' use of the new Archimedes with the Archimedeanism of Alberti and Cusanus, which he sees as lying wholly within the medieval tradition; *Archimedes*, vol. 3/3, chap. 1.

[147] Jervis, "Mathematics," esp. 9-10; Vignaud, *Toscanelli and Columbus*, 277-92; Wagner, "Rekonstruktion," 303-12; Durand, *Map Corpus*, 258. The sources of the perspective treatise attributed doubtfully to Toscanelli are equally traditional; Parronchi, *Studi*, 583.

[148] See above, note 138.

[149] Jervis, "Toscanelli's Cometary Observations," 19; Warner, *Sky Explored;* ix-x.

nineteenth century—than in its sources. Florence was one of the principal centers of the new mathematical cartography developed in the fifteenth century on the basis of new Greek sources and new observations. Like his friend Alberti, Toscanelli was very much involved in this enterprise.[150] He collected maps and owned a copy of Claudius Clavus's map of Scandinavia, the first of the "new maps" drawn to supplement the classical canon in Ptolemy's *Cosmography*, which Clavus had brought to Florence from Denmark in 1424. Furthermore, as his letter to Martins and his notebook show, he tried his own hand at mapmaking.[151]

Toscanelli's work in geography and astronomy is important above all for its concern with mathematical accuracy combined with systematic observation, neither of which had been a signal feature of medieval contributions.[152] In his empiricism Toscanelli recalls Ugolino da Montecatini. Not only did he regularly interrogate travelers to Florence from exotic lands about local geography and topography;[153] he also engaged in a demanding program of astronomical observations, recorded in his notebook as "the immense labors and painful vigils of Maestro Paolo dal Pozzo Toscanelli regarding the measure of the comet."[154] With Alberti, he was recognized by Regiomontanus as one of the few contemporary astronomers who did not, like "credulous women," accept the astronomical parameters found in books but insisted on verifying them empirically. (Regiomontanus was referring specifically to Toscanelli's attempts to determine the obliquity of the ecliptic and the time of the summer solstice using a special meridian installed in the cupola of Brunelleschi's dome.)[155]

Toscanelli was unusual among both doctors and humanists. Educated in medicine, he rejected it for mathematics, geography, astron-

---

[150] Durand, *Map Corpus*, 252-73; Gadol, *Alberti*, 164-78; Bagrow, *History of Cartography*, 77-82. The most important Florentine workshops were those of Niccolò Germano, his student Henricus Martellus (also German), and Pietro del Massaio.

[151] See Vignaud, *Toscanelli and Columbus*, 295; Diller, "Geographical Treatise," 447; and ASF: CS-S. Veridiana, 134. The map enclosed with the letter to Martins is missing; for the numerous early attempts to reconstruct it see Wagner, "Rekonstruktion."

[152] Cf. Durand, *Map Corpus*, chaps. 5-6.

[153] See Landino, Commentary on Vergil, in *Scritti*, 2:309: "Nostro tamen tempore cum Florentia homines viderit qui circa initia Tanais habitent, omnia de illa regione vera novit. Ego autem interfui cum illos Paulus Physicus diligenter quaeque interrogaret"; also Toscanelli's letter to Martins in Vignaud, *Toscanelli and Columbus*, 299 and 285-86n.

[154] BNF: Banco rari 30, fol. 244v: "immensi labores et graves vigilie magistri Pauli de Puteo Toscanelli super mensura comete." Cf. Vespasiano da Bisticci, *Vite*, 2:73-74.

[155] Jervis, "Mathematics," 7-8, 10; Saalman, *Brunelleschi*, 294.

omy, and astrology. An intimate associate of Niccoli, Traversari, and their circle, he never succeeded fully in integrating the new classical learning into his own studies. Nonetheless, he exemplifies the importance of ties between university science and early humanist literary inquiry—ties also demonstrated in the career of his colleague Alberti. He shows, too, how doctors trained in technical scholastic disciplines could serve as mediators and interpreters for the vast corpus of Greek scientific texts which was beginning to be reconstructed. These studies were still inchoate in the first half of the fifteenth century; it was not until the generation of Angelo Poliziano, the 1480s and 1490s, that Greek philology began to reach a level which permitted real progress. But men like Poliziano, Ficino (also trained in medicine), and Giovanni Pico acknowledged their debt to the first efforts of Toscanelli.[156]

If a doctor like Toscanelli had so much to offer, why then were so few Florentine physicians involved with the new Renaissance movements of the early fifteenth century? To a large degree the obstacles were social and economic. There was in the first place the simple problem of time. Medicine was a demanding career and left its practitioners little leisure to cultivate other fields. Toscanelli was highly privileged in this respect: he came from the wealthiest medical family in Florence and never had to engage in regular practice.[157] Far more typical were Lorenzo Sassoli da Prato, forced by financial worries to abandon a cherished scholarly career, or Giovanni Fontana, who studied mathematics and medicine in Padua at the same time as Toscanelli.[158] In the epilogue to his work on mensuration, Fontana apologized to its addressee, Domenico Bragadino, for not having produced a richer book. His time and energies, he explained, had been taken up by his practice as communal physician in Udine:

> You know that I have been salaried here and devoted to serving the sick, who require such constant care that waking and studying and eating, I seem to hear always their weary sighs and meet them daily crying in the streets, and even sleeping I seem to dream of them in distorted and unclear images, and I feel as if I must al-

---

[156] See Perosa, "Codici," 75-78; Marsiglio Ficino, *Disputatio contra iudicium astrologorum*, in Kristeller, *Supplementum ficinianum*, 2:66; and Pico della Mirandola, *Disputationes*, 2:310.

[157] See Vespasiano da Bisticci, *Vite*, 2:75. Toscanelli's practice was confined to his friends; he is known to have treated Niccoli (Traversari, *Epistolae*, VIII, 19, and XII, 24; vol. 2, cols. 381 and 587), Traversari's brother (Mercati, *Ultimi contributi*, 10-11), and Nicholas of Cusa (Meuthen, *Die letzten Jahre*, 99, 246).

[158] On Sassoli see above, Chapter Four; on Fontana, Clagett, *Archimedes*, 3/1-2: 239-59, and Thorndike, *History of Magic*, 4:150-82.

ways be considering and reflecting and reading about what I can give them to assure them health or forbid them to prevent them from dying of their illnesses. The care of the sick is demanding and requires great strength of mind and body and ultimately all the doctor's energy. Thus it is only with many interruptions and distractions from my studies and with many obstacles to my project ... that I have completed my book on the triangular ballista.[159]

Toscanelli was also atypical among contemporary Florentine physicians in that he was a Florentine citizen, while most of his peers were immigrants from the countryside or foreign towns. As we have seen, the social and economic position of these immigrants was more precarious than that of citizens of similar wealth and standing, and they were under greater constraints when it came to mapping out their professional and personal lives. We can sense these constraints when we look at the relationship between Maestro Lorenzo Sassoli and his son Sassolo. As we have already seen, Maestro Lorenzo had immigrated from Prato in the early fifteenth century and married into the Cavalcanti. He also appears to have had connections with the new learning in Florence. Praised by Poggio as "the most excellent and cultivated among the city's doctors," he sent his son to study Greek and Latin with Francesco Filelfo, who according to Vespasiano "taught all the sons of the leading men [*uomini da bene*] at his lessons."[160] But Maestro Lorenzo almost broke with Sassolo when his son, not satisfied with the aristocratic patina of a classical education, chose to continue his studies and become a humanist himself. There is an autobiographical ring to Sassolo's letter castigating parents who, "blinded" by love of money and security, push their children into the professions rather than the humanities: "They all hate letters," he wrote, "while they

---

[159] Cited in Clagett, *Archimedes*, 3/1-2: 242-43n: "Scis me huius loci salario deditum et ut ita dixerim quodammodo famulatui infirmorum assiduo, quibus tam solicitum me oportuit et continuum esse, ut vigilans et studens et comedens videar audire semper subspiria ipsorum languentium et per vias cotidie et ubique clamantibus illis occurrere, dormiens quoque in sompnis concipere ymagines eorum deformes et obscuras. Adde quod non parum existimandum censeo semper examinare cogi[tare?] aut legere quod pro eorum salute sit offerendum illis vel prohibendum ne malo ipso pereant.

Noscis profato quantam [*sic*] esse debeat ipsa cura infirmantium que mentis et corporis omnem valitudinem at denique omnes medici vires cons[tanter?] requirit. Multis itaque cum intervallis temporum studiorumque diversionibus et adversantibus multis huic intentioni et librum prolixum et hunc abreviatum quos de trigono balistario concepi ad finem duxi."

[160] Poggio Bracciolini, *Epistolae*, VI, 15, in *Opera omnia*, 3:114-15. Vespasiano da Bisticci, *Vite*, 2:54.

respect and love law and medicine as the most convenient ways to wealth; they claim that to study the others is the most expeditious way to ruin."[161]

Maestro Lorenzo, like Ugolino da Montecatini and many other doctors, had a strong sense of the limited options open to those of immigrant stock—Sassolo's short life in fact bore out his father's fears[162]—and this sense of limitation may have kept him from full participation in the literary culture of the day. It is worth noting, in comparison, that the Florentine citizens involved in early humanist circles were overwhelmingly men from native patrician families, who could afford to live off rents, business proceeds, and patrimony, whereas their immigrant counterparts (Salutati, Bruni, Poggio) were trained in law or *notaria*.[163] For the latter, like immigrant doctors, a professional degree was necessary for security and as an entrée into Florentine society, although law and the notariate seem to have mixed more easily with humanist study than the practice of medicine.[164]

Successful Florentine physicians had more money than time, and it is probably for this reason that the majority of those with ties to the new Renaissance culture appear not as participants in the literary movement, which required a time-consuming study of Greek and Latin philology, but as patrons and arbiters of the new art. Maestro Tommaso di Baccio da Arezzo, for example, was involved in his family's project for the decoration of the main chapel of the church of San Francesco, a project ultimately executed by Piero della Francesca, who covered its walls with the fresco cycle *The Story of the True Cross*.[165] Maestro Giovanni Chellini da San Miniato, the book collector, cultivated close ties with Donatello, Antonio Rossellino, and Bernardo Rossellino, and his portrait bust by Antonio is one of the earliest and finest of its kind.[166] On a smaller scale Maestro Galileo Galilei, Ma-

---

[161] Letter to Lionardo Dati, in Guasti, *Intorno alla vita*, 27: "Litteras bonas oderunt omnes, leges ac medicinam admirantur et amant, ut instrumenta videlicet quaestus et pecuniae commodissima: Artium vero ceterarum studium compendiariam esse viam ad calamitatem contendunt." See also Guasti, "Sassolo Pratese," 578.

[162] He died a suicide at the age of 32; Guasti, *Intorno alla vita*, 20-21.

[163] Statement based on the humanists studied by Lauro Martines in *Social World*, chap. 3. The only two immigrants who did not fit this pattern were Traversari, a monk, and Marsuppini, who came from a very rich Aretine family.

[164] On the symbiotic relationship between law, the notariate, and humanism, see Martines, *Lawyers*, 72, 107-12, 387-96.

[165] Borsook, *Mural Painters*, 91-102.

[166] Pope-Hennessy, with Lightbown, *Catalogue of Italian Sculpture*, 1:126. Chellini also owned a roundel by Donatello, given him in return for medical care; see Lightbown, "Giovanni Chellini," and Pope-Hennessy, "Madonna Reliefs." Chelini's tomb

estro Ugolino da Montecatini, Maestro Niccolò Falcucci, and Maestro
Agostino di Stefano Santucci invested in tomb sculpture and paint-
ings.[167] In addition doctors were sometimes consulted as arbiters and
advisers in communal artistic projects: Toscanelli, for example, was
called on in 1442 to help decide on the decoration of the Florentine
cathedral, and Maestro Lorenzo Sassoli was asked to determine the
price of the outdoor pulpit which Donatello sculpted for the Cathedral
of Prato.[168]

It would be wrong to claim, however, that only social and economic
pressures confined most doctors to the more passive roles of patron,
arbiter, and collector. No institutional barriers prevented a physician
trained in the scholastic fields of logic, natural philosophy, and medicine from participating in the recovery of classical culture; rather, as I
have already mentioned, the literary and ethical interests of the leading
Florentine humanists during the first decades of the fifteenth century
led in a different direction from those of the city's physicians. In the
second half of the century, however, the situation changed, as Florentine scholars turned toward science and philosophy and began to
examine the Greek works of Aristotle, Galen, Hippocrates, and the
Platonic tradition in the light of the new philology.

Many explanations have been given for the shift: the declining vitality of Florentine republicanism, continuing improvement in the
mastery of Greek, the arrival of Byzantine émigrés like Argyropoulos,
who were steeped in the traditions of Greek philosophy rather than
Latin rhetoric.[169] The result, however, is clear: the intellectual atmos-
phere in humanist circles of the later fifteenth century was much more
congenial to medical men, while the increasingly centralized patronage
of the Medici, initiated by Cosimo and continued by his son Piero and
grandson Lorenzo, could offer a reasonable livelihood to immigrant
intellectuals in the form of outright subsidies, ecclesiastical benefices,
chancery positions, and university chairs. Thus, if we look at the groups
which set the tone of cultural life in Florence in these years, we find a
disproportionate number of doctors and men with medical training:

and funerary chapel in the church of San Iacopo in San Miniato (two of his numerous
building projects there) have been attributed to Bernardo Rossellino, Donatello, Mino
da Fiesole, and others; see Schulz, *Sculpture of Bernardo Rossellino*, chap. 9; Battistini,
"Giovanni Chellini"; and Lightbown, "Giovanni Chellini," 103.

[167] Ristori, "Niccolò Falcucci," 263-65; Battistini, "Contributo," 129-30, where
Ugolino's tomb is attributed to Michelozzo. The tombs of M° Galileo and M° Agostino
are still visible in the floor of the center aisle of the church of Santa Croce.

[168] See note 2 above.

[169] For example George Holmes, *Florentine Enlightenment*, chap. 8, and Garin, *Italian
Humanism*, chap. 3.

Niccolò Tignosi da Foligno, Antonio Benivieni, Pierleone Leoni da Spoleto, Bernardo Torni, and—most influential of all—Marsiglio Ficino, whose father had been an immigrant surgeon.[170]

By the 1460s, then, doctors began increasingly to participate in humanist circles, but it took several more decades for humanist learning to begin to penetrate the discipline of medicine itself. This lag is not difficult to understand. Late medieval medicine, as shown in the works of Tommaso Del Garbo, Niccolò Falcucci, and Ugolino da Montecatini, was a complex and sophisticated discipline with its own highly developed modes of analysis and standards of argument and inquiry. This initally made it less able to assimilate new texts and new approaches rapidly—a difficulty not felt in other, less developed disciplines such as history, ethics, and political theory. Furthermore, the reform of medical learning was contingent on reforms in teaching and study in the medical faculties of the Italian universities, a system which had been in place for two centuries. It is for all these reasons that no coherent school of medical humanism or Renaissance medicine emerged until the early sixteenth century and that when it did, it found its center not in Florence but at the new academic powerhouse of Italian medicine: the University of Padua.[171]

[170] On Medici patronage of these doctors see Brown, "Humanist Portrait," 197-98, 201-4, 210; Garin, *Cultura filosofica*, 274-75, 392; Thorndike, *Science and Thought*, chaps. 6, 10. The literature on Ficino is enormous. The classic study of his thought is Kristeller, *Philosophy of Ficino*. The lists of teaching faculty at the University of Florence at Pisa after 1473 appear in Verde, *Studio fiorentino*, 1:296-383.

[171] Bylebyl, "School of Padua." Richard Palmer of the Wellcome Institute for the History of Medicine in London is also working on this topic.

Conclusion

IF FLORENCE did not assume a leading role in the sixteenth-century movement to reform medical learning, Florentines nonetheless participated in this endeavor; by the 1530s the city had produced a New Galenic Academy devoted to criticizing the works of the Arabs and to publicizing the new classical scholarship in medicine.[1] The most striking change in Florentine medicine in this period, however, concerned not the content of medical learning but the composition and organization of the medical profession. The mid-sixteenth century saw the resumption and intensification of efforts by university-educated physicians to establish a hierarchical structure within their guild's branch of doctors and to subordinate other groups of practitioners to their authority.

Threatened by the influx of immigrants and empirics in the decades after the plague of 1348, as we have already seen, Florentine physicians had taken the first steps to create such a hierarchy in the 1380s by founding the College of Doctors as a separate corporation within the Guild of Doctors, Apothecaries, and Grocers. The collapse of the native medical profession and the disappearance of physicians from social prominence and political power in the late fourteenth and the fifteenth centuries robbed these reforms of meaning; the college remained a shadowy and ineffective body throughout the early Renaissance. In the mid-sixteenth century, however, the process began to reverse itself. Physicians once again sat among the guild consuls, and the College of Doctors emerged as a powerful force within the profession. Reconstituted in 1560 as an elite body of twelve physicians, the college assumed most of the control over medicine which had previously been invested in the guild as a whole. It oversaw the licensing of all practitioners, regulated all forms of practice, and advised the state

---

[1] See Antonioli, *Rabelais et la médecine*, 45n. I have not examined the texts by Landi and others in *Novae academiae florentinae opuscula*.

on matters of public health. The increased stratification of the profession appeared in the new format of the guild's matriculation lists, which after 1560 differentiated among physicians, surgeons, and empirics instead of listing them indiscriminately as before.[2]

The change reflected in part the increasing stratification of Florentine society in these years and the growing social gap between physicians and lower practitioners, as Cipolla has argued. It also mirrored the centralization of political authority in the hands of the Medici dukes after the fall of the Florentine republic in 1532 and the increasingly close ties between collegiate physicians and the state.[3] Above all, however, it testified to a dramatic change in the composition of the medical profession, as the rate of immigration slowed and native Florentines of good family began once more to choose careers as physicians. Of the ninety-four doctors who matriculated in the guild between 1548 and 1565, almost 40 percent were native to the city, and of those the majority were physicians; most of the immigrants, in contrast, were surgeons and empirics.[4] Thus, as the waves of plague decreased in severity and frequency over the course of the sixteenth century, medicine again attracted well-born citizens who could use social and political connections to reassert their authority over the profession as a whole. This process of exclusion, stratification, and control—in other words, of professionalization—represents the resumption of an evolution begun more than two hundred years earlier but temporarily halted by the coming of plague and the resultant disruption of patterns of medical recruitment.

The period after 1348 was anomalous for doctors and medicine not only in Florence but in other parts of Europe as well. The long medical crisis ushered in by the Black Death was neither a typical nor a predictable episode in the life of the medical profession. But it is precisely

---

[2] Details of this reform in Cipolla, *Public Health*, 72-73, and Mannelli, "Il Collegio medico fiorentino." See also the new statutes in AMS-4, esp. fols. 58v-59r. Only in the 1590s did doctors begin to be elected to the guild consulate in large numbers: AMS-46, *ad annum*.

[3] See Cochrane, *Florence in the Forgotten Centuries*, esp. introduction and book I; Palmer, "Physicians and the State," 54-57; and Cipolla, *Public Health*, 72. Cipolla certainly overstates the former change; there is evidence that surgery retained social and intellectual respectability into the seventeenth century.

[4] These figures are drawn from the index to the list in AMS-12. Of the 94 new doctors, 37 (39%) were natives of the city, 24 (26%) were natives of the Florentine territories, and 33 (35%) were foreigners. Of the 34 new physicians, 19 were natives of the city, 10 were natives of the territories, and only 5 were foreigners. This trend continued into the seventeenth century; see Cipolla's analysis of the profession in 1630 in *Public Health*, chap. 2.

because of its anomaly that this period reveals so much about the consolidation of the medical profession and the institutional order of medical practice. In the first place, it shows that although the consolidation of medicine as an academic discipline may have been a necessary condition for the development of medicine as a profession, it was not a sufficient one. The new university curriculum of the late thirteenth century provided the justification for a new system of medical licensing and control, but university-educated doctors could not enforce that system by intellectual authority alone; they needed political influence both within their guild and within the state as a whole. Access to power depended on membership in the republic's oligarchical elite in early Renaissance Florence and on ducal patronage after 1532. Thus the process of professionalization was highly sensitive to changes in the political order as well as to shifting demographic and epidemiological conditions. The history of the medical profession cannot be written without taking such factors into account.

In the second place, the evolution of Florentine medical institutions shows a different pattern than is often portrayed. It is commonly assumed that although the outlines of a powerful medical profession were visible by the end of the Middle Ages, it took much longer to develop a system of medical practice sophisticated enough to meet the needs of the population as a whole. The experience of Florence suggests that the case was the reverse. At least in northern Italy, the institutional order of medical practice seems to have constituted itself more quickly than the profession and to have been less disrupted by the Black Death. If anything, the plague acted to strengthen the corporate structures of medical patronage by giving new urgency to the problem of caring for the vulnerable and the disadvantaged. In the years after 1348, while the medical profession struggled unsuccessfully to regain its lost authority and prestige, public and private money poured into other medical institutions. Citizens founded hospitals by the score and joined confraternities which insured them and their families in case of illness. The cities salaried public doctors, constructed their own hospitals, and established ever more powerful health boards—institutions later diffused and imitated elsewhere in Europe. From this point of view, Florentine medicine was a collective creation; its real heroes were less the scholars who codified its theory than the citizens who shaped and subsidized it and the physicians, surgeons, and empirics who, in the words of Michele Pianellari, were "always there when needed."[5]

[5] See Chapter 2, note 22.

APPENDIX I

Names, Dates, Places, and Money

NAMES

A typical Florentine name in the fourteenth and fifteenth centuries contained a number of different pieces of information, corresponding to its various elements as follows.

Maestro	Niccolò	di Francesco
/	/	/
honorific title	given name	father's name

di Gialdo . . .	Falcucci	da Borgo San Lorenzo
/	/	/
grandfather's name (etc.)	family name	place of origin (usually of birth)

Not all names included all elements. Only certain classes of citizens, for example, had honorifics: *Messer* (knights and lawyers); *Maestro*, abbreviated M° (doctors, students, teachers, and a few master craftsmen); and *Ser* (notaries and some thirteenth- and early fourteenth-century doctors). Only the more established families had acquired family names, and only a foreigner would have been regularly known by a toponymic. I have in general retained the Tuscan forms of names like Agnolo or Lionardo.

DATES

The Florentine year began on the day of the Incarnation (March 24), and the dates of days between January 1 and March 23 must be adjusted accordingly. Thus 18 February 1422 by Florentine reckoning corresponds to our 18 February 1423. It would be abbreviated in the notes and appendices to this book as 18.ii.1422/3.

PLACES

The territories of early Renaissance Florence were divided into three parts—the city (*civitas, città*), countryside (*comitatus, contado*), and district (*districtus, distretto*). The city proper corresponded to the land enclosed by the most recent circle of walls. Its basic administrative divisions after 1346 were the four quarters of Santo Spirito, Santa Croce, Santa Maria Novella, and San Giovanni, each of which was further divided into four *gonfaloni*.[1] The city was also divided according to parish.[2]

The *contado* corresponded to the original Florentine territory and enjoyed the closest ties to the city. Composed of the bishoprics of Florence and Fiesole in the thirteenth century, it was enlarged by accretion in the fourteenth. Its principal towns were either previously independent cities like Prato or San Miniato al Tedesco, acquired or conquered by Florence, or *castelli* like Borgo San Lorenzo or Montevarchi, fortified by the Florentine government for defense.[3] For administrative purposes the *contado* was divided into quarters corresponding to those of the city.[4]

The district was composed of the neighboring cities which had been conquered, bought, or otherwise assimilated by Florence, together with their *contadi*.[5]

MONEY (CURRENCY, WAGES, PRICES, TAXES)

The economic life of Florence operated on two separate monetary systems, one based on the gold florin (abbreviated fl.) and the other on the silver lira (abbreviated £), a money of account.[6] Most wages and prices were established in lire, while dowries, inheritances, transactions

---

[1] See, in general, Greppi and Massa, "Città e territorio," and Herlihy and Klapisch-Zuber, *Les toscans*, chap. 4. Before the transition to quarters the city had been divided into six *sesti*.

[2] For a list of the city parishes in the mid-fourteenth century and the *gonfaloni* to which they corresponded see Herlihy and Klapisch-Zuber, *Les toscans*, 123.

[3] See Plesner, *L'émigration*, chap. 1.

[4] See Plesner, "Una rivoluzione," 76-83.

[5] See Herlihy and Klapisch-Zuber, *Les toscans*, 114-21 and maps on 113 and 296.

[6] More details in de Roover, *Medici Bank*, 31-33.

of international merchants, salaries of important officials, and so forth were calculated in florins. Like the old English pound, the lira was equivalent to twenty shillings (soldi, abbreviated s.) or 240 pence (denari, abbreviated d.). The relationship between the lira and the florin was not fixed but fluctuated between £3 and £4 to the florin; the relative value of the lira tended downward in the later fourteenth and the fifteenth centuries.

Most prices remained fairly stable in this period, although the cost of food fluctuated according to conditions. Wages rose immediately after the plague of 1348 but fell again and seem to have stabilized by the end of the fourteenth century. A manual laborer might have earned fl. 2½ to fl. 3 a month (fl. 30 to fl. 36 a year), while the annual salary of a master mason might have amounted to fl. 50 to fl. 60, that of a minor communal official fl. 70, and that of an important officer or prominent university lecturer fl. 200 to fl. 300. It is always difficult to establish equivalences, given changes in the relative cost of food, housing, fuel, and clothing; recent work on wages and prices in Florence of this period has tended to show that the master mason's salary was probably adequate to support a family of four but that the laborer with dependents would have been living in conditions close to poverty and malnutrition.[7]

The communal government used three principal means of collecting money from its subjects: indirect taxes (*gabelle*); direct taxes; and loans, forced and voluntary. Only the last two concern us here.[8] In this study I have used the records of three different kinds of taxes:[9]

1. *Sega* of 1352 and 1355. The *sega* was a hearth tax assessed on nearly ten thousand city households, each registered under the name of its head, by quarter and *gonfalone*.

2. *Prestanza*. The *prestanza* was a forced loan levied on all but the poorest city households. *Prestanze* were collected regularly and frequently between 1359 and 1427. Householders could pay only part of their assessment *ad perdendum* (without return); those who paid in full received interest-bearing shares in the *Monte*, or funded communal debt, established in 1345.

3. *Catasto*. The *catasto* replaced *prestanze* as the principal direct citizen tax in 1427. The net wealth of each household was calculated by subtracting its obligations (*incarichi*) from the sum of its assets, or

[7] De la Roncière, "Pauvres et pauvreté," 672-85; Pinto, "Personale," 143-57.

[8] On the first see de la Roncière, "Indirect Taxes," 160-92.

[9] See Barbadoro, "Finanza e demografia" (on the *sega*); Becker, *Florence in Transition*, 1:170-81 (on the *prestanze*); and Herlihy and Klapisch-Zuber, *Les toscans*, chaps. 1-3 (on the *catasto*).

raw wealth. After a standard deduction for dependents, the household's tax was calculated on a progressive scale. The first and most comprehensive *catasto* was assessed in 1427-28. *Catasti* were also collected from institutions like monasteries, hospitals, and guilds, and in the *contado* and district as well as in the city.

Medical Curriculum at
the University of Bologna (1405)[1]

THEORETICAL MEDICINE[2]

First Year

MORNING

FIRST LECTURE

Avicenna, *Canon*, I (excluding chapters on anatomy in fen 1 and chapters on the seasons in fen 2; including only chapters in fen 3 on the necessity of death, diseases of infants, regimen of eating and drinking, regimen of water and wine, and sleep and waking)

SECOND LECTURE

Galen, *De differentiis febrium*

Galen, *De complexionibus*

Galen, *De mala complexione*

Galen, *De simplicibus medicinis* (excluding book VI)

Galen, *De diebus criticis*, I

AFTERNOON

Avicenna, *Canon*, IV, fen 2 (on prognostication), and II (on medicines)

Galen, *De interioribus* (excluding book II)

Galen, *De regimine sanitatis*, VI

Galen, *De diebus criticis*, II

Hippocrates, *Aphorismata* (excluding part 7)

---

[1] The University of Florence modeled its medical curriculum on that of Bologna; see Alessandro Gherardi, *Statuti*, 161.

[2] University of Medicine and Arts of Bologna: statute of 1405, 78; in Malagola, *Statuti*, 274-76. The program seems very ambitious; it is possible that not all books were read each year. Compare the list of medical books available at the university stationers (Malagola, *Statuti*, 284) and the subjects listed in the roll of lecturers at Bologna for 1466/7, in Dallari, *Rotuli*, 4:71-74. Lynn Thorndike included this information in his *University Records*, 280-81, although in incomplete form.

Second Year

MORNING   FIRST LECTURE

Galen, *Tegni*

Hippocrates, *Prognostica* (without commentary)

Hippocrates, *De morbis acutis* (without commentary and excluding book IV)

Avicenna, *De viribus cordis* (to "postquam locuti sumus")

SECOND LECTURE

Galen, *De accidenti et morbo*

Galen, *De crisi*

Galen, *De diebus criticis*

Galen, *De febribus ad Glauconem*, I

Galen, *De tabe*

Galen, *De utilitate respirationis*

AFTERNOON   FIRST LECTURE

Avicenna, *Canon* (as in morning of first year)

SECOND LECTURE

Galen, *De differentiis febrium*

Avicenna, *Canon*, IV, fen 2

Galen, *De mala complexione*

Galen, *De simplicibus medicinis* (excluding book VI)

Galen, *De diebus criticis*, I

Third Year

MORNING   FIRST LECTURE

Hippocrates, *Aphorismata* (excluding part 7)

SECOND LECTURE

Galen, *Therapeutica*, VII-XII

Averroës, *Colliget*, proemium; I, 2; II; V (up to section on simple medicines and from last section to end)

Galen, *De virtutibus naturalibus*, I (to chapter 7); III

Galen, *De diebus criticis*, II

AFTERNOON   FIRST LECTURE

As in morning of second year, first lecture

SECOND LECTURE

Galen, *De accidenti et morbo*

Galen, *De crisi*

Galen, *De diebus criticis*, III
Galen, *De complexionibus*
Galen, *De febribus ad Glauconem*, I

Fourth Year

MORNING
    FIRST LECTURE
    Avicenna, *Canon* (as in morning lecture of first year)
    SECOND LECTURE
    Avicenna, *Canon*, IV, fen 1 (on fevers); II, canones
    Galen, *De interioribus* (excluding book II)
    Galen, *Regimen sanitatis*
    Hippocrates, *De natura*

AFTERNOON
    FIRST LECTURE
    Hippocrates, *Aphorismata* (excluding part 7)
    SECOND LECTURE
    Galen, *Therapeutica*, VII-XII
    Averroës, *Colliget* (as in morning of third year)
    Galen, *De virtutibus naturalibus*, I, 1-12; III

PRACTICAL MEDICINE[3]
(All classes held in the evening)

First Year

Avicenna, *Canon*, III, 1-3 (on the anatomy, physiology, and diseases of the brain and eye; excluding the ears, nose, mouth, tongue, teeth, and gums)

Second Year

Avicenna, *Canon*, III, 9-12 (throat, chest and lungs, heart, breasts)

Third Year

Avicenna, *Canon*, III, 13-16 (stomach, liver, spleen, intestines)

[3] University of Medicine and Arts of Bologna: statute of 1405, 78; in Malagola, *Statuti*, 276-77.

Fourth Year

Avicenna, *Canon*, III, 18-21 (kidneys, bladder, genitals—including conception and birth; omit anus, extremities)
Other sections of *Canon*, III, to be read in a second lecture or otherwise, at the discretion of the rector of the university.

SURGERY[4]
(All classes held in the afternoon)

FIRST LECTURE	SECOND LECTURE
Bruno da Longoburgo, *Chirurgia*	Avicenna, *Chirurgia* (apostemata,
Galen, *Chirurgia*	fractures and dislocations,
	wounds, bruises, ulcers)[5]
	Rhazes, *Ad Almansorem*, VII

Surgery lectures were given on a one-year cycle, and the same readings were repeated from year to year.

[4] Ibid., 35; in Malagola, *Statuti*, 247-48.

[5] Avicenna, *Canon*, IV, 3-6, was known as Avicenna's *Chirurgia* in this period.

APPENDIX III
Doctors in the *Catasto* of 1427

Name[a]	Type of Doctor	Age[b]	"Mouths"[c]	Value of Books (fl.)	Wealth (fl.)[d]		Composition[e]
					Raw	Net	
1. M° Agnolo di Cristofano dal contado di Arezzo	hospital doctor	44	8	25	742	401	s. 10
2. M° Antonio di Giovanni da Norcia	hernia doctor	60	10	—	1,668	1,304	exempt
3. M° Luca di m° Antonio	hernia doctor	30					
4. M° Bartolomeo di m° Antonio	hernia doctor	28					
5. M° Giovanni di m° Antonio	hernia doctor	24					
6. M° Antonio di m° Guccio da Scarperia	physician	75	6	50	5,339	4,675	
7. M° Bandino di m° Giovanni Banducci	physician	45	4	100	441	441	fl. 1
8. M° Bartolomeo di Cambio	physician	53	5	60	2,111	1,832	
9. M° Benedetto di Francesco	shoemaker and eye doctor	52	3	—	147	0	s. 4
10. M° Domenico d'Agnolo Accennati da Montegonzio	surgeon	85	3	—	150	61	s. 3
11. M° Domenico di m° Giovanni	bone doctor and physician	48	4	49	923	667	fl. 1
12. M° Domenico di Piero	physician?	67	8	160	8,927	8,737	
13. M° Piero di m° Domenico	physician	31					

APPENDIX III (cont'd.)

Name[a]	Type of Doctor	Age[b]	"Months"[c]	Value of Books (fl.)	Wealth (fl.)[d]		Composition[e]
					Raw	Net	
14. M° Paolo di m° Domenico	physician	30					
15. M° Francesco di ser Conte Mini	surgeon	67	5	—	277	216	s. 5
16. M° Francesco di Giovanni da Norcia	hernia doctor	48	6	—	599	571	exempt
17. M° Galileo di Giovanni Galilei	physician	57	9	30	4,816	4,454	
18. M° Giorgio di Niccolò da Arencio di Mugello	surgeon?	67	1	—	73	19	s. 3
19. M° Giovanni di m° Antonio Chellini da San Miniato	physician	ca.50	4	20	9,448	7,613	
20. M° Giovanni di ser Bartolo da Radda	surgeon	70	3	—	4,852	4,819	
21. M° Giovanni di Bartolomeo da Montecatini	physician	50	4	—	45	−102	s. 4
22. M° Giovanni di m° Piero da Norcia	surgeon	60	3	—	23	18	s. 4
23. M° Guasparre di ser Matteo da Radda (dependant of brother)	physician	34	7	30	1,176	954	fl. 1 s. 10
24. M° Iacopo di m° Antonio da Montecatini	physician	?	1	—	164	104	s. 5

25. M° Iacopo di ser Antonio da Poppi	physician?	47	5	16	416	374	s. 10
26. M° Iacopo di Martino da Spoleto	physician	57	1	30	254	254	
27. M° Lionardo di m° Agnolo da Bibbiena	physician	54	1	24	7,795	5,142	
28. M° Lorenzo d'Agnolo Sassoli da Prato	physician	51	15	150	6,404	6,119	
29. M° Niccolò di ser Niccolò Leonardi[f]	physician				5,500	5,500	
30. M° Piero di Feo dal Pozzo di Arezzo[g]	surgeon	65	2	10 (pawned)	70	50	
31. M° Ridolfo di Francesco da Cortona	physician	31	2	80	936	530	
32. M° Rinieri di m° Lionardo	physician	ca.70	7	20	883	577	s. 13 d. 4
33. M° Salvadore di m° Niccolò da Catania di Sicilia	empiric	42	5	—	47	–45	s. 3
34. M° Simone di Pacino da San Martino[g]	dentist/ herbalist	45	4	—	101	101	s. 19 d. 1
35. M° Stefano di m° Lodovico, called Scappuccino	poultice doctor	40	2	—	758	491	
36. M° Taddeo di Cambino di Giovanni Ghini	surgeon?	27	3	—	390	244	s. 4
37. M° Tommaso di Baccio da Arezzo	physician	60	8	25	3,786	2,359	

APPENDIX III (cont'd.)

NOTE: This table includes doctors appearing in the city *catasto* of 1427 and those resident just outside the city in parishes with boundaries that extended outside the gates, from the *catasto* for the countryside of 1429. (Unless noted, doctors are from the city *catasto*.) Sources for city doctors are Catasto-17 to 62 (for individual declarations or *portate*) and Catasto-65 to 83 and Catasto-Campioni del Monte-S. Giovanni-1427 (for official summaries or *campioni*). The *contado* references come from Catasto-88 (*portate*) and Catasto-307 (*campioni*).

a For the form of Italian names in this period see Appendix I.

b Declarations of age are not always reliable in the *catasto* and other early sources; see Herlihy and Klapisch-Zuber, *Les toscans*, 353-70.

c This figure represents the number of people in the household, including the declarer but excluding salaried servants.

d On the distinction between raw and net wealth, see discussion of the *catasto* in Appendix I.

e An exemption of fl. 200 was given for each "mouth." If the total of exemptions and debts exceeded the household's assets, a "composition" or agreement was made between the declarer and the tax officials as to a fair payment. Such payments probably give a good idea of the relative wealth of these households.

f M° Niccolò was permanently resident in Venice and had no property in Florence except for fl. 5,500 invested in the *Monte*; see his declaration in Catasto-55, fol. 517.

g M° Piero and M° Simone were residents of the section of the parish of S. Frediano which lay outside the city walls. As such they were counted in the *catasto* of the countryside (for S. Spirito) and assessed at a different rate from inhabitants of the city.

APPENDIX IV

Index to Doctors' Letters

A. LETTERS OF Mᵒ NADDINO DI ALDOBRANDINO DA PRATO TO
MONTE D'ANDREA ANGIOLINI AND FRANCESCO DI MARCO
DATINI DA PRATO

*ASP: Archivio Datini, Carteggio privato-1091*₂

FROM PRATO
1. 9.vi.1385, to F.
2. 15.v.1386, to F.

FROM PAVIA
3. 8.x.1386, to F.
4. 8.x.1386, to M.

FROM AVIGNON
5. 26.x.1386, to M.
6. 20.xii.1386, to M.
7. 7.i.1386/7, to F.
8. 7.i.1386/7, to M.
9. 21.i.1386/7, to M.
10. 11.iv.1387, to F.
11. 11.iv.1387, to M.
12. 30.v.1387, to M.
13. ?.vii.1387, to M.
14. 21.xi.1387, to M.
15. 3.iv.1388, to M.
16. 16.iv.1388, to M.
17. 18.iv.1388, to F.
18. 6.v.1388, to M.
19. 5.ix.1388, to M.
20. 29.i.1388/9, to M.
21. 4.iii.1388/9, to M.

22. 21.iii.1388/9, to F.
23. 21.iii.1388/9, to M.
24. 30.iv.1389, to M.

FROM PRATO
25. 18.vii.1389, to F.

FROM PISA
26. 20.x.1389, to F.

FROM GENOA
27. 13.iv.1390, to F.
28. 16.iv.1390, to F.

FROM AVIGNON
29. 18.iii.1391/2, to F.
30. 19.ix.1392, to F.
31. 29.ix.1392, to F.
32. 2.i.1392/3, to F.
33. 1.v.1393, to F.
34. 27.vii.1393, to F.
35. 28.x.1394, to F.
36. 6.xi.1394, to F.
37. 11.ii.1394/5, to F.
38. 15.viii.1395, to F.
39. received 20.ix.1395, to F.
40. 31.ix.1396, to F.

ASP: Archivio Datini, Carteggi privati diversi-cartella A

41. 9.ii.1407, to F.   42. 26.viii.1407, to F.

B. Letters of Mᵒ Lorenzo d'Agnolo Sassoli da Prato to Francesco di Marco Datini da Prato

ASP: Archivio Datini, Carteggio privato-1102 (Busta)

FROM BOLOGNA
1. 2.ix.1400, to Matteo di Matteo Toffi

FROM PADUA
2. 8.ii.1400/1 (Mazzei, 2:362-63)[1]
3. 26.ii.1400/1
4. 5.iii.[1400/1]
5. 28.iii.1401
6. 18.iv.1401
7. 1.iv.1401 (Mazzei, 2:363-64)
8. 8.viii.1401
9. 12.xi.1401
10. 27.x.1401
11. 15.xi.1401
12. 5.xii.[1401]
13. 12.ii.1401/2
14. 8.vi.1402 (Mazzei, 2, 365-66)
15. 3.viii.1402
16. 30.viii.1402 (Mazzei, 2:366-67)
17. 7.ix.1402
18. 18.ix.1402
19. 7.x.1402
20. 10.x.1402
21. 15.x.1402 (Mazzei, 2:367-68)

FROM FERRARA
22. 25.x.1402
23. 24.xi.1402

24. 10.i.1402/3
25. 7.ii.1402/3
26. 20.vii.1403
27. 2.viii.1403

FROM VENICE
28. 10.ix.1403
29. 28.x.1403
30. 8.xii.1403
31. 15.xii.1403 (Mazzei, 2:369)
32. 20.i.1403/4
33. 15.iii.1403/4

FROM PRATO
34. 16.v.1404 (Mazzei, 2, 370)
35. 28.v.1404
36. 2.vi.1404 (Mazzei, 2:374-75)
37. 6.vi.1404
38. 13.vi.1404
39. 19.vi.1404
40. 25.vi.1404
41. 1.vii. 1404
42. 12.vii.1404
43. 4.viii.1404 (Mazzei, 2:375-76)
44. 18.viii.1404
45. 27.viii.1404
46. 20.ix.1404
47. 22.ix.1404
48. 18.x.1404
49. 27.x.1404
50. 4.xi.1404
51. 4.xi.1404

52. 6.xi.1404
53. 12.xi.1404 (Mazzei, 2:376)
54. 19.xi.1404
55. 25.xi.1404

FROM FLORENCE
56. 3.vi.[1405?]
57. 3.viii.1406

FROM PRATO
58. 8.xii.1406

FROM FLORENCE
59. 14.vi.1407 (Mazzei, 2:377)
60. 12.i.1407/8 (Mazzei, 2:378)
61. 30.i.1407/8

62. 2.iii.1407/8
63. 13.iii.1407/8
64. 31.iii.1408
65. 18.iv.1408 (Mazzei, 2:378-79)
66. 24.iv.1408
67. 14.xi.1408
68. 24.viii.?

PRESCRIPTIONS FOR FRANCESCO
1. Olio d'ameto
2. Pillole a sordità, 1404
3. Pillole a sordità
4. Reggimento, 13.iii.[1404?] (Mazzei, 2:370-74)

C. LETTERS TO AND FROM ANTONIO DI M° MARCO DI M° ANTONIO DA PISTOIA

ASPist: Collectio rerum antiquarum, Documenti vari-15 and 22

ANTONIO TO M° MARCO
1. Montale, 14.xi.1457 (15, no. 102)
2. Prato, 27.vii.1458 (22, no. 219)
3. Prato, 30.vii.1458 (22, no. 224)
4. Prato, 15.viii.1458 (22, no. 225)
5. Florence, 21.x.1458 (22, no. 229)
6. Florence, ?.[xii].1458 (22, no. 230)
7. Florence, [xii?.1459] (22, no. 244)
8. Florence, 22.xi.[1459] (22, no. 242)

M° MARCO TO ANTONIO (FROM PISTOIA)
1. 29.vii.1458 (22, no. 303)
2. 12.viii.1458 (22, no. 304)

3. 27.[viii or ix.1458] (22, no. 305)
4. 3.ix.1458 (22, no. 306)
5. 26.ix.1458 (22, no. 305bis)
6. 7.x.1458 (22, no. 307)
7. 12.x.1458 (22, no. 308)
8. 21.x.1458 (22, no. 310)
9. 24.xi.[1458] (22, no. 309)
10. 15.xii.1458 (22, no. 311)
11. 22.xii.1458 (22, no. 312)
12. 28.xii.1458 (22, no. 313)
13. 2.i.1459 (22, no. 314)
14. ?.i.1459 (22, no. 315)
15. 19.i.1459 (22, no. 316)
16. 3.ii.1459 (22, no. 317)
17. 19.ii.1459 (22, no. 318)
18. 1.iii.1459 (22, no. 319)
19. 4.iv.1459 (22, no. 320)
20. 8.v.1459 (22, no. 321)
21. 15.iii or v.[1459] (22, no. 341)

22. 17.iii or v.[1459] (22, no. 302)
23. 9.vii.1459 (22, no. 322)
24. 18.vii.1459 (22, no. 323)
25. 12.viii.1459 (22, no. 324)
26. 1.xi.1459 (22, no. 325)
27. 19.xi.1459 (22, no. 326)
28. 27.xi.1459 (22, no. 327)
29. 13.xii.1459 (22, no. 328)
30. 11.i.1460 (22, no. 328bis)
31. 24.iii.1460 (22, no. 330)
32. 27.iii.1460 (22, no. 331)
33. 31.iii.1460 (22, no. 332)
34. 12.iv.1460 (22, no. 333)
35. 24.iv.1460 (22, no. 334)
36. 1.v.1460 (22, no. 335)
37. 9.vi.1460 (22, no. 336)
38. 17.vi.1460 (22, no. 337)
39. 2.vii.1460 (22, no. 338)
40. 6.vii.1460 (22, no. 329)
41. 11.vii.1460 (22, no. 339)
42. 19.vii.1460 (22, no. 340)

Mº BARTOLOMEO DI Mº
ANTONIO, ANTONIO'S UNCLE,
TO ANTONIO (FROM PISTOIA)
1. 8.[vi?].1459 (15, no. 107)

2. 1.vii.[1459] (15, no. 105)
3. 23.i.1460 (22, no. 343)
4. 1.ii.1460 (15, no. 106)
5. 27. iv. 1460 (15, no. 112)

MONNA LUCIA, ANTONIO'S
MOTHER, TO ANTONIO (FROM
PISTOIA)
1. 1.iii.1459 (15, no. 108)
2. 20.v.1459 (15, no. 109)
3. n.d. (15, no. 110)

BENEDETTO COLUCCIO, FAMILY
FRIEND, TO ANTONIO (FROM
PISTOIA)
1. 1.vi.1459 (15, no. 111)

TALENTO DI SIMONE LAINI,
ANTONIO'S FRIEND, TO
ANTONIO (FROM PISTOIA)
1. 27.viii.1458 (22, no. 270)
2. 7.xi.1459 (22, no. 271)
3. 14.xi.1459 (22, no. 272)
4. 19.xi.1459 (22, no. 273)
5. 23.xi.[1459] (22, no. 274)
6. 2.i.1460 (22, no. 276)
7. 17.?.? (22, no. 275)

[1] References to the letters of Mº Lorenzo as edited in Mazzei, *Lettere*.

Bibliography

ARCHIVAL AND MANUSCRIPT SOURCES

Florence: Archivio di Stato di Firenze (ASF)

Archivi della repubblica
   Capitoli
   Consulte e pratiche (CP)
   Libri fabarum (LF)
   Miscellanea repubblicana
   Otto di guardia (OG)
   Provvisioni-Registri (PR)
   Statuti del comune di Firenze (Statuti)
   Tratte
Archivio Galilei
Arti
   Arte dei medici e speziali (AMS)
   Arte della lana (Lana)
   Arte della seta (Seta)
Atti del podestà
Camerlinghi della camera del comune-Uscita (CCCU)
Carte Del Bene
Carte Strozziane
Catasto
Compagnie religiose soppresse
Compagnie religiose soppresse, Capitoli
Conventi soppressi (CS)
Diplomatico
Estimo
Medici avanti il principato (MAP)
Mercanzia
Monte comune (Monte)

Notarile antecosimiano (Notarile)
Prestanze
Pupilli
Spedale di Messer Bonifazio
Spedale di Santa Maria Nuova (SMN)
Uffiziali di sanità

Florence: Biblioteca Medicea Laurentiana (BLF)

Ashburnham 644: Benedetto Dei, *Memorie.*
Ashburnham 970: Statuto della compagnia di San Lorenzo in Piano.
Gadd. 74, fols. 97-101: Giovanni Baldi da Faenza, *De temporibus partus*; fols. 102-5: idem, *Disputatio an medicina sit legibus politicis praeferenda.*
Laur. 19, 30, fols. 1-30: Giovanni Baldi, *Utrum naturalis phylosophya, ut aliqua gentilium scientia* . . . ; fols. 30-31: idem, ed., *Extirpatio ire*; fols. 31-38: idem, Consolation for the Count of Montegarneli; fols. 38-44: idem, *De temporibus partus*; fols. 44-45: idem, *De electione medici.*
Laur. 39, 40, fols. 50-51: Ugolino Verino, epigraph on Paolo Toscanelli.
Laur. 77, 22, fols. 5-27: Giovanni da Arezzo, *De medicinae et legum praestantia.*

Florence: Biblioteca Nazionale di Firenze (BNF)

Banco rari 30: Paolo Toscanelli, notebook of mathematical, geographical, and astronomical fragments.
Conventi soppressi C.4.895: Priorista of Pietro Pietribuoni.
MS II, I, 138: Notizie e memorie della compagnia di S. Maria della Croce al Tempio di Firenze.
Pal. 811, fols. 1-25: Iacopo da Prato, *Liber in medicina de operatione manuali*; fol. 26: *Responsio ad quandam lecteram quam misit michi Magister Nerius de Senis* . . . ; fol. 27: *Quae complexio humana sit longioris vite.*

Florence: Biblioteca Riccardiana (BR)

Ricc. 1853: Benedetto Dei, *Memorie.*
Ricc. 2153, fols. 61-101: Antonio di maestro Guccio da Scarperia, *De signis febrium.*
Ricc. 2353: Statuto della compagnia della Vergine Maria delle Laudesi di Santa Croce.

London: Wellcome Institute for the History of Medicine

Wellcome MS. 375, fols. 1-73: Iacopo da Prato, *De operatione manuali*.

Wellcome MS. 540, fols. 151-76: Iacopo da Prato, *De operatione manuali*.

Lucca: Archivio di Stato di Lucca (ASL)

Ospedale di San Luca-180: Ricordi di Maestro Iacopo di Coluccino Bonavia.

Milan: Università Bocconi, Istituto di storia economica

Cod. 2 (new numeration), fols. 1-201: Ricordi di Giovanni di maestro Antonio Chellini da San Miniato.

Pistoia: Archivio di Stato di Pistoia (ASPist)

Archivio del comune di Pistoia (Collectio rerum antiquarum).
Ricordi di Maestro Polidoro d'Antonio Bracali (uninventoried: Sala C, 2° piano, scaff. 238-39, filza 2a, no. 18).

Prato: Archivio di Stato di Prato (ASP)

Archivio Datini-Carteggio privato (Datini CP).

Vatican City: Biblioteca Apostolica Vaticana (BVA)

Chigiano L.VII.262, no. 23: Tommaso Del Garbo, letter to Francesco Petrarca (not consulted).
Pal. lat. 1131, fols. 1-168: Lodovico di Bartolo da Gubbio, Commentary on Avicenna, *Canon*, IV, 3.
Pal. lat. 1260, fols. 35-36, 77-79, 88-89: Tommaso Del Garbo, *consilia*.
Pal. lat. 1265, fols. 13-21: Antonio di maestro Guccio da Scarperia, *De signis febrium*.
Pal. lat. 1284, fol. 121: Tommaso Del Garbo, *recepta*.
Pal. lat. 1295, fols. 118, 156: Tommaso Del Garbo, *receptae*.
Vat. lat. 2484, fols. 195-96: Tomaso Del Garbo, *Utrum sanitas membri consimilis* . . . ; fols. 211-12: *An fetus in octavo mense sit vitalis*; fols. 212-14: *Verbum cedidit inter querentes scientia quid est*.
Vat. lat. 3144, fol. 11: Tommaso Del Garbo, *Utrum solutio continuitatis sit per se* . . . ; fols. 15-16: *An per solam digestionem materie putride*. . . .

Vat. lat. 4440, fols. 90-107: Antonio di maestro Guccio da Scarperia, *Summa de causis et curis febrium*.

Vat. lat. 4445, fols. 66-90: Antonio di maestro Guccio da Scarperia, *Questio de contraoperantiis*; fol. 242: Tommaso Del Garbo, *Utrum solutio continuitatis sit per se*. . . .

Vat. lat. 4446, fols. 147-49: Tommaso Del Garbo, *Utrum solutio continuitatis sit per se*. . . .

Vat. lat. 4447, fols. 2-24: Antonio di maestro Guccio da Scarperia, *Questio de contraoperantiis*; fols. 25-32: *Questio utrum digestio et evacuatio que fiunt in morbo* . . . ; fols. 33-98: Commentary on Hippocrates, *Prognostics*; fols. 99-157: Commentary on Hippocrates, *De regimine acutorum*; fols. 257-94: Thirty-three questions on natural philosophy and medicine.

Vat. lat. 4448: Antonio di maestro Guccio da Scarperia, Commentary on Galen, *Tegni*.

PRIMARY SOURCES

Note: Names with the prefixes de, del, della, etc. are listed under the principal element.

Alberti, Leon Battista. *The Albertis of Florence: Leon Battista Alberti's Della famiglia*. Tr. Guido A. Guarino. Lewisburg, Pa., 1971.

———. *I libri della famiglia*. Ed. Girolamo Mancini. Florence, 1908.

Badia, Iodoco del, ed. *Miscellanea fiorentina*. 2 vols. Florence, 1902.

Baldasseroni, F., and G. Degli Azzi. "Consiglio medico di Maestr'Ugolino da Montecatini ad Averardo de' Medici." *ASI*, ser. 5, 38(1906): 140-52.

Benivieni, Antonio. *De abditis nonnullis ac mirandis morborum et sanationum causis*. Tr. Charles Singer. Springfield, Ill., 1954.

———. Unpublished sections of *De abditis*. In A. Costa and G. Weber, *L'inizio dell'anatomia patologica nel Quattrocento fiorentino, sui testi di Antonio Benivieni, Bernardo Torni, Leonardo da Vinci*. Florence, 1952.

[Bernardi, Ruberto di Guido.] *Una curiosa raccolta di segreti e di pratiche superstiziose fatta da un popolano fiorentino del secolo XIV*. Ed. Giovanni Giannini. Città di Castello, 1898.

Bernardino da Siena. *Le prediche volgari*. Ed. Piero Bargellini. Milan/Rome, 1936.

Boccaccio, Giovanni. *Decameron, Filocolo, Ameto, Fiammetta*. Ed. Enrico Bianchi, Carlo Salinari, and Natalino Sapegno. Milan/Naples, 1952.

Bracciolini, Poggio. See also Gordan.

―――. *Opera omnia*. 4 vols. Basel, 1538; repr. Turin, 1964-69.

Caggese, Romolo, ed. *Statuti della repubblica fiorentina*. 2 vols. Florence, 1910-21.

Cambi, Giovanni. *Istorie*. Ed. Ildefonso di San Luigi. In *Delizie*, vols. 20-21.

I capitoli del comune di Firenze. Ed. Cesare Guasti and A. Gherardi. 2 vols. Florence, 1866-93.

Cavalcanti, Giovanni. *Istorie fiorentine*. 2 vols. Florence, 1838-39.

Chiappelli, Alberto, ed. "Gli ordinamenti sanitari del comune di Pistoia contro la pestilenza del 1348." *ASI*, ser. 4, 20(1887): 3-24.

Ciasca, Raffaele, ed. *Statuti dell'arte dei medici e speziali*. Florence, 1922.

Cusanus, Nicolaus. *Die mathematischen Schriften*. Ed. Joseph Ehrenreich Hofmann. Tr. Josepha Hofmann. Hamburg, 1952.

Dallari, Umberto, ed. *I rotuli dei lettori legisti e artisti dello studio bolognese dal 1384 al 1799*. 4 vols. Bologna, 1888-1924.

Dati, Gregorio. *L'istoria di Firenze . . . dal 1380 al 1405*. Ed. Luigi Pratesi. Norcia, 1902.

Delizie degli eruditi toscani. Ed. Ildefonso di San Luigi. 24 vols. in 25. Florence, 1770-89.

Dominici, Giovanni. *Regola del governo di cura familiare*. Florence, 1926.

Falcucci, Niccolò. *Consilium contra pestilentiam*. In Karl Sudhoff, "Pestschriften aus den ersten 150 Jahren nach der Epidemie des 'Schwarzen Todes' 1348, IV: Italienische des 14. Jahrhunderts." *Archiv für Geschichte der Medizin* 5(1912): 367-84.

―――. *Sermones medicinales*. 4 vols. Venice, 1490-91.

Ficino, Marsilio. See Kristeller.

Francesco da Conegliano. *Consilium contra pestilentiam*. In Karl Sudhoff, "Pestschriften aus den ersten 150 Jahren nach der Epidemie des 'Schwarzen Todes' 1348, IV: Italienische des 14. Jahrhunderts." *Archiv für Geschichte der Medizin* 5(1912): 354-67.

Garbo, Tommaso Del. *Consiglio contro a pistolenza*. Ed. Pietro Ferrato. Bologna, 1866.

―――. *De generatione embryonis*. In Iacopo da Forlì et al., *Expositio de generatione foetus*, fols. 33-45. Venice, 1502.

―――. *In libros de differentiis febrium Galeni commentum*. Venice, 1521.

―――. *Summa medicinalis, De reductione medicinarum ad actum, De gradibus medicinarum, De restauratione humidi radicalis*. Lyon, 1529.

Garin, Eugenio, ed. *La disputà delle arti nel Quattrocento: testi editi ed inediti di Giovanni Baldi, Leonardo Bruni, Poggio Bracciolini, Giovanni d'Arezzo, Bernardo Ilicino, Niccoletto Vernia, Antonio de' Ferrariis detto il Galateo*. Florence, 1947.

Gherardi, Alessandro, ed. *Statuti della università e studio fiorentino dal anno 1387, seguiti da un'appendice di documenti dal 1320 al 1472.* Florence, 1881.

Gherardi, Giovanni, da Prato. *Il paradiso degli Alberti.* Ed. Alessandro Wesselofsky. 3 vols. Bologna, 1867.

Gloria, Andrea, ed. *Monumenti della università di Padova (1318-1415).* 2 vols. Padua, 1888.

Gordan, Phyllis Walter Goodhart, tr. *Two Renaissance Book Hunters: The Letters of Poggius Bracciolini to Nicolaus de Niccolis.* New York/London, 1974.

Guasti, Cesare, ed. *Commissioni di Rinaldo degli Albizzi per il comune di Firenze dal 1399 al 1433.* 3 vols. Florence, 1893.

––––––. *Intorno alla vita e all'insegnamento di Vittorino da Feltre: lettere di Sassolo Pratese.* Florence, 1869.

Kristeller, Paul Oskar. *Supplementum ficinianum.* 2 vols. Florence, 1937.

Landino, Cristoforo. *Scritti critici et teorici.* Ed. Roberto Cardini. 2 vols. Rome, 1974.

Landucci, Luca. *Diario fiorentino dal 1450 al 1516.* Ed. Iodoco del Badia. Florence, 1883.

Il libro di Montaperti. Ed. Cesare Paoli. Florence, 1889.

Il libro di ricordanze dei Corsini (1362-1457). Ed. Armando Petrucci. Rome, 1965.

Malagola, Carlo, ed. *Statuti delle università e dei collegi dello studio bolognese.* Bologna, 1888.

Manetti, Antonio di Tuccio. *The Life of Brunelleschi.* Ed. Howard Saalman. Tr. Catherine Enggass. London, 1970.

Marri, Giulia Camerani, ed. *Statuti delle arti dei correggiai, tavolacciai e scudai, dei vaiai e pellicciai (1338-1386).* Florence, 1960.

Mazzei, Lapo. *Lettere di un notaro a un mercante del secolo XIV.* Ed. Cesare Guasti. 2 vols. Florence, 1880.

Morandini, Francesca, ed. *Statuti dell'arte dei legnaioli di Firenze (1301-1346).* Florence, 1958.

Morelli, Giovanni di Pagolo. *Ricordi.* Ed. Vittore Branca. Florence, 1956.

Müller, Johannes, von Königsberg. See Regiomontanus.

Novae academiae florentinae opuscula. Venice, 1553.

Nuovo receptario composto dal famosissimo Chollegio degli eximii doctori della arte e medicina della inclita ciptà di Firenze. Florence, 1499.

Paolo di ser Pace da Certaldo. *Libro di buoni costumi.* Ed. Alfredo Schiaffini. Florence, 1945.

Petrarca, Francesco. *Le familiari.* Ed. Vittorio Rossi. 4 vols. Florence, 1933-42.

————. *Invective contra medicum: testo latino e volgarizzamento di Ser Domenico Silvestri*. Ed. Pier Giorgio Ricci. Rome, 1950.

————. *Lettere delle cose familiari*. Tr. Giuseppe Fracassetti. 5 vols. Florence, 1863-67.

————. *Lettere senili*. Tr. Giuseppe Fracassetti. 2 vols. Florence, 1869-70.

Pico della Mirandola, Giovanni. *Disputationes adversus astrologiam divinatricem*. Ed. Eugenio Garin. 2 vols. Florence, 1946-52.

Regiomontanus, Joannes. *De triangulis*. Nuremberg, 1533.

Salutati, Coluccio. *De nobilitate legum et medicinae e De verecundia*. Ed. Eugenio Garin. Florence, 1947.

————. *Epistolario*. Ed. Francesco Novati. 4 vols. Rome, 1891-1911.

Sassolo da Prato. See Guasti.

Sozomeno da Pistoia. *Chronicon universale (1411-1455)*. Ed. Guido Zaccagnini. In *RIS* 16/1.

Statuta dominorum artistarum achademiae patavinae. Padua, [ca. 1520].

Statuta populi et communis Florentiae publica auctoritate collecta, castigata et praeposita anno salutis MCCCCXV. 3 vols. Freiburg, 1778-83.

Statuti e ordinamenti della università di Pavia dall'anno 1361 all'anno 1859. Pavia, 1925.

Stefani, Marchionne di Coppo. *Cronaca fiorentina*. Ed. Niccolò Rodolico. In *RIS* 30/1.

Traversari, Ambrogio. *Latinae epistolae*. Ed. Lorenzo Mehus. 2 vols. Florence, 1759.

Ugolino da Montecatini. See also Baldasseroni.

————. *Tractatus de balneis*. Ed. and tr. Michele Giuseppe Nardi. Florence, 1950.

Vergerio, Pier Paolo. *Epistolario*. Ed. Leonardo Smith. Rome, 1934.

Vespasiano da Bisticci. *Vite di uomini illustri del secolo XV*. Ed. Aulo Greco. 2 vols. Florence, 1970-76.

Villani, Filippo. *Le vite d'uomini illustri fiorentini*. 2d ed. Ed. Giammaria Mazzuchelli. Florence, 1826.

Villani, Giovanni. *Cronica*. Ed. Francesco Gherardi Dragomanni. 4 vols. Milan, 1848.

Villani, Matteo. *Cronica*. Ed. Francesco Gherardi Dragomanni. 2 vols. Florence, 1846.

Zerbi, Gabriele. *De cautelis medicorum*. Tr. Clodomiro Mancini. In Mancini, *Un codice deontologico del secolo XV*. Scientia veterum, 44. Pisa, 1963.

————. *Opus perutile de cautelis medicorum*. In Pantaleone de Confluentia, *Pillularium omnibus medicis quamnecessarium*. Lyon, 1528.

Zonta, Gasparo, and Giovanni Brotto, eds. *Acta graduum academicorum gymnasii patavini, 1406-1450*. 2d ed. 3 vols. Padua, 1970.

SECONDARY STUDIES

Note: Names with the prefixes de, del, della, etc. are listed under the principal element.

Abbondanza, Roberto. "Gli atti degli ufficiali dello studio fiorentino dal maggio al settembre 1388." *ASI* 117(1959): 80-110.

Addario, Arnaldo d'. *Aspetti della contrariforma in Firenze*. Rome, 1972.

Agrimi, Jole, and Chiara Crisciani. "Medici e 'vetulae' dal Dugento al Quattrocento: problemi di una ricerca." In Paolo Rossi et al., *Cultura popolare e cultura dotta nel Seicento*, 144-59. Milan, 1983.

Amundsen, Darrel W. "Medical Deontology and Pestilential Disease in the Late Middle Ages." *JHM* 32(1977): 403-21.

———. "Medieval Canon Law on Medical and Surgical Practice by the Clergy." *BHM* 52(1978): 22-44.

Amundsen, Darrel W., and Gary B. Ferngren. "The Forensic Role of Physicians in Roman Law." *BHM* 53(1979): 39-56.

Antonioli, R. *Rabelais et la médecine*. Geneva, 1976.

Ariès, Philippe. *Centuries of Childhood*. Tr. Robert Baldick. London, 1962.

Baader, Gerhard. "Die Bibliothek des Giovanni Marco da Rimini: eine Quelle zur medizinischen Bildung im Humanismus." In Kurt Treu et al., eds., *Studia codicologica*, 43-97. Berlin, 1977.

Baccini, Giovanni. "Maestro Antonio di Guccio da Scarperia." *Giotto: bollettino storico, letterario, artistico del Mugello* 2(1903): 339-416, 441-42.

Bagrow, Leo. *History of Cartography*. Tr. D. L. Paisley. Revised and enlarged by R. A. Skelton. Cambridge, Mass., 1966.

Barbadoro, Bernardino. "Finanza e demografia nei ruoli d'imposta del 1352-55." In Corrado Gini, ed., *Atti del congresso internazionale per gli studi sulla popolazione*, 10 vols., 9:614-45. Rome, 1933-34.

Barduzzi, Domenico. *Ugolino da Montecatini*. Florence, 1915.

Bargellini, Piero. *Scoperta di palazzo vecchio*. Florence, 1968.

Baron, Hans. *The Crisis of the Early Italian Renaissance*. 2d ed. Princeton, 1966.

———. *Humanistic and Political Literature in Florence and Venice at the Beginning of the Quattrocento*. Cambridge, Mass., 1955.

Battisti, Eugenio. *Filippo Brunelleschi: The Complete Work*. Tr. Robert Erich Wolf. New York, 1981.

Battistini, Mario. "Contributo alla vita di Ugolino da Montecatini." *RSSMN* 14(1923): 125-47.

――――. "Giovanni Chellini, medico di S. Miniato." *RSSMN* 18(1927): 106-17.

――――. *I medici e la medicina in Volterra nel medioevo*. Castelfiorentino, 1923.

Bec, Christian. *Les marchands écrivains: affaires et humanisme à Florence, 1375-1434*. Paris, 1967.

Becker, Marvin B. "Aspects of Lay Piety in Early Renaissance Florence." In Charles Trinkaus and Heiko A. Oberman, eds., *The Pursuit of Holiness in Late Medieval and Renaissance Religion*, 177-99. Leiden, 1974.

――――. "An Essay on the 'Novi Cives' and Florentine Politics, 1343-1382." *Mediaeval Studies*, 24(1962): 35-82.

――――. *Florence in Transition*. 2 vols. Baltimore, 1967-68.

――――. "Florentine 'Libertas': Political Independents and 'Novi Cives,' 1372-1378." *Traditio* 18(1962): 393-407.

――――. "Florentine Politics and the Diffusion of Heresy in the Trecento: A Socioeconomic Inquiry." *Speculum* 34(1959): 60-75.

Belloni, Luigi. *La medicina a Milano fino al Seicento*. In Fondazione Treccani degli Alfieri, *Storia di Milano*, 16 vols., 11:595-696. Milan, 1953-62.

Biadego, Giuseppe. "Medici veronesi e una libreria medica del secolo XIV." *Atti del Reale istituto veneto di scienze, lettere ed arti* 75(1915-16): 565-85.

Billanovich, M. C. Ganguzza. "Giacomo Zanetini (m. 1402), professore di medicina: il patrimonio, la biblioteca." *Quaderni per la storia dell'università di Padova* 5(1972): 1-44.

Biraben, Jean Noël. *Les hommes et la peste en France et dans les pays européens et méditerranéens*. 2 vols. Paris, 1975-76.

Björnbo, Axel Anthon. "Die mathematischen San Marco Handschriften in Florenz." *Bibliotheca mathematica*, ser. 3, 4(1903): 238-45; 6(1905): 230-38; 12(1911-12): 97-132, 193-224.

Bombe, Walter. "Hausinventar und Bibliothek Ugolinos da Montecatini." *Archiv für Geschichte der Medizin* 5(1912): 225-39.

Borsook, Eve. *The Mural Painters of Tuscany from Cimabue to Andrea del Sarto*. 2d ed. Oxford, 1980.

Bowsky, William M. "The Impact of the Black Death upon Sienese Government and Society." *Speculum* 39(1964): 1-34.

Brentano-Keller, Nelly. "Il libretto di spese e di ricordi di un monaco vallombrosano per libri dati o avuti in prestito." *La bibliofilia* 41(1939): 129-58.

Bresciano, Giovanni. "Inventarii inediti del secolo XV continenti libri a stampa e manoscritti." *Archivio storico per le province napoletane* 26(1901): 3-32.

Brown, Alison M. "The Humanist Portrait of Cosimo de' Medici, *Pater Patriae*." *Journal of the Warburg and Courtauld Institutes* 24(1961): 186-221.

Brucker, Gene. *The Civic World of Early Renaissance Florence*. Princeton, 1977.

———. "Florence and Its University, 1348-1434." In Theodore K. Rabb and Jerrold Seigel, eds., *Action and Conviction in Early Modern Europe*, 220-36. Princeton, 1969.

———. *Florentine Politics and Society, 1343-1378*. Princeton, 1962.

———. *Renaissance Florence*. London, 1969.

———, ed. *The Society of Renaissance Florence: A Documentary Study*. New York, 1971.

Brugaro, A. "Contributo alla storia dei medici pisani dal XII al XIV secolo." *Studi storici* 18(1909): 209-63.

Brun, Robert. "Quelques italiens d'Avignon au XIVᵉ siècle, II: Naddino de Prato, médecin de la cour pontificale." *Mélanges d'archéologie et d'histoire* 40(1923): 219-36.

Brunetti, Mario. "Venezia durante la peste del 1348." *Ateneo veneto* 32/1(1909): 289-311; 2:5-42.

Bullough, Vern L. *The Development of Medicine as a Profession: The Contribution of the Medieval University to Modern Medicine*. Basel/New York, 1966.

———. "Medieval Bologna and the Development of Medical Education." *BHM* 32(1958): 201-15.

———. "A Note on Medical Care in Medieval English Hospitals." *BHM* 35(1961): 74-77.

———. "Population and the Study and Practice of Medieval Medicine." *BHM* 36(1962): 62-69.

———. "Training of the Nonuniversity-Educated Medical Practitioners in the Later Middle Ages." *JHM* 14(1959): 446-58.

Bylebyl, Jerome J. "The School of Padua: Humanistic Medicine in the Sixteenth Century." In Charles Webster, ed., *Health, Medicine and Mortality in the Sixteenth Century*, 335-70. Cambridge, 1979.

Cagni, Giuseppe M. *Vespasiano da Bisticci e il suo epistolario*. Rome, 1969.

Calleri, Santi. *L'arte dei giudici e notai di Firenze nell'età comunale e nel suo statuto del 1344*. Milan, 1966.

Camagna, Anna. "L'organizzazione interna delle arti maggiori di Firenze." *ASI*, ser. 7, 18/2(1932): 165-203.

Campbell, Anna Montgomery. *The Black Death and Men of Learning.* New York, 1931.

Capanna, Gian Piero Della. *Studi sull'umanesimo e rinascimento medico: gli archiatri pontefici toscani dal secolo XIII al secolo XVI.* Scientia veterum, 123. Montecatini, 1968.

Capasso, R. "Baldi, Giovanni dei Tambeni." *Dizionario biografico degli italiani* 5:468-69. Rome, 1963.

Cappellini, Icilio. "Ancora di Maestro Tommaso Del Garbo: la data precisa della morte; la tomba." *RSSMN* 43(1952): 247-77.

―――. "Date importanti per la biografia di Maestro Tommaso Del Garbo e per gli inizi dell'insegnamento medico nello studio fiorentino desunte da codici del Fondo Vaticano latino." *RSSMN* 41(1950): 212-18.

―――. "I medici fiorentini alla battaglia di Montaperti (4 settembre, 1260)." *RSSMN* 41(1950): 15-50.

Carabellese, Francesco. "La compagnia di Orsanmichele e il mercato dei libri in Firenze nel secolo XIV." *ASI*, ser. 5, 16(1895): 267-73.

―――. *La peste del 1348 e le condizioni della sanità pubblica in Toscana.* Rocca San Casciano, 1897.

Carmichael, Ann Gayton. "Epidemic Diseases in Early Renaissance Florence." Ph.D. diss., Duke University, 1978.

Carpentier, Elisabeth. "Autour de la peste noire: famine et épidémies dans l'histoire du XIVᵉ siècle." *Annales* 17(1962): 1062-92.

―――. *Une ville devant la peste: Orvieto et la peste noire de 1348.* Paris, 1962.

Carr-Saunders, A. M., and P. A. Wilson. *The Professions.* Oxford, 1933.

Casanova, Eugenio. "L'astrologia e la consegna del bastone al capitano generale della repubblica fiorentina." *ASI*, ser. 5, 7(1891): 134-44.

Casarini, A. *Storia della medicina militare.* Milan/Rome, 1943.

Cassuto, Umberto. *Gli ebrei a Firenze nell'età del rinascimento.* Florence, 1918.

Castellani, Carlo. "Un capitolo di storia della medicina: medicazione delle ferite." *Castalia* 19(1963): 3-9.

Castiglioni, Arturo. "Ugo Benzi di Siena ed il 'Trattato utilissimo circa la conservazione della sanitade.'" *RSSMN* 12(1921): 75-102.

Ceccarelli, Ubaldo. *La tradizione medico-chirurgica lucchese.* Scientia veterum, 16. Pisa, 1961.

Ceccarelli, Ubaldo, and Ruggero Manara. "Il livello di cultura di quattro medici toscani desunto dalle loro ricche biblioteche di testi di medicina." *Atti XXI* 1:83-90.

Cecchetti, B. *Per la storia della medicina in Venezia: spigolature d'archivio*. Venice, 1886.

Chiappelli, Alberto. "Antichi medici pistoiesi, pesciatini e della Valdinievole." *Bullettino storico pistoiese* 30(1928): 81-104.

———. "Di un singolare procedimento medico-legale in Pistoia nell'anno 1375." *RSSMN* 10(1919): 129-35.

———. "Maestro Iacopo di Coluccino da Lucca medico ed il giornale delle sue ricordanze (1364-1402)." *RSSMN* 12(1921): 121-33.

———. *Medici e chirurghi pistoiesi nel medioevo*. Pistoia, 1909.

———. "Note storiche sull'esercizio professionale medico in Italia nell'alto medioevo." *RSSMN* 15(1924): 151-72.

———. "Gli ordinamenti sanitari del comune di Pistoia contro la pestilenza del 1348." *ASI*, ser. 4, 20(1887): 3-24.

———. "Studi sull'esercizio della medicina in Italia negli ultimi tre secoli del medioevo." *Giornale della società italiana d'igiene* 7(1885): 611-48, 785-815.

Chiappelli, Alberto, and Andrea Corsini. "Un antico inventario dello spedale di S. M. Nuova in Firenze (a. 1376)." *Rivista delle biblioteche e degli archivi* 32(1921): 1-37.

Chiti, Alfredo. "Di Marco Carafantoni medico pistoiese e della sua famiglia." *Bullettino storico pistoiese* 3(1901): 13-20.

Ciasca, Raffaele. *L'arte dei medici e speziali nella storia e nel commercio fiorentino dal secolo XII al XV*. Florence, 1927.

Cipolla, Carlo. "Il valore di alcune biblioteche nel Trecento." *Bollettino storico pavese* 7(1944): 5-20.

Cipolla, Carlo Maria. *Before the Industrial Revolution: European Society and Economy, 1000-1700*. New York, 1976.

———. "The Professions: The Long View." *The Journal of European Economic History* 2(1973): 37-52.

———. *Public Health and the Medical Profession in the Renaissance*. Cambridge, 1976.

Ciscato, Antonio. *Gli ebrei a Padova (1300-1800): monografia storica documentata*. Bologna, 1967.

Clagett, Marshall. *Archimedes in the Middle Ages*. 4 vols. in 8. Madison, 1964-80.

———. "Some Novel Trends in the Science of the Fourteenth Century." In C. S. Singleton, ed., *Art, Science and History in the Renaissance*, 275-303. Baltimore, 1968.

Cochrane, Eric. *Florence in the Forgotten Centuries, 1527-1800: A History of Florence and the Florentines in the Age of the Grand Dukes*. Chicago, 1973.

Cohn, Samuel Kline, Jr. *The Laboring Classes in Renaissance Florence.* New York, 1980.

Corradi, Alfonso. *Annali delle epidemie occorse in Italia dalle prime memorie fino al 1850.* Pt. I (to 1500). Bologna, 1865.

————. "Biblioteca di un medico marchigiano del secolo XIV." *Annali universali di medicina* 272(1885): 312-17.

Corsini, Andrea. *Il costume del medico nelle pitture fiorentine del rinascimento.* Florence, 1912.

————. *Medici ciarlatani e ciarlatani medici.* Bologna, n.d.

————. "Nuovo contributo di notizie intorno alla vita di Maestro Tommaso del Garbo." *RSSMN* 7(1925): 268-78.

Cosenza, Mario. *Biographical and Bibliographical Dictionary of the Italian Humanists and of the World of Classical Scholarship in Italy, 1300-1800.* 6 vols. Boston, 1962-67.

Coturri, Enrico. "L'ospedale così detto 'di Bonifazio' in Firenze." *Pagine di storia della medicina* 3/2(1959): 15-33.

————. "I più antichi provvedimenti adottati in Firenze per l'isolamento degli appestati." *Castalia* 15(1959): 73-78.

————. "Vi furono, nella Toscana settentrionale, nell'alto medioevo, scuole nelle quali si insegnò la medicina?" In Mario Santoro, ed., *Atti della IV Biennale della Marca per la storia della medicina.* Fermo, 1961.

Davis, Charles T. "Education in Dante's Florence." *Speculum* 40(1965): 415-35.

Demaitre, Luke. "Scholasticism in Compendia of Practical Medicine, 1250-1450." *Manuscripta* 20(1976): 81-95.

————. "Theory and Practice in Medical Education at the University of Montpellier in the Thirteenth and Fourteenth Centuries." *JHM* 30(1975): 103-23.

Diepgen, Paul. *Die Theologie und der ärztliche Stand.* Berlin, 1922.

Diller, Aubrey. "A Geographical Treatise by Georgius Gemistus Pletho." *Isis* 27(1937): 441-51.

Dols, Michael W. *The Black Death in the Middle East.* Princeton, 1977.

Dominici, Cristiano. "La scuola chirurgica preciana." *Rivista di storia della medicina* 9(1965): 198-210.

Doren, Alfred. *Le arti fiorentine.* Tr. G. B. Klein. 2 vols. Florence, 1940.

————. *Entwicklung und Organisation der Florentiner Zünfte im 13. und 14. Jahrhundert.* Leipzig, 1897.

Dorez, Léon. "Recherches sur la bibliothèque de Pier di Leone Leoni, médecin de Laurent de Médicis." *Revue des bibliothèques* 7(1897): 81-106.

Durand, Dana B. *The Vienna-Klosterneuberg Map Corpus of the Fifteenth Century: A Study in the Transition from Medieval to Modern Science*. Leiden, 1939.

Eckstein, Harry. *Division and Cohesion in Democracy: A Study of Norway*. Princeton, 1966.

Edgerton, Samuel. *The Renaissance Rediscovery of Linear Perspective*. New York, 1975.

Egmond, Warren von. "New Light on Paolo dell'Abbaco." *AIMSSF* 2/1(1977): 1-21.

Emery, Richard W. "The Black Death of 1348 in Perpignan." *Speculum* 42(1967): 611-23.

Ermini, Giuseppe. *Storia dell'università di Perugia*. 2 vols. Florence, 1971.

Fabbi, Ansano. "Il lebbrosario della Valnerina e la scuola chirurgica di Preci." *BDSPU* 61(1964): 5-55.

———. "The *Norcini* and their Families." *Medicina nei secoli* 9/3(1972): 67-89.

Fabbri, G. B. "Della litotomia antica e dei litotomi ed oculisti norcini e preciani." *Memorie dell'accademia delle scienze dell'istituto di Bologna*, ser. 2, 9/2(1870): 239-66.

Favaro, Antonio. "Ascendenti e collaterali di Galileo Galilei." *ASI*, ser. 5, 47(1911): 346-78.

———. "Intorno alla vita ed alle opere di Prosdocimo de' Beldomandi." *Bullettino di bibliografia e di storia delle scienze matematiche e fisiche* 12(1879): 1-74, 115-251; 18(1885): 405-23.

———. "I lettori di matematiche nella università di Padova dal principio del secolo XIV alla fine del XVI." *Memorie e documenti per la storia dell'università di Padova*, 6-31. Padua, 1922.

Febvre, Lucien, and Henri-Jean Martin. *The Coming of the Book: The Impact of Printing, 1450-1800*. Ed. Geoffrey Nowell-Smith and David Wootton. Tr. David Gerard. London, 1976.

Feigenbaum, Aryeh. "Early History of Cataract and the Ancient Operation for Cataract." *American Journal of Ophthalmology* 49(1960): 305-26.

Ferrari da Grado, Henri-Maxime. *Une chaire de médecine au XVᵉ siècle: un professeur à l'université de Pavie de 1432 à 1472*. Paris, 1899.

Fiumi, Enrico. "La demografia fiorentina nelle pagine di Giovanni Villani." *ASI* 108(1950): 78-158.

———. *Demografia, movimento urbanistico e classi sociali in Prato dall'età comunale ai tempi moderni*. Florence, 1968.

———. "Fioritura e decadenza dell'economia fiorentina." *ASI* 115(1957): 385-439; 116(1958): 443-510; 117(1959): 427-502.

———. "Sui rapporti economici tra città e contado nell'età comunale." *ASI* 114(1956): 18-68.

Freidson, Eliot. *Profession of Medicine: A Study in the Sociology of Applied Knowledge*. New York, 1970.

Friedenwald, Harry. *The Jews and Medicine*. 2 vols. Baltimore, 1944.

Gadol, Joan Kelly. *Leon Battista Alberti: Universal Man of the Early Renaissance*. Chicago/London, 1969.

Garin, Eugenio. *La cultura filosofica del rinascimento italiano*. Florence, 1961.

———. "La cultura fiorentina nella seconda metà del '300 e i 'barbari britanni.'" *La rassegna della letteratura italiana*, ser. 7, 64(1960): 181-95.

———. *Italian Humanism: Philosophy and Civic Life in the Renaissance*. Tr. Peter Munz. New York, 1965.

———. "Paolo Toscanelli." In his *Portraits from the Quattrocento*, tr. Victor A. Velen and Elizabeth Velen, 118-41. New York, 1972.

———. "Petrarca e la polemica contro i 'moderni.'" In his *Rinascite e rivoluzioni: movimenti culturali dal XIV al XVIII secolo*, 71-88. Bari, 1975.

———. "Gli umanisti e la scienza." *Rivista di filosofia* 52(1961): 259-79.

Garosi, Alcide. "Alcuni documenti e rilievi sulla vita di Ugo Benzi." *RSSMN* 24(1933), Appendix (Atti del IV congresso nazionale): 89-135.

———. "I codici di medicina del Maestro Alessandro Sermoneta." *RSSMN* 28(1937): 225-32.

———. *Inter artium et medicinae doctores*. Florence, 1963.

———. *Siena nella storia della medicina (1240-1555)*. Florence, 1958.

———. "Spunti di organizzazione sanitaria di guerra in documenti senesi del Dugento." *RSSMN* 27(1930): 233-42.

Garrison, Fielding H. *Notes on the History of Military Medicine*. Washington, 1922.

Gatti, Gerolamo. "Il Collegio medico fiorentino." *Annuario della R. università degli studi di Firenze*, 1927-28. Reprinted separately, Florence, 1928.

Getz, Faye. "Gilbertus Anglicus Anglicized." *Medical History* 26(1982): 436-42.

Goldthwaite, Richard A. *The Building of Renaissance Florence: An Economic and Social History*. Baltimore, 1980.

———. *Private Wealth in Renaissance Florence: A Study of Four Families*. Princeton, 1968.

———. "Schools and Teachers of Commercial Arithmetic in Renaissance Florence." *Journal of European Economic History* 1(1972): 418-33.

Goode, William J. "Encroachment, Charlatanism and the Emerging Profession: Psychology, Sociology and Medicine." *American Sociological Review* 25(1960): 902-14.

Gottfried, Robert S. *The Black Death: Natural and Human Disaster in Medieval Europe*. New York, 1983.

———. *Epidemic Diseases in Fifteenth Century England: The Medical Response and the Demographic Consequences*. New Brunswick, N.J., 1978.

Grant, Edward. *Physical Science in the Middle Ages*. Cambridge, 1977.

Greppi, Claudio, and Marco Massa. "Città e territorio nella repubblica fiorentina." In *Un'altra Firenze: l'epoca di Cosimo il Vecchio, riscontri tra cultura e società nella storia fiorentina*, 3-58. Florence, 1971.

Guasti, Cesare. *La cupola di Santa Maria del Fiore*. Florence, 1857.

———. *Intorno alla vita e all'insegnamento di Vittorino da Feltre: lettere di Sassolo Pratese*. Florence, 1869.

———. "Sassolo Pratese e la sua apologia di Vittorino da Feltre." In his *Opere*, 5/2 (*Letteratura, storia, critica*), 565-94. Prato, 1899.

Guerra-Coppioli, L. *Il Bagno a Morba nel Volterrano e Maestro Pierleone Leoni da Spoleto, medico di Lorenzo il magnifico*. Siena, 1915.

Guido, Francesco. "Cenni biografici su Dino e Tommaso Del Garbo." *Atti XXI* 1:156-63.

Hammond, E. A. "Physicians in Medieval English Religious Houses." *BHM* 32(1958): 105-20.

———. "The Westminster Abbey Infirmarers' Rolls as a Source of Medical History." *BHM* 39(1965): 261-76.

Haskell, Thomas L. *The Emergence of Professional Social Science: The American Social Science Association and the Nineteenth-Century Crisis of Authority*. Urbana, 1977.

Herlihy, David. *Medieval and Renaissance Pistoia: The Social History of an Italian Town, 1200-1430*. New Haven, 1967.

———. "Population, Plague and Social Change in Rural Pistoia." *The Economic History Review*, ser. 2, 18(1965): 225-44.

———. "Three Patterns of Social Mobility in Medieval History." *Journal of Interdisciplinary History* 3/4(1973): 623-47.

Herlihy, David, and Christiane Klapisch-Zuber. *Les toscans et leurs familles: une étude du catasto florentin de 1427*. Paris, 1978.

Holmes, Geoffrey. *Augustan England: Professions, State and Society, 1680-1730*. London/Boston, 1982.

Holmes, George. *The Florentine Enlightenment, 1400-1450*. New York, 1969.

Hopkins, Keith. "Elite Mobility in the Roman Empire." *Past and Present* 32(1965): 12-26.

Jacquart, Danielle. *Le milieu médical en France du XIIe au XVe siècle.* Geneva, 1981.

————. *Supplément au Dictionnaire biographique de Wickersheimer.* Geneva, 1979.

Jandolo. "Storia della chirurgia dell'ernia inguinale." *Castalia* 15(1959): 59-70.

Janson, H. W. "Giovanni Chellini's *Libro* e Donatello." In *Studien zur toskanischen Kunst: Festschrift für Ludwig Heinrich Heydenreich,* 131-38. Munich, 1964.

————. *The Sculpture of Donatello.* 2 vols. Princeton, 1957.

Jervis, Jane R. "The Mathematics of Paolo Toscanelli." *AIMSSF* 4/1 (1979): 3-14.

————. "Toscanelli's Cometary Observations: Some New Evidence." *AIMSSF* 2/1(1977): 15-20.

Johnson, Terence J. *Professions and Power.* London, 1972.

Kealey, Edward J. *Medieval Medicus: A Social History of Anglo-Norman Medicine.* Baltimore, 1981.

Kent, Dale M. "The Florentine *Reggimento* in the Fifteenth Century." *Renaissance Quarterly* 28(1975): 575-638.

————. *The Rise of the Medici: Faction in Florence, 1426-1434.* Oxford, 1978.

Kent, Francis William. *Household and Lineage in Renaissance Florence: The Family Life of the Capponi, Ginori, and Rucellai.* Princeton, 1977.

Kibre, Pearl. "The Faculty of Medicine at Paris, Charlatanism and Unlicensed Medical Practice in the Later Middle Ages." *BHM* 27 (1953): 1-20.

————. *Scholarly Privileges in the Middle Ages: The Rights, Privileges, and Immunities of Scholars and Universities at Bologna, Padua, Paris and Oxford.* Cambridge, Mass., 1962.

Kirshner, Julius. "Paolo di Castro on *Cives ex privilegio*: A Controversy over the Legal Qualification for Public Office in Early Fifteenth-Century Florence." In Anthony Molho and John A. Tedeschi, eds., *Renaissance Studies in Honor of Hans Baron,* 227-64. Florence, 1971.

Klein, Robert. "Les humanistes et la science." *Bibliothèque d'humanisme et renaissance* 23(1961): 7-15.

————. "Studies on Perspective in the Renaissance." In his *Form and Meaning: Essays on the Renaissance and Modern Art,* tr. Madeline Jay and Leon Wieseltier, 129-40. New York, 1979.

Kristeller, Paul Oskar. "Bartholomaeus, Musandinus, and Maurus of Salerno and Other Early Commentators on the 'Articella,' with a

Tentative List of Texts and Manuscripts." *Italia medioevale e umanistica* 19(1976): 57-87.

———. "Humanism and Scholasticism in the Italian Renaissance." *Byzantion* 7(1944-45): 346-74.

———. *Iter italicum.* 2 vols. London/Leiden, 1963-67.

———. "Philosophy and Medicine in Medieval and Renaissance Italy." In Stuart F. Spicker, ed., *Organism, Medicine and Metaphysics*, 29-40. Dordrecht, 1978.

———. *The Philosophy of Marsilio Ficino.* New York, 1943.

———. "The School of Salerno: Its Development and Its Contribution to the History of Learning." In his *Studies in Renaissance Thought and Letters*, 495-551. Rome, 1956.

Larson, Margali Sarfatti. *The Rise of Professionalism: A Sociological Analysis.* Berkeley, 1977.

La Sorsa, Saverio. *L'arte dei medici, speziali e merciai a Firenze e negli altri comuni italiani.* Molfetta, 1907.

———. *La compagnia d'Or San Michele nel secolo XIV.* Trani, 1902.

Lazzareschi, Eugenio. "Le ricchezze di due medici lucchesi della rinascenza." *RSSMN* 16(1925): 112-39.

Lazzarino, Vittorio. "I libri, gli argenti, le vesti di Giovanni Dondi dall'Orologio." *Bollettino del museo civico di Padova* 1(1925): 11-36.

Lecce, Michele. "Un maestro di arte chirurgica a Verona nel Quattrocento." *Economia e storia* 7(1960): 746-50.

Le Goff, Jacques. "Academic Expenses at Padua in the Fifteenth Century." In his *Time, Work, and Culture in the Middle Ages*, tr. Arthur Goldhammer, 101-6. Chicago, 1982.

Lehoux, Françoise. *Le cadre de vie de médicins parisiens au XVIe et XVIIe siècles.* Paris, 1976.

Leporace, Tullia Gasparrini. "Due biblioteche mediche del Quattrocento." *La bibliofilia* 52(1950): 205-20.

Levati, Ambrogio. *I viaggi di Francesco Petrarca in Francia, in Germania ed in Italia.* 5 vols. Milan, 1820.

Lightbown, R. W. "Giovanni Chellini, Donatello, and Antonio Rossellino." *Burlington Magazine* 104(1962): 102-4.

Lind, Levi Robert. *Studies in Pre-Vesalian Anatomy: Biography, Translations, Documents.* Philadelphia, 1975.

———. "Il tema di deontologia medica: il 'De cautelis medicorum' di Gabriele Zerbi." *RSSMN* 46(1956): 60-83.

Litta, Pompeo. *Famiglie celebri italiane.* Ser. 1. 11 vols. Milan, 1819-74.

Lockwood, Dean Putnam. *Ugo Benzi, Medieval Philosopher and Physician, 1376-1439.* Chicago, 1951.

Lopez, Robert S. *The Commercial Revolution of the Middle Ages, 950-1350*. Englewood Cliffs, N.J., 1971.

Lungo, Isidoro Del. *Dino Compagni e la sua cronica*. 3 vols. in 4. Florence, 1879-87.

Luzzato, Gino. "L'inurbamento delle popolazioni rurali in Italia nei secoli XII e XIII." In *Studi di storia e diritto in onore di Enrico Besta*, 2 vols., 2:185-203. Milan, 1939.

MacKinney, Loren C. *Medical Illustrations in Medieval Manuscripts*. London, 1965.

McVaugh, Michael R. *The Development of Medieval Pharmaceutical Theory*. In Arnaldo de Villanova, *Aphorismi de gradibus*, ed. McVaugh, 1-136. Granada/Barcelona, 1975.

―――. "The *Experimenta* of Arnald of Villanova." *Journal of Medieval and Renaissance Studies* 1(1971): 107-18.

―――. "The '*Humidum Radicale*' in Thirteenth-Century Medicine." *Traditio* 30(1974): 259-83.

―――. "Quantified Medical Theory and Practice at Fourteenth-Century Montpellier." *BHM* 43(1969): 397-413.

Maddalena, Aldo de. "Les archives Saminiati: de l'économie à l'histoire de l'art." *Annales* 14(1959): 738-44.

Maguire, Yvonne. *The Women of the Medici*. London, 1927.

Maier, Anneliese. "Das Problem der *Species sensibiles in Medio* und die neue Naturphilosophie des 14. Jahrhunderts." In her *Ausgehendes Mittelalter: gesammelte Aufsätze zur Geistesgeschichte des 14. Jahrhunderts*, 2 vols., 2:419-52. Rome, 1967.

Mannelli, Maria Assunta. "Il Collegio medico fiorentino ed i 'matricolati' presso il collegio stesso dal 28 agosto 1560 al 30 agosto 1561 (anno fiorentino)." *Ospedali d'Italia, Chirurgia* 14(1967): 209-22.

―――. "Istituzione e soppressione degli ospedali minori in Firenze." *Studi di storia ospitaliera* 3(1956): 171-82.

―――. "L'ospedale di San Matteo in Firenze." *Ospedali d'Italia, Chirurgia* 11(1964): 730-32.

―――. "L'ospedale di Sant'Antonio in Firenze." *Ospedali d'Italia, Chirurgia*, 12(1965): 505-8.

―――. "Lo spedale di San Paolo dei convalescenti in Firenze." *Ospedali d'Italia, Chirurgia* 12(1965): 241-45.

―――. "Tommaso Del Garbo ed Ugo Benzi da Siena, lettori di medicina nello *studium generale* di Firenze." *Rivista di storia della medicina* 8(1964): 183-90.

Marangon, Tiziana Pesenti. "La miscellanea astrologica del prototipografo padovano Bartolomeo Valdizocco e la diffusione dei testi astrologici e medici tra i lettori padovani del '400." *Quaderni per la storia dell'università di Padova* 11(1978): 87-106.

——. " 'Professores chirugie,' 'medici ciroici' e 'barbitonsores' a Padova nell'età di Leonardo Buffi da Bertipaglia (+ dopo il 1448)." *Quaderni per la storia dell'università di Padova* 11(1978): 1-38.

Mare, Albinia De la. "Messer Piero Strozzi, a Florentine Scribe." In A. S. Osley, ed., *Calligraphy and Paleography: Essays presented to A. J. Fairbank*, 55-68. London, 1965.

——. "The Shop of a Florentine 'Cartolaio' in 1427." In Berta Maracchi Biagiarelli and Dennis E. Rhodes, eds., *Studi offerti a Roberto Ridolfi*, 237-48. Florence, 1973.

Mariani, Ugo. *Il Petrarca e gli agostiniani.* Rome, 1946.

Marini, Luigi Gaetano. *Degli archiatri pontifici.* 2 vols. Rome, 1784.

Martinelli, Bortolo. "Il Petrarca e la medicina." In Francesco Petrarca, *Invective contra medicum: testo latino e volgarizzamento di Ser Domenico Silvestri*, ed. Pier Giorgio Ricci, 205-49. Rome, 1978.

Martines, Lauro. *Lawyers and Statecraft in Renaissance Florence.* Princeton, 1968.

——. *The Social World of the Florentine Humanists, 1390-1460.* Princeton, 1963.

Mattesini, Francesco. "La biblioteca francescana di Santa Croce e Fra Tedaldo Della Casa." *Studi francescani* 57(1960): 254-316.

Mazzi, Curzio. "L'inventario quattrocentesco della biblioteca di Santa Croce in Firenze." *Rivista delle biblioteche e degli archivi* 8(1897): 16-31, 99-113, 130-47.

——. "Lo studio di un medico senese del secolo XV." *Rivista delle biblioteche e degli archivi* 5(1892): 27-48.

Mecatti, Giuseppe Maria. *Storia genealogica della nobiltà e cittadinanza di Firenze.* Naples, 1754.

Meiss, Millard. *Painting in Florence and Siena after the Black Death.* Princeton, 1951.

Mercati, Giovanni. *Ultimi contributi alla storia degli umanisti*, vol. 1, *Traversariana.* Vatican City, 1939.

Meuthen, Erich. *Die letzten Jahre des Nikolaus von Kues: biographische Untersuchungen nach neuen Quellen.* Cologne/Opladen, 1958.

Michaud-Quantin, Pierre. *Universitas: expressions du mouvement communautaire dans le Moyen Age latin.* Paris, 1970.

Millerson, Geoffrey. *The Qualifying Associations: A Study in Professionalization.* London, 1964.

Molho, Anthony. *Florentine Public Finances in the Early Renaissance, 1400-1433.* Cambridge, Mass., 1971.

————. "Politics and the Ruling Class in Early Renaissance Florence." *Nuova rivista storica* 52(1968): 401-20.

Molho, Anthony, and Julius Kirshner, "The Dowry Fund and the Marriage Market in Early Quattrocento Florence." *Journal of Modern History* 50(1978): 403-38.

Molho, Anthony, and John A. Tedeschi, eds. *Renaissance Studies in Honor of Hans Baron*. Florence, 1971.

Monti, Gennaro Maria. *Le confraternite medievali dell'alta e media Italia*. 2 vols. Venice, 1927.

Moody, Ernest. *The Logic of William of Ockham*. New York, 1935.

————. "Ockham, Buridan, and Nicholas of Autrecourt." In his *Studies in Medieval Philosophy, Science, and Logic*, 127-60. Berkeley, 1975.

Morçay, Raoul. *Saint Antonin, fondateur du couvent de Saint-Marc, archévêque de Florence (1389-1459)*. Tours, 1914.

Münster, Ladislao. "Alcuni episodi sconosciuti o poco noti sulla vita e sull'attività di Bartolomeo da Varignana." *Castalia* 10(1954): 207-15.

Münster, Ladislao, and Mirko Malavolti. "Su alcuni documenti relativi a medici ebrei conservati nell'archivo di stato di Firenze." *Medicina nei secoli* 8/3(1971): 22-53.

Murdoch, John E. "From Social into Intellectual Factors: An Aspect of the Unitary Character of Late Medieval Learning." In John E. Murdoch and Edith Dudley Sylla, eds., *The Cultural Context of Medieval Learning*, 276-312. Dordrecht/Boston, 1975.

————, and Edith Dudley Sylla. "The Science of Motion." In David C. Lindberg, ed., *Science in the Middle Ages*, chap. 7. Chicago, 1978.

Najemy, John M. *"Audiant omnes artes*: Corporate Origins of the Ciompi Revolution." In *Il tumulto dei Ciompi: un momento di storia fiorentina ed europea*, 59-93. Florence, 1981.

————. *Corporatism and Consensus in Florentine Electoral Politics, 1280-1400*. Chapel Hill, 1982.

————. "Guild Republicanism in Trecento Florence: The Successes and Ultimate Failure of Corporate Politics." *The American Historical Review* 84(1979): 53-71.

Nardi, Bruno. "L'averroismo bolognese nel secolo XIII e Taddeo Alderotto." *Rivista di storia della filosofia* 4(1949): 11-22.

Nardi, M. G. "Statuti e documenti riflettenti la dissezione anatomica umana e la nomina di alcuni lettori di medicina nell'antico 'studium generale' fiorentino." *RSSMN* 47(1956): 237-49.

Nicholas, David. "Patterns of Social Mobility." In Richard L. De-Molen, ed., *One Thousand Years: Western Europe in the Middle Ages*, 45-105. Boston, 1974.

Novati, Francesco. "Sul riordinamento dello studio fiorentino nel 1385." *Rassegna bibliografica della letteratura italiana* 4(1896): 318-23.

Nutton, Vivian. "Continuity or Rediscovery? The City Physician in Classical Antiquity and Medieval Italy." In Andrew W. Russell, ed., *The Town and State Physician in Europe from the Middle Ages to the Enlightenment*, 9-46. Wolfenbüttel, 1981.

Origo, Iris. *The Merchant of Prato: Francesco di Marco Datini, 1335-1410*. London. 1960.

Os, Henk Van. "The Black Death and Sienese Painting: A Problem of Interpretation." *Art History* 4(1981): 237-49.

Dall'Osso, Eugenio. *L'organizzazione medico-legale a Bologna e a Venezia nei secoli XII-XIV*. Cesena, 1956.

Pagallo, Giulio. "Nuovi testi per la 'disputà delle arti' nel Quattrocento: La 'Quaestio' di Bernardo da Firenze e la 'Disputatio' di Domenico Bianchelli." *Italia medioevale e umanistica* 2(1959): 467-81.

Palmer, Richard John. "The Control of the Plague in Venice and Northern Italy 1348-1600." Ph.D. diss., University of Kent, 1978.

————. "Physicians and Surgeons in Sixteenth-Century Venice." *Medical History* 23(1979): 451-60.

————. "Physicians and The State in Post-Medieval Italy." In Andrew W. Russell, ed., *The Town and State Physician in Europe from the Middle Ages to the Enlightenment*, 47-61. Wolfenbüttel, 1981.

Pampaloni, Guido. *Lo spedale di Santa Maria Nuova*. Florence, 1961.

Panebianco, Domenico. "Contributo alla storia del collegio medico fiorentino (secoli XIII-XIX)." *Rassegna storica toscana* 15(1969): 3-13.

Panizza, L. A. "Textual Interpretation in Italy, 1350-1450: Seneca's Letter I to Lucilius." *Journal of the Warburg and Courtauld Institutes* 46(1983): 40-62.

Park, Katharine. "Albert's Influence on Late Medieval Psychology." In James A. Weisheipl, ed., *Albertus Magnus and the Sciences*, 501-35. Toronto, 1980.

————. "The Readers at The Florentine *Studio* according to Comunal Fiscal Records." *Rinascimento*, n.s., 20(1980): 249-310.

Parronchi, Alessandro. *Studi sulla dolce prospettiva*. Milan, 1964.

Passerini, Luigi. *Storia degli stabilimenti di beneficenza e d'istruzione elementare gratuita della città di Firenze*. Florence, 1853.

Pelling, Margaret, and Charles Webster. "Medical Practitioners." In Charles Webster, ed., *Health, Medicine and Mortality in the Sixteenth Century*, 165-235. Cambridge, 1979.

Perosa, A. "Codici di Galeno postillati dal Poliziano." In *Umanesimo e rinascimento: studi offerti a Paul Oskar Kristeller da V. Branca, A. Frugoni et al.*, 75-109. Florence, 1980.

Peruzzi, S. L. *Storia del commercio e dei banchieri di Firenze . . . dal 1200 al 1345.* Florence, 1868.

Pieraccini, Gaetano. *La stirpe de' Medici di Cafaggiolo.* 2d ed. 3 vols. Florence, 1947.

Pieri, Pier Felice. "Maestro Ugolino da Montecatini." *Castalia* 18(1962): 132-33.

Pinto, G. "Firenze e la carestia del 1346-47: aspetti e problemi delle crisi annonarie alla metà del '300." *ASI* 130(1972): 3-84.

―――. "Il personale, le balie e i salariati dell'ospedale di San Gallo di Firenze negli anni 1395-1406: note per la storia del salariato nelle città medievali." *Ricerche storiche* 4(1974): 113-68.

Pizzoni, Pietro. "La litotomia e i litotomi Norcini." *BDSPU* 48(1951): 202-11.

―――. "I medici umbri lettori presso l'università di Perugia." *BDSPU* 47(1950): 5-208.

Plesner, Johan. *L'émigration de la campagne à la ville libre de Florence au XIIIe siècle.* Tr. F. Gleizal. Copenhagen, 1934.

―――. "Una rivoluzione stradale del Dugento." *Acta jutlandica* 10(1938): 1-103.

Pope-Hennessy, John. "The Madonna Reliefs of Donatello." *Apollo* 103(March 1976): 172-91.

Pope-Hennessy, John, with Ronald Lightbown. *Catalogue of Italian Sculpture in the Victoria and Albert Museum.* 3 vols. London, 1964.

Premuda, L., and F. Ongaro. "I primordi della dissezione anatomica in Padova." *Acta medicae historiae patavina* 12(1965): 117-42.

Puccinotti, Francesco. *Storia della medicina.* 3 vols. Livorno, 1850-59; Prato, 1866.

Radcliffe, Anthony, and Charles Avery. "The 'Chellini Madonna' by Donatello." *Burlington Magazine* 118(1976): 377-87.

Rajna, Pio. "Una lettera di Averardo de' Medici al medico Galileo Galilei." *ASI* 75(1971): 149-65.

Rashdall, Hastings. *The Universities of Europe in the Middle Ages.* 2d ed. Ed. F. M. Powicke and A. B. Emden. 3 vols. Oxford, 1936.

Raspadori, Francesco. "Legislazioni termali senesi nel Medioevo." *Atti XXI*, 1:35-39.

Reader, W. J. *Professional Men: The Rise of the Professional Classes in Nineteenth-Century England.* London, 1966.

Reguardati, Fausto M. de'. *Benedetto de' Reguardati da Norcia.* Trieste, 1977.

Riddle, John M. "Theory and Practice in Medieval Medicine." *Viator*, 5(1974): 157-84.

Ristori, G. B. "Libreria del Maestro Agostino Santucci." *Rivista delle biblioteche* 15(1904): 35-37.

———. "Niccolò Falcucci, medico del secolo XIV." *Giotto: bollettino storico, letterario, artistico del Mugello* 2 (1903): 259-88.

Rizzi, Guido. "Un contratto notarile quattrocentesco per operazione di cataratta." *Atti del II convegno della Marca per la storia della medicina*, 59-61. Fermo, 1958.

Roberts, R. S. "The Personnel and Practice of Medicine in Tudor and Stuart England, I: The Provinces." *Medical History* 6(1962): 363-82.

———. "The Personnel and Practice of Medicine in Tudor and Stuart England, II: London." *Medical History* 8(1964): 217-34.

Rodolico, Niccolò. *Il popolo minuto: note di storia fiorentina, 1343-1378*. Bologna, 1899.

Roncière, Charles-M. de la. *Florence, centre économique régional au XIVᵉ siècle: le marché des denrées de première nécessité à Florence et dans sa campagne et les conditions de vie des salariés (1320-1380)*. 5 vols. Aix-en-Provence, 1977.

———. "Indirect Taxes or 'Gabelles' at Florence in the Fourteenth Century: The Evolution of Tariffs and Problems of Collection." In N. Rubinstein, ed., *Florentine Studies*, 140-92. Evanston, Ill., 1968.

———. "Pauvres et pauvreté à Florence au XIVᵉ siècle." In Michel Mollat, ed., *Etudes sur l'histoire de la pauvreté*, 2 vols., 2:661-745. Paris, 1974.

Roover, Raymond de. *The Rise and Decline of the Medici Bank, 1397-1494*. Cambridge, Mass., 1963.

Rose, Paul Lawrence. "Humanist Culture and Renaissance Mathematics: The Italian Libraries of the Quattrocento." *Studies in the Renaissance* 20(1973): 46-105.

———. *The Italian Renaissance of Mathematics: Studies on Humanists and Mathematicians from Petrarch to Galileo*. Geneva, 1975.

Rosenberg, Hans. *Bureaucracy, Aristocracy and Autocracy: The Prussian Experience, 1660-1815*. Cambridge, Mass., 1958.

Ross, Janet. *The Lives of the Early Medici as told in their Correspondence*. London, 1910.

Roth, Cecil. *The Jews in the Renaissance*. Philadelphia, 1959.

———. "Qualifications of Jewish Physicians in the Middle Ages." *Speculum* 28(1953): 834-43.

Rubinstein, Nicolai. *The Government of Florence under the Medici (1434-1494)*. Oxford, 1966.

Ruggiero, Guido. "The Cooperation of Physicians and the State in the Control of Violence in Renaissance Venice." *JHM* 33(1978): 156-66.

——. "The Status of Physicians and Surgeons in Renaissance Venice." *JHM* 36(1981): 168-84.

Saalman, Howard. *Filippo Brunelleschi: The Cupola of Santa Maria del Fiore*. London, 1980.

Sabbadini, Remigio. *Giovanni da Ravenna, insigne figura d'umanista (1343-1408) da documenti inediti*. Como, 1924.

——. *Le scoperte dei codici latini e greci ne' secoli XIV e XV*. 2d ed. Ed. Eugenio Garin. 2 vols. Florence, 1967.

Sacino, Giovanni. "Primi albori de specializzazione nell'esercizio della medicina toscana nel medioevo." *Atti XXI*, 1:100-5.

Sambin, Paolo. "Cristoforo Barzizza e i suoi libri." *Bollettino del museo civico di Padova* 44(1955): 145-64.

Santillana, Giorgio de. "Paolo Toscanelli and his Friends." In his *Reflections on Men and Ideas*, 33-47. Cambridge, Mass., 1968.

Sarti, M., and M. Fattorini. *De claris archigymnasii bononiensis professoribus a saeculo XI usque ad saeculum XIV*. Ed. C. Albicini and C. Malagola. 2 vols. Bologna, 1888-96.

Schulz, Anne Markham. *The Sculpture of Bernardo Rossellino and his Workshop*. Princeton, 1977.

Shapiro, Herman. *Motion, Time and Place according to William Ockham*. St. Bonaventure, N.Y., 1957.

Singer, Charles. "The Early Treatment of Gunshot Wounds." *The Quarterly Review* 226(1916): 452-69.

Siraisi, Nancy. *Arts and Sciences at Padua: The Studium of Padua before 1350*. Toronto, 1973.

——. "Some Recent Work on Western European Medical Learning, ca. 1200-ca. 1500." *History of Universities* 2(1982): 226-38.

——. "Taddeo Alderotti and Bartolomeo da Varignana on the Nature of Medical Learning." *Isis* 68(1977): 27-39.

——. *Taddeo Alderotti and his Pupils: Two Generations of Italian Medical Learning*. Princeton, 1981.

Slack, Paul. "Mirrors of Health and Treasures of Poor Men: The Uses of the Vernacular Medical Literature of Tudor England." In Charles Webster, ed., *Health, Medicine and Mortality in the Sixteenth Century*, 237-73. Cambridge, 1979.

Smith, Edward Griffin. "A Disagreement on the Need of a Sensible Species in the Writings of Some Medical Doctors in the Late Middle Ages." Ph.D. diss., St. Louis University, 1974; University Microfilms, 74-24, 144.

Somerville, Robert. *The Savoy: Manor, Hospital, Chapel*. London, 1960.

Stephens, John N. "Heresy in Medieval and Renaissance Florence." *Past and Present* 54(1972): 25-60.

Stinger, Charles L. *Humanism and the Church Fathers: Ambrogio Traversari (1386-1439) and Christian Antiquity in the Italian Renaissance*. Albany, N.Y., 1977.

Stone, Lawrence. "Social Mobility in England, 1500-1700." *Past and Present* 33(April 1966): 16-55.

Sudhoff, Karl. *Beiträge zur Geschichte der Chirurgie im Mittelalter*. 2 vols. Leipzig, 1914-18.

————. "Pestschriften aus den ersten 150 Jahren nach der Epidemie des 'schwarzen Todes' 1348, IV: Italienische des 14. Jahrhunderts." *Archiv für Geschichte der Medizin* 5(1912): 332-96.

Sylla, Edith, "Medieval Concepts of the Latitude of Forms: The Oxford Calculators." *Archive d'histoire doctrinale et littéraire du moyen âge* 40(1973): 223-83.

Tabanelli, Mario. *La chirurgia italiana nell'alto medioevo*. 2 vols. Florence, 1965.

Talbot, C. H., and E. A. Hammond. *The Medical Practitioners in Medieval England: A Biographical Register*. London, 1965.

Targioni-Tozzetti, Giovanni. *Notizie sulla storia delle scienze fisiche in Toscana*. Florence, 1852.

Temkin, Owsei. *Galenism: Rise and Decline of a Medical Philosophy*. Ithaca, N.Y., 1973.

Thorndike, Lynn. *A History of Magic and Experimental Science*. 8 vols. New York, 1923-58.

————. *Science and Thought in the Fifteenth Century*. New York, 1929.

————. "Some Minor Medical Works of the Florentine Renaissance." *Isis* 9(1927): 29-43.

————. *University Records and Life in the Middle Ages*. New York, 1944.

Thorndike, Lynn, and Pearl Kibre. *A Catalogue of Incipits of Mediaeval Scientific Writing in Latin*. 2d ed. Cambridge, Mass., 1963.

Thrupp, Silvia L. "The Gilds." In *The Cambridge Economic History of Europe*, ed. M. M. Postan and H. J. Habakkuk, 7 vols., vol. 3, chap. 5. Cambridge, 1941-78.

————. "Plague Effects in Medieval Europe." *Comparative Studies in Society and History* 8(1965-66): 474-83.

Toaff, Ariel. *Gli ebrei a Perugia*. Perugia, 1975.

Torre, Arnaldo della. *Storia dell'accademia platonica di Firenze*. Florence, 1902.

Ullman, Berthold L. *The Humanism of Coluccio Salutati*. Padua, 1963.

Ullman, Berthold L., and Philip A. Stadter. *The Public Library of Ren-*

aissance Florence: Niccolò Niccoli, Cosimo de' Medici and the Library of San Marco. Padua, 1972.

Uzielli, Gustavo. *La vita e i tempi di Paolo dal Pozzo Toscanelli*. Rome, 1894.

Vansteenberghe, Edmond. *Le cardinal Nicolas de Cues (1401-1464)*. Paris, 1920.

Vasoli, Cesare. "Polemiche occamiste." *Rinascimento* 3(1952): 119-41.

Vecchi, Bindo de. "I libri di un medico umanista fiorentino del secolo XV, dai 'ricordi' di Maestro Antonio Benivieni." *La bibliofilia* 34(1932): 297-301.

Verde, Armando F. *Lo studio fiorentino, 1473-1503: ricerche e documenti*. 3 vols. Florence/Pistoia, 1973-77.

Vignaud, Henry. *Toscanelli and Columbus*. New York, 1902.

Vitelleschi, G. degli Azzi. *Le relazioni tra la repubblica di Firenze e l'Umbria nel secolo XIV*. 2 vols. Perugia, 1964-69.

Wagner, Hermann. "Die Rekonstruktion der Toscanelli-Karte vom J. 1471 und die Pseudo-Faksimilia des Behaim-Globus vom J. 1492." *Nachrichten von der Königlichen Gesellschaft der Wissenschaften zu Göttingen*, phil.-hist Klasse, 1894: 208-312.

Walker, D. P. *Spiritual and Demonic Magic from Ficino to Campanella*. London, 1958.

Warner, Deborah. *The Sky Explored: Celestial Cartography, 1500-1800*. New York/Amsterdam, 1979.

Webster, Charles. "Thomas Linacre and the Foundation of the College of Physicans." In Francis Maddison, Margaret Pelling and Charles Webster, eds., *Essays on the Life and Work of Thomas Linacre, c. 1460-1524*, 198-222. Oxford, 1977.

Weiss, Roberto. "Jacopo Angeli da Scarperia (c. 1360-1410/11)." In *Medioevo e rinascimento: studi in onore di Bruno Nardi*, 2 vols., 2:801-27. Florence, 1955.

Weissman, Ronald F. E. *Ritual Brotherhood in Renaissance Florence*. New York, 1982.

Wellborn, Mary Catherine. "The Long Tradition: A Study in Fourteenth-Century Medical Deontology." In James Lea Cate and Eugene N. Anderson, eds., *Medieval and Historiographical Essays in Honor of James Westfall Thompson*, 344-57. Chicago, 1938.

Wickersheimer, E. *Dictionnaire biographique des médecins en France au Moyen Age*. Paris, 1936.

———. "Médecins et chirurgiens dans les hôpitaux du moyen âge." *Janus* 32(1928): 1-11.

Wilson, Curtis. *William Heytesbury: Medieval Logic and the Rise of Mathematical Physics*. Madison, 1956.

Witt, Ronald G. "Florentine Politics and the Ruling Class, 1382-1407." *Journal of Medieval and Renaissance Studies* 6(1976): 243-67.

Zaccagnini, Guido. "L'insegnamento privato a Bologna e altrove nei secoli XIII e XIV." *Atti e memorie della R. deputazione di storia patria per le provincie di Romagna*, ser. 4, 14(1923-24): 254-301.

Ziegler, Philip. *The Black Death*. New York, 1969.

Zinner, Ernst. *Leben und Wirken des Johannes Müller von Königsberg, genannt Regiomontanus*. Munich, 1938.

General Index

Rossellino, Antonio, 234; Bernardo, 234, 235n
Rucellai, 165; Carlo di Bernardo, 166n; Giovanni, 113

Sacchetti, Andreolo di Niccolò, 165
Saint Anthony's Fire, 103, 104n
Salutati, Coluccio, 98, 145, 215, 234; attitude toward doctors, 98, 145, 215; *On the Nobility of Law and Medicine*, 222-23
San Gimignano, 79, 138
San Miniato, 81, 165
Sassolo di maestro Lorenzo Sassoli da Prato, 164n, 175n, 233-34
Scholasticism: and humanism, 190-91, 221-23, 225; importance and vitality, 189-90, 201, 205, 209
schools, 123, 189
Sebastian, St., 212
Seneca, 224
Serapion, *Practica*, 194
Sercambi, Giovanni, da Lucca, apoth, 157
Sforza, Francesco, 115
Sicily, 80
Siena, 79, 80, 87, 88, 90n, 94
Siraisi, Nancy, 11
social mobility, 151, 170-86
Sozomeno da Pistoia, 134
Spain, 72, 74, 80
specialization, medical, 8, 47-48, 67-71, 92, 93, 104
species in vision, 208-209
spice and drug trade, 29, 146, 157, 168, 176
Stefani, Marchionne di Coppo, 35, 169; Vanni, 36
Stinche, 89, 90. *See also* prison doctors
stones, 68, 214
Strozzi, 165
studio fiorentino, see University of Florence
surgeons, 8, 33-34, 37; education and training, 62-66; in employ of hospitals, 104, 106; numbers, 75-76; relations with other doctors, 19-20, 22, 70, 115; social position, 167-70, 175, 183; use of books by, 192, 195; wealth and income, 153, 155, 157

surgery, 52; as university discipline, 60, 62-65, 95, 199; curriculum at Bologna, 248; Florentine writing on, 201-202
Swineshead, Richard, 194, 201

Talbot, C. H., 11
Talento di Simone da Pistoia, 121n, 256
taxes, 55, 147, 152-53, 243-44; tax exemptions for doctors, 55, 56, 57, 70, 71, 74, 91, 92, 93. *See also catasto*
Theophrastus, 226
theorica, 60, 95; curriculum at Bologna, 245-47
theory and practice, 206, 211-12
Tolosini, 166n
toothache, 49
tooth doctors, 68
torture, 90
Traversari, Ambrogio, 190, 226-27, 229, 232

universities: and medical licencing, 13, 21-22; attractions of, 149; cost, 125-26; medical examinations and degrees, 8, 58, 62, 122, 125, 126; teaching of medicine at, 38, 59-66, 128-32, 198-209, 236
University of Bologna, 130n, 199; Florentines at, 95, 131, 203, 211; medical curriculum at, 60-62, 64-65, 68n, 245-48; power and reputation of medical faculty, 7n, 59, 123-24, 199; ties with Florence, 59, 209
University of Ferrara, 123, 130, 144
University of Florence, 7n, 59, 131, 199; and Guild of Doctors, Apothecaries, and Grocers, 23, 38-41; and humanism, 10, 223; and immigration, 80, 143-44; Antonio di maestro Marco da Pistoia at 120, 123-27; a center of medical scholarship, 199-209; as cultural center, 188, 189, 200-201; origins, 57, 94-95, 199; readers in medicine at, 27, 32, 62, 94, 128-29, 131, 132, 162, 198-209; teaching of medicine at, 59-64, 65, 194
University of Oxford, 209
University of Padua: and medical humanism, 236; center for astronomy and

Index of Doctors and Their Families

Library of Congress Cataloging in Publication Data

Park, Katharine, 1950-
Doctors and medicine in early Renaissance Florence.

Bibliography: p.   Includes index.

1. Medicine, Medieval—Italy—Florence. 2. Physicians—
Italy—Florence. 3. Gilds—Italy—Florence. 4. Florence
(Italy)—Gilds. 5. Florence (Italy)—Social life and customs.
I. Title. [DNLM: 1. History of Medicine, Medieval—Italy.
2. Physicians—history—Italy. WZ 70 GI8 P2d]

R519.F6P37 1985   362.1′0945′51   84-42898
ISBN 0-691-08373-8 (alk. paper)

Katharine Park is Assistant Professor of History at
Wellesley College in Wellesley, Massachusetts.